Emergency and Intensive Care Medicine

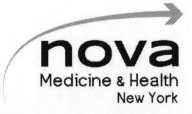

nova
Medicine & Health
New York

Emergency and Intensive Care Medicine

Peritonitis: Causes, Diagnosis and Treatment
David F. Walker (Editor)
2021. ISBN: 978-1-53619-624-5 (Softcover)
2021. ISBN: 978-1-53619-641-2 (eBook)

Pediatric Critical Care: A Primer for All Clinicians
Jason Kane, MD (Editor), Joseph R. Hageman, MD (Editor), Rachel Wolfson, MD (Editor) and
Stuart Berger, MD (Editor)
2019. ISBN: 978-1-53614-837-4 (Hardcover)
2019. ISBN: 978-1-53614-838-1 (eBook)

Gastrointestinal Bleeding: Symptoms, Treatment and Prognosis
Ahmed Kamel Abdel Aal, MD, PhD and Souheil Saddekni, MD (Editors)
2014. ISBN: 978-1-63117-333-2 (Hardcover)
2014. ISBN: 978-1-63117-334-9 (eBook)

Recent Advances in Stroke Therapeutics
Manzoor Ahmad Mir, PhD (Editor)
Raid Saleem Albaradie, PhD (Editor)
Malik D. Alhussainawi (Editor)
2014. ISBN: 978-1-63117-754-5 (Hardcover)
2014. ISBN: 978-1-63117-756-9 (eBook)

**Communications and Planning for the Disabled in Emergencies and Disasters:
Considerations and Effective Practice**
Lindsay Anderson (Editor)
2014. ISBN: 978-1-63321-574-0 (Hardcover)
2014. ISBN: 978-1-63321-607-5 (eBook)

Appendicitis: Risk Factors, Management Strategies and Clinical Implications
Angela S. Marmo (Editor)
2014. ISBN: 978-1-63321-526-9 (Hardcover)
2014. ISBN: 978-1-63321-541-2 (eBook)

More information about this series can be found at https://novapublishers.com/shop/peritonitis-causes-diagnosis-and-treatment/

Murat Yücel, Murat Güzel and İbrahim İkizceli
Editors

Environmental Emergencies and Injuries in Nature

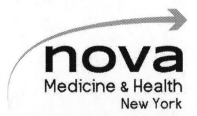

nova
Medicine & Health
New York

Library of Congress Cataloging-in-Publication Data

ISBN: 978-1-68507-833-1

Published by Nova Science Publishers, Inc. † New York

Contents

Preface

The interaction of human beings with the environment can cause unwanted injuries. The damage to the environment from people is a big problem carried from the past to the future. The healthy living of both parties in harmony is associated with "environmental awareness" and "preparedness." Lives can be saved with the rapid recognition and treatment of environmental emergencies such as disasters, injuries, and poisonings, which occur with increasing frequency, and with the right first aid.

The book *Environmental Emergencies and Injuries in Nature* contains up-to-date information to help manage many emergencies that every person may suddenly encounter. It has been prepared as a resource book that can be used by everyone interested, especially health professionals, medical students, and first aid volunteers. The common purpose of all chapters in this book is to provide the reader with theoretical and practical information for early recognition of the clinical situation in the prehospital setting and emergency departments and the rapid initiation of appropriate treatment. Effective and safe interventions in environmental emergencies will reduce the risk of bad outcomes as in every emergency.

We hope you will enjoy reading our book, a ready source covering basic and recent literature information in its field.

Associate Professor Murat Yücel, MD
Associate Professor Murat Güzel, MD
Professor İbrahim İkizceli, MD

Chapter 1

Drownings

Necip Gökhan Güner[1], MD, Nuray Aslan[1], MD and Yusuf Yürümez[2,*], MD

[1]Clinic of Emergency Medicine Sakarya Training and Research Hospital Sakarya, Turkey
[2]Department of Emergency Medicine Sakarya Univesity Sakarya, Turkey

Abstract

Drowning is an environmental emergency caused by immersion or submersion. According to the World Health Organization, drowning cases have an important place among the causes of death. The approach to drowning cases is a multidisciplinary process that includes crime scene, pre-hospital, emergency room, and intensive care. Early and correct intervention is directly related to prognosis after a careful rescue process without putting anyone in danger. The prognosis of unconscious cases after drowning is not good, and they need to be followed up in intensive care units. Drowning cases are preventable, due care must be exercised, and recommendations must be followed.

Keywords: drowning, acute lung injury, aspiration, hypothermia, immersion, submersion

Introduction

Drowning is the process of impaired breathing due to immersion or submersion. As a result of the drowning event, the person may die or be saved. Therefore, regardless of the outcome, all such events are defined as drowning (Hausser and Niquelle, 2007).

Around the world, approximately 42 people die every hour due to suffocation, and the majority of these are victims under the age of 25 (maximum 1-4 age group) (World Health Organization, 2014). 91% of deaths from drowning occur in low- and middle-income societies. It has been reported that death due to drowning is 30 times higher in Thailand and 10 to 20 times higher in many countries in Africa and Central America compared to the United States (Hausser and Niquelle, 2007; Linnan et al., 2007, Szpilman et al., 2012).

Causes of drowning vary with age. According to this;

---

* Corresponding Author's Email: yyurumez@sakarya.edu.tr.

In: Environmental Emergencies and Injuries in Nature
Editors: Murat Yücel, Murat Güzel and İbrahim İkizceli
ISBN: 978-1-68507-833-1
© 2022 Nova Science Publishers, Inc.

- Children under 12 months are more inactive and need more care than other age groups. They can drown very quickly, even in small amounts of water or in water containers that cannot be perceived as deep (for example, buckets or toilets) due to a momentary distraction of their parents/caregivers.
- Areas with insufficient supervision and unprotected pools constitute the most significant risk factor for active children who are too young to perceive the dangers and get out of the water by their own efforts.
- As age progresses, especially in adolescence, the most common cause of drowning in this age group is that children move away from the parent/caregiver's control and engage in dangerous behaviors such as consuming alcohol by the water's edge.
- In the elderly, drowning in the bathtub is more common, often due to concomitant diseases or medications (Hausser and Niquille, 2007; Peden et al., 2016).

Other drowning causes include travel on overcrowded or neglected ships, heavy rainfall, storm surges, tsunamis, or flooding from cyclones. The factors that increase the risk of drowning are shown in Table 1.

Table 1. Factors that increase the risk of drowning

Male gender
Aged under 14
Alcohol use
Low-income level
Insufficient education
Residing in rural areas
Water-borne disasters
Dangerous behavior
Lack of control
Epilepsy

Pathophysiology

The drowning person deliberately tries to spit out or swallows the water that enters the airway. The following conscious response he can do is to hold his breath. However, the breath-holding action cannot last for more than one minute due to the great urge to breathe in humans (Sterba and Lundgren, 1985). Water is aspirated into the airways with the first effort to breathe, and cough develops in response. In the next stage, people develop laryngospasm. This situation only ends with the onset of brain hypoxia. At this stage;

- *If the person cannot be rescued:* Aspiration continues, and unconsciousness and apnea occur within seconds/minutes. This is followed by the development of hypoxia and acidosis in vital tissues. Afterward, tachycardia, bradycardia, pulseless electrical activity, and asystole are seen, respectively.

- *If the person is rescued:* The clinical picture is related to the amount of aspirated water. Aspirated fluid may cause dysfunction of the surfactant in the lungs, increased membrane permeability, decreased compliance, and ventilation/perfusion ratio mismatch. As a result, a picture similar to acute respiratory distress syndrome (ARDS) and noncardiogenic pulmonary edema may develop. Morbidity and mortality in the process of drowning are associated with central nervous system (CNS) damage due to cerebral hypoxia (Buzzacott and Mease, 2018; Smith et al., 2018).

Electrolyte disturbances due to suffocation are only seen when huge amounts of fluid are aspirated and resolved unless there is significant hypoxia, CNS, and kidney damage. Whether the fluid is contaminated or not is much more important than the possibility of developing an electrolyte disorder. As the possibility of developing a pulmonary infection in these patients is very high, prophylactic antibiotics may be required. In addition, drowning cases should be approached like a trauma patient unless proven otherwise by history, examination, and imaging methods, and cervical stabilization must be ensured (McCall and Sternard, 2021).

The risk of neurological damage associated with cardiopulmonary resuscitation (CPR) in drowning cases is similar to other cases of cardiac arrest. However, hypothermia associated with immersion reduces the oxygen consumption of the CNS. This may lead to a delay in cellular anoxia and ATP consumption and a reduced risk of neurological damage (Szpilman et al., 2012).

Story and Physical Examination

The history should be questioned in detail to learn the details of the drowning. Is it an accident? Suicide? Is it murder? Or additional trauma history should be questioned. Especially the mother is depressed, the child is born out of wedlock, the young mother is in financial crisis are the situations that need to be carefully considered relating to newborn murders (Rougé-Maillart et al., 2005).

In drowning cases, the physical examination may reveal difficulty in breathing, apnea or shallow breathing, and decreased consciousness, confusion, or other neurological findings, mainly due to prolonged immersion in water. Due to hypoxia, the skin may appear blue and pale (McCall and Sternard, 2021).

Evaluation

A routine laboratory or imaging examination is not recommended for patients in good general condition who do not have symptoms of hypoxia. The examinations should be made according to the history taken about the event and the physical examination findings obtained, e.g., thoracic imaging (thorax imaging is not required in all cases of drowning) and blood gas evaluation may be performed for ongoing hypoxia. Brain computed tomography (CT), blood glucose, blood gas, toxicological analysis, and/or ethanol level can be checked for altered mental status. The most common laboratory abnormality seen in drowning cases is metabolic acidosis secondary to lactic acidosis. In contrast, electrolyte abnormalities are usually rare in non-fatal drowning cases, regardless of the type of fluid the drowning occurred in (McCall and Sternard, 2021).

Rescue at the Scene

In cases of drowning, rescuers are usually professionals. Studies have shown that fewer than 6% of drowning cases occur in an area where permanent lifeguards require intervention, while only 0.5% of them apply CPR (Borse et al., 2008; Szpilman, 1997).

During the rescue process, the first thing to do is to keep the victim above water, thus ending the drowning process. During this process, the rescuer should not make inappropriate and dangerous interventions because this may cause an increase in the number of affected people (Venema et al., 2010). In cases where the suffocation process cannot be terminated, cardiac arrest may develop after apnea and loss of consciousness. Therefore, if possible, respiratory support should be started with rescue breathing while the victim is in the water. Respiratory support initiated in water can triple the rate of post-hospital discharge without sequelae. Breathing may return even after a few rescue breaths, usually performed only in cases where breathing has stopped. However, if there is no response despite rescue breaths, the victim should be considered to be in cardiac arrest, and CPR should be started immediately after being safely removed from the water (Szpilman and Soares, 2004).

Pre-Hospital Care

CPR procedures, which are started immediately in drowning cases, are critical in clinical outcomes. Therefore, it is recommended to start CPR as soon as possible in cases of cardiac arrest (Grenfell, 2003).

Cervical injury risk is low (0.5%) in patients who do not have a history of motor vehicle accident before diving, falling from a height, or drowning.

Oxygen support can be provided with a face mask in cases that can breathe. However, in cases without respiration, high flow oxygen should be given with a balloon-valve-mask without wasting time. If spontaneous breathing does not return despite this, the victim should be intubated and connected to a mechanical ventilator, and positive pressure ventilation should be applied (European Resuscitation Council, 2000).

Intravenous and intraosseous routes should be preferred for drug administration before reaching the hospital. Endotracheal applications are recommended (Vanden et al., 2010). If the victim's hemodynamics cannot be improved despite oxygen administration, infusion of crystalloids should be started quickly (Orlowski et al., 1989).

Emergency Care

The first thing to do in the emergency room is to evaluate the airway and, if necessary, to ensure airway patency. At this stage, the victim should be started on oxygen and ventilated, and the core body temperature should be measured. In the presence of hypothermia, heated IV crystalloid fluids and warming devices such as blankets should be used. Primary and secondary evaluations should be made in detail and evaluated in trauma. Routine imaging for trauma is not recommended. However, if findings related to cervical trauma, diving, or prior motor vehicle accidents are detected, appropriate imaging methods should be preferred (Watson et al., 2001).

Toxicological examination, brain, and cervical CT should be considered in unresponsive cases without any reason (Rafaat et al., 2008). Measurement of electrolytes, blood urea nitrogen, creatinine, and hematocrit is often useless, and abnormalities are rarely observed (Modell et al., 1976).

Patients with good arterial oxygenation and no other morbidity can be discharged without supportive treatment. However, discharged cases; should be instructed to seek immediate medical attention if fever, altered consciousness, or respiratory symptoms occur. Oxygen demand, auscultation findings, and/or cases whose condition worsens despite oxygen therapy should be monitored and hospitalized. Patients who need intubation and mechanical ventilation should be admitted to the intensive care unit (Szpilman, 1997).

Treatment in Intensive Care

The Respiratory System

In cases where oxygenation is impaired, and mechanical ventilators are needed, treatment should be started with 100% oxygen, but this rate should be reduced as soon as possible. During mechanical ventilation, positive end-expiratory pressure (PEEP) should be started with 5 cm H2O, and if necessary, 2-3 cm H2O increments should be made. PEEP should be used until the intrapulmonary shunt drops below 20% or PaO2:FiO2 is 250 or more (Orlowski et al., 1989).

Drowning cases can be confused with pneumonia due to the radiographic appearance of water in the early period. A study showed that only 12% of drowning cases needed antibiotics (Berkel et al., 1996). Therefore, these cases should be followed up for resistant fever, leukocytosis, pulmonary infiltration, and leukocyte response in the tracheal aspirate. Bronchoscopy can be performed in selected cases for lung infection and clearing mucus plugs or solid material (Kapur et al., 2009). If drowning occurs in contaminated water (e.g., sewage), it is recommended to immediately initiate a broad-spectrum antibiotic therapy, including gram-positive and gram-negative (Orlowski, 1987).

In some cases, pulmonary function is impaired so dramatically that adequate oxygenation can only be achieved by using extracorporeal membrane oxygenation (ECMO) (Szpilman, 2012). Intubated cases should be weaned from the mechanical ventilator at least 24 hours later. This is because, in case of early extubation, pulmonary damage may not be adequately resolved, and pulmonary edema may recur. This condition may lead to reintubation, a prolonged hospital stay, and increased morbidity (Eggink and Bruining, 1977).

The Circulatory System

In most cases, circulatory oxygen support, rapid infusion of crystalloids, and elimination of hypothermia improve after drowning. There is a high probability of developing low-output cardiac dysfunction in severe cases. Significantly the increase in pulmonary capillary occlusion pressure, high central venous pressure, and increase in pulmonary vascular resistance are the leading causes of low cardiac output. Therefore, noncardiogenic pulmonary edema may be added to the cardiogenic component (Szpilman et al., 2012).

In cases of persistent hypotension despite crystalloid replacement, inotropes should be added to the treatment. In cases of resistant hypotension despite inotropes, vasopressors can be used in the treatment. In addition, routine echocardiography is recommended to evaluate cardiac functions (Orlowski, 1987). There is no evidence in the literature to support the use of diuretics, water restriction, or any specific fluid therapy after drowning, regardless of water content (Szpilman, 1997).

Neurological System

Late sequelae and deaths secondary to drowning are of neurological origin. Although the primary purpose of CPR in drowning cases is to restore spontaneous circulation, all procedures performed in the early stages are to prevent neurological damage (Topijan et al., 2012; Finfer et al., 2009). The procedures are aimed at providing brain perfusion with adequate oxygenation. In cases where spontaneous circulation returns after the intervention and in coma, the goal should be to manage the body temperature to correct the damage after brain hypoxia. Indeed, maintaining body temperature between 32 and 34^{0}C in the first 24 hours after CPR has been associated with better neurological outcomes (Nolan et al., 2015; Abdul Aziz and Meduye, 2010).

Unusual Complications

In severe cases, resuscitation hypoxia and hypoperfusion may initiate a systemic inflammatory response syndrome. This condition can progress from isolated cardiac, renal, and hepatic failure to sepsis and multiorgan failure. The most important markers for predicting the patient outcome after resuscitation are shown in Table 2. In patients with a normal chest X-ray after drowning, fulminant pulmonary edema may rarely develop up to 12 hours later. It is unclear whether delayed pulmonary edema is caused by delayed ARDS, hypoxia-induced neurogenic pulmonary edema, or airway hyperactivity due to aspirated water (Szpilman et al., 2012; Dyson et al., 2013).

Table 2. Important factors and outcome markers influencing
the resuscitation of a drowning patient

Early initiation of basic and advanced life support improves clinical outcome.
Every 10°C decrease in brain temperature reduces the amount of ATP the brain spends by approximately 50% during drowning.
There is a linear relationship between drowning time and death and neurologic damage after discharge (0-5 min – 10%; 6-10 min – 56%; 11-25 min – 88%; > 25 min – 99%).
Brain stem damage findings are markers for death or severe neurological sequelae.

Prognosis

The prognosis is generally good for patients who are conscious at admission and have mild confusion. The prognosis of patients in coma is poor. Severe brain damage and hypoxic encephalopathy are usually seen in comatose patients whose spontaneous circulation returns after CPR. After brain damage in children, long-term rehabilitation will likely be needed. Hypothermia can protect the brain. Serious risks for death include aspiration and ARDS (McCall and Sternard, 2021).

Prevention

Precautions to be taken to prevent drowning and death after drowning are as important as the prognosis after drowning. The ten preventive actions in the drowning guide published by the WHO on this subject are summarized in Table 3 (World Health Organization, 2014).

Table 3. Ten actions to be taken to prevent drowning according to the World Health
Organization guidelines (World Health Organization, 2014)

Build barriers to control access to water
Give preschoolers a place that is competent in care and where they can stay away from water (such as a nursery)
Teach school-age children basic swimming, water safety, and safe rescue skills
Educate bystanders on safe rescue and resuscitation
Raise public awareness and highlight children's vulnerability
Use watercraft with regulated safety and enforced precautions
Reinforce structures, and manage flood risks and other hazards at the local and national level
Coordinate drowning prevention efforts with other industries and agendas
Develop a national water security plan
Address priority research questions with well-designed studies

Conclusion

Drowning is an environmental emergency caused by fluids escaping the airway. Asphyxia is the most important factor in the drowning process, as it can cause cerebral and pulmonary damage. Hypothermia may be associated with drowning and may improve patient survival. Early and correct intervention is directly related to the prognosis after a careful rescue process without putting anyone in danger. The prognosis of unconscious cases after drowning is not good, and they need to be followed up in intensive care units. Drowning cases are preventable, due care must be exercised, and recommendations must be followed.

References

Abdul Aziz, K. A., & Meduoye, A. (2010). Is pH-stat or alpha-stat the best technique to follow in patients undergoing deep hypothermic circulatory arrest? *Interactive Cardiovascular and Thoracic Surgery*, 10, 271–282.

Borse N. N., Gilchrist J, Dellinger A. M., Rudd R. A., Ballesteros M. F, Sleet D. A., (2008). *CDC childhood injury report: patterns of unintentional Injuries among 0–19 year olds in the United States, 2000–2006*. Atlanta: Centers for Disease Control and Prevention.

Buzzacott, P., & Mease, A. (2018). Pediatric and adolescent injury in aquatic adventure sports. *Research in Sports Medicine* (Print), 26, 20–37.

Claesson, A., Svensson, L., Silfverstolpe, J., & Herlitz, J. (2008). Characteristics and outcome among patients suffering out-of-hospital cardiac arrest due to drowning. *Resuscitation*, 76, 381-7.

Dyson, K., Morgans, A., Bray, J. E., Matthews, B. L., & Smith, K. (2013). Drowning related out-of-hospital cardiac arrests: characteristics and outcomes. *Resuscitation, 84*, 1114-8.

Eggink W. F., Bruining H. A. (1977). Respiratory distress syndrome caused by near- or secondary drowning and treatment by positive end-expiratory pressure ventilation. *Neth. J. Med.*, 20:162-167.

European Resuscitation Council. (2000). Part 6: Advanced Cardiovascular Life Support. Section 3: adjuncts for oxygenation, ventilation, and airway control. *Resuscitation*, 46, 115–125.

Grenfell R. (2003). Drowning management and prevention. *Australian Family Physician*, 32(12), 990–993.

Hausser, J., & Niquille, M. (2007). La noyade [Drowning]. *Revue Medicale Suisse*, 3, 1834–38.

Kapur N., Slater A., McEniery J., Greer M. L., Masters I. B., Chang A. B. (2009) Therapeutic bronchoscopy in a child with sand aspiration and respiratory failure from near drowning - case report and literature review. *Pediatr. Pulmonol.*, 44:1043-1047

Linnan M., Anh L. V., Cuong P. V., et al., (2007). *Special series on child injury: child mortality and injury in Asia: survey results and evidence*. Florence, Italy: UNICEF Innocenti Research Center.

Manolios, N., & Mackie, I. (1988). Drowning and near-drowning on Australian beaches patrolled by life-savers: a 10-year study, 1973-1983. *The Medical Journal of Australia*, 148, 165–171.

McCall, J. D., & Sternard, B. T. (2021). *Drowning*. In *StatPearls*. StatPearls Publishing.

Modell J. H., Graves S. A., Ketover A. (1976) Clinical course of 91 consecutive near-drowning victims. *Chest*, 70:231-238.

NICE-SUGAR Study Investigators, Finfer, S., Chittock, D. R., Su, S. Y., Blair, D., Foster, D., Dhingra, V., Bellomo, R., Cook, D., Dodek, P., Henderson, W. R., Hébert, P. C., Heritier, S., Heyland, D. K., McArthur, C., McDonald, E., Mitchell, I., Myburgh, J. A., Norton, R., Potter, J., … Ronco, J. J. (2009). Intensive versus conventional glucose control in critically ill patients. *The New England Journal of Medicine*, 360, 1283–1297.

Nolan, J. P., Soar, J., Cariou, A., Cronberg, T., Moulaert, V. R., Deakin, C. D., Bottiger, B. W., Friberg, H., Sunde, K., & Sandroni, C. (2015). European Resuscitation Council and European Society of Intensive Care Medicine Guidelines for Post-resuscitation Care 2015: Section 5 of the European Resuscitation Council Guidelines for Resuscitation 2015. *Resuscitation*, 95, 202–222.

Orlowski J. P. (1987). Drowning, near-drowning, and ice-water submersions. *Pediatric Clinics of North America*, 34, 75–92.

Orlowski, J. P., Abulleil, M. M., & Phillips, J. M. (1989). The hemodynamic and cardiovascular effects of near-drowning in hypotonic, isotonic, or hypertonic solutions. *Annals of Emergency Medicine*, 18, 1044–1049.

Peden, A. E., Franklin, R. C., & Leggat, P. A. (2016). The Hidden Tragedy of Rivers: A Decade of Unintentional Fatal Drowning in Australia. *PloS one*, 11(8), e0160709.

Rafaat, K. T., Spear, R. M., Kuelbs, C., Parsapour, K., & Peterson, B. (2008). Cranial computed tomographic findings in a large group of children with drowning: diagnostic, prognostic, and forensic implications. *Pediatric critical care medicine*: a journal of the Society of Critical Care Medicine and the World Federation of Pediatric Intensive and Critical Care Societies, 9, 567–572.

Rougé-Maillart, C., Jousset, N., Gaudin, A., Bouju, B., & Penneau, M. (2005). Women who kill their children. *The American Journal of Forensic Medicine And Pathology*, 26, 320–326.

Smith, R., Ormerod, J., Sabharwal, N., & Kipps, C. (2018). Swimming-induced pulmonary edema: current perspectives. *Open Access Journal of Sports Medicine*, 9, 131–137.

Sterba J. A, Lundgren C. E. (1985). Diving bradycardia and breath-holding time in man. *Undersea Biomed. Res.*, 12, 139-50.

Szpilman, D., Bierens, J. J., Handley, A. J., & Orlowski, J. P. (2012). Drowning. *The New England Journal of Medicine*, 366(22), 2102–2110.

Szpilman D, Soares M. (2004) In-water resuscitation--is it worthwhile? *Resuscitation*, 63, 25-31.

Szpilman D. (1997). Near-drowning and drowning classification: a proposal to stratify mortality based on the analysis of 1831 cases. *Chest,* 112:660-665.

Tipton, M. J., & Golden, F. S. (2011). A proposed decision-making guide for the search, rescue and resuscitation of submersion (head under) victims based on expert opinion. *Resuscitation*, 82, 819–824.

Topjian, A. A., Berg, R. A., Bierens, J. J., Branche, C. M., Clark, R. S., Friberg, H., Hoedemaekers, C. W., Holzer, M., Katz, L. M., Knape, J. T., Kochanek, P. M., Nadkarni, V., van der Hoeven, J. G., & Warner, D. S. (2012). Brain resuscitation in the drowning victim. *Neurocritical Care*, 17, 441–467.

Vanden Hoek, T. L., Morrison, L. J., Shuster, M., Donnino, M., Sinz, E., Lavonas, E. J., Jeejeebhoy, F. M., & Gabrielli, A. (2010). Part 12: cardiac arrest in special situations: 2010 American Heart Association Guidelines for Cardiopulmonary Resuscitation and Emergency Cardiovascular Care. *Circulation*, 122, 829–861.

Van Berkel, M., Bierens, J. J., Lie, R. L., de Rooy, T. P., Kool, L. J., van de Velde, E. A., & Meinders, A. E. (1996). Pulmonary oedema, pneumonia and mortality in submersion victims; a retrospective study in 125 patients. *Intensive Care Medicine*, 22, 101–107.

Venema, A. M., Groothoff, J. W., & Bierens, J. J. (2010). The role of bystanders during rescue and resuscitation of drowning victims. *Resuscitation*, 81, 434–439.

Wood C. (2010). Towards evidence based emergency medicine: best BETs from the Manchester Royal Infirmary. BET 1: prophylactic antibiotics in near-drowning. *Emergency Medicine Journal*, 27, 393–394.

World Health Organization (2014). *Global Report on Drowning: Preventing a Leading Killer*. Geneva, Switzerland: World Health Organization.

Chapter 2

Hypothermia

Onur Karakayalı*, MD and Murat Özsaraç, MD

Department of Emergency Medicine, Sakarya University Faculty of Medicine,
Sakarya, Turkey

Abstract

Morbidity and mortality due to hypothermia still account for a significant percentage among all environmental emergencies. Hypothermia can be defined as a decrease of body core temperature or a "core" temperature below 35°C. Ambient air temperature of 18°C or water temperatures up to 22°C can easily cause hypothermia, especially in patients with underlying abnormal physiology. Predisposing factors are physiological, mechanical, psychological, environmental and cardiovascular factors. First, shivering begins when the core temperature of the patient is at the level of mild hypothermia. Tachycardia develops and blood pressure rises with a sympathomimetic response. However, when the core temperature drops below 32°C, the shivering ceases, heart rate and blood pressure decrease, and an irreversible deterioration occurs. Mental functions slowdown, and the cough and gag reflex disappear. Diffuse intravascular coagulation, DIC, is the last to develop and causes mortality in patients. Severe hypothermia is associated with high mortality due to progressive systemic edema, respiratory failure and neurological complications. Central arrangements planned according to guidelines and specific protocols allow for a shorter intervention time and effective treatment. Signs of hypothermia require quick treatment. Treatments should be initiated at the site and wet, cold clothing should be changed for dry, warm clothing. If the patient is cardiovascularly unstable, aggressive intervention is required. Today, successful management of severe accidental hypothermia can be achieved with extracorporeal membrane oxygenation (ECMO) using early rewarming techniques. ECMO provides continuous oxygenation and hemodynamic support with rapid and safe rewarming. It is necessary to increase the body temperature of the patient with gastric, bladder, peritoneal, and pleural lavage routes with heated fluids. Even prolonged cardio-pulmonary resuscitation does not usually lead to hypoxic brain damage in severe hypothermia. In cases of severe hypothermia, CPR can be performed intermittently during transport if continuous CPR is not possible due to environmental conditions. All precautions should be taken to prevent hypothermia in the prehospital care of trauma and non-trauma patients and in the emergency department.

---

* Corresponding Author's Email: onurkarakayali@sakarya.edu.tr.

In: Environmental Emergencies and Injuries in Nature
Editors: Murat Yücel, Murat Güzel and İbrahim İkizceli
ISBN: 978-1-68507-833-1
© 2022 Nova Science Publishers, Inc.

Keywords: hypothermia, environmental emergencies, cold emergencies

Introduction

Morbidity and mortality due to hypothermia still account for a significant percentage among all environmental emergencies. In the United States alone, approximately 1500 deaths are reported annually due to hypothermia. Although most of the deaths are the homeless living in uncovered areas, these deaths also increase in times of disasters. The majority of hypothermia patients due to freezing are people who have taken alcohol or drugs, and substance addicts. A few cases are patients who enter hypothermia due to water immersion (from the book of Disaster) Ambient air temperatures of 18°C or water temperatures up to 22°C can easily cause hypothermia, especially in patients with underlying abnormal physiology. Disease conditions which may cause impairment in thermoregulation and vasodilation including alcohol consumption, and inappropriate clothing choices can cause a rapid decrease in body temperature in the external environment (Robert, 2020).

Definition of Hypothermia

Hypothermia can be defined as a decrease of body core temperature or a "core" temperature below 35°C. For a sustainable life with normal physiological conditions, the core temperature should be above 35°C. In the case of mild hypothermia, the core temperature is between 32°C and 35°C. Clinical classifications have been made according to the severity of hypothermia, and the Swiss classification is the most well-known (Table 1).

Table.1. Swiss hypothermia classification

Hypothermia stage	Core temperature	Clinic
HT1	35-32 ºC	Conscious, shivering
HT2	32-28 ºC	Fuzzy consciousness, no shivering
HT3	28-24 ºC	No consciousness
HT4	24-13.7 ºC	Death
HT5	< 13.7 ºC	Death (no CPR response)

It is not possible to measure these temperatures with the standard thermometers used today. For this purpose, special thermometers that can measure at lower degrees are used. Tympanic and axillary measurements made with the classical method may give out erroneous results. Accordingly, gold standard measurement methods should be made from rectal, intravesical and esophageal area.

It will be useful to know the heat loss mechanisms in terms of protection from cold diseases and understand the main principles.

Radiation: Radiation is direct heat transfer that causes the body to lose the most heat. As the external environment gets colder, the heat lost by radiation also increases. It is a way of heat loss that is difficult to prevent or reduce.

Evaporation: Water evaporates from the skin and respiratory tract with sweating. Approximately 0.6 kcal of heat is lost with the evaporation of 1 g of water. Heat is also lost in order to heat the air we breathe and make it 100% relative humidity. There is no practical way to reduce the heat lost through the respiratory tract. It is also practically impossible to prevent the loss of heat from sweat which is not felt as in breathing.

Convection: The air in contact with the skin is heated to the temperature of the skin. When this warm air is displaced, the cold air that comes in its place is also heated again. Since the energy that warms the air comes from the body, heat is lost as the air moves. Heat loss by convection is a dynamic process and this loss is very low in normal temperatures, but in cold weather, more energy is required to heat the air, so the heat loss is high. The heat stolen by the moving air is proportional to the square of the speed of the wind. Therefore, wind is directly related to heat loss. Since convective heat loss increases rapidly, it is the biggest cause of hypothermia cases in nature (Guyatt, 2006; Zafren et al., 2014).

Clinical Findings of Hypothermia

First, shivering begins when the core temperature of the patient is at the level of mild hypothermia, 32-35°C. Tachycardia develops and blood pressure rises with the sympathomimetic response. However, when the core temperature drops below 32°C, the shivering ceases, the heart rate and blood pressure decrease, and an irreversible deterioration occurs due to the neuronergic conduction disorder in the temperature regulation center in the central nervous system. Mental functions slow down, and cough and gag reflex disappear. In addition, the patient develops dehydration due to cold diuresis. Diffuse intravascular coagulation, DIC, is the last to develop and causes mortality in patients.

In patients, clinically, superficial damage, i.e., edema, burning, erythema and small bullae, is present in 1st and 2nd degree frostbite, while deep damage develops in 3rd and 4th degree frostbite. Necrosis of the skin and subcutaneous tissue develop in 3rd degree injuries and muscle, tendon and bone necrosis in 4th degree injuries. Finally, there is extensive cyanosis, loss of tissue sensation, hemorrhagic bullae, and soft tissue necrosis. A table called mummification necrosis is seen in patients (Zafren and Danzl, 2018).

Predisposing Factors in Hypothermia

The degree of peripheral cold injuries is proportional to the type of injury and the duration of cold contact. Predisposing factors are physiological, mechanical, psychological, environmental and cardiovascular factors.

Physiological reasons: Genetics, previous history of cold injury, acclimatization, dehydration, overexertion, trauma, skin diseases, sweating, hypoxia.

Mechanical causes: Tight or wet clothing, tight boots, insufficient insulation, immobilization.

Psychological reasons: Mental state, fear, panic, fatigue, intense concentration on task, hunger, malnutrition, intoxication.

Environmental: Ambient temperature, humidity, duration of exposure, wind chill factor, altitude and associated conditions.

Cardiovascular: Hypotension, atherosclerosis, Raynaud's phenomenon, anemia, diabetes mellitus (Marx A, 2014).

Table 2. Hypothermia classification (Danzl D F, 1994)

According to time	Acute hypothermia	Freezing time < 6 hours
	Chronic hypothermia	Freezing time > 6 hours
According to temperature	Mild hypothermia	32 ^{0}C-35 ^{0}C
	Moderate hypothermia	28 ^{0}C-32 ^{0}C
	Severe hypothermia	< 28 ^{0}C
According to etiological reason	1^0 hypothermia	Direct exposure to cold
	2^0 hypothermia	Chronic diseases, advanced age, secondary to poisoning

Clinic

The response of different organ systems to low temperatures varies between individuals (3, 4). It is considered as mild hypothermia between 32 and 35°C. In the mild hypothermia stage, the patient is in the excitation (responding) phase. Physiological compensation is active. The body makes physiological adjustments by attempting to retain and produce the body temperature. During the initial phase of the excitation stage, blood pressure, heart rate, and cardiac output increase. In the following stages, all of these tend to decrease with the temperature (Marx, 2014). The first symptom of hypothermia is chills. At the end of the process, which starts with painful coldness in the hands and feet, muscle coordination decreases as the temperature drops. Coordination difficulties and consciousness changes may develop at 34°C-35°C.

Moderate hypothermia: The excitation leaves its place to the deceleration stage at 30°C-32°C. Oxygen use and carbon dioxide production decrease, and metabolism slows down in general. Below these temperatures, the shivering stops, and the suppression increases with concomitant hypovolemia. The circulating volume is reduced to one-third of the normal blood volume.

Severe hypothermia: Syncope and fatal cardiac rhythms occur below 28°C. Death occurs with sudden cardiac arrest below 20°C. One of the most common symptoms of severe hypothermia is that the shivering stops so the person does not try to protect himself from the cold.

Cardiovascular system: The main cause of mortality in hypothermia is rhythm disorders. ECG changes are often diagnostic in hypothermia which can cause a wide range of dysrhythmias from ventricular dysrhythmia to sinus bradycardia (Wittmers LE, 2001). The Osborn or J wave (slow, positive deflection at the end of the QRS complexes) is characteristic of hypothermia, although not pathognomonic.

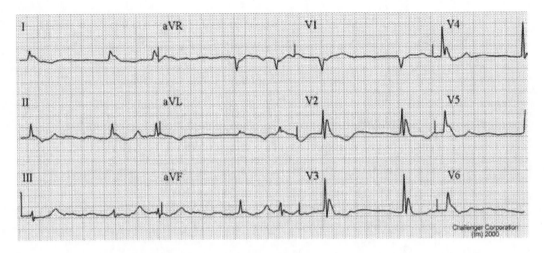

Figure 1. Osborn wave in positive deflection after QRS in V2, V3, V4, V4 derivations.

ECG findings in hypothermia:

I.   T-wave inversion
II.   PR, QRS, QT prolongation
III. Muscle tremor artifacts
IV.   Osborn wave.

Dysrhythmias:

I.   Sinus bradycardia
II.   Atrial fibrillation or flutter
III. Nodal rhythm
IV.   Atrioventricular block
V.   Ventricular fibrillation
VI.   Asystole.

Pulmonary System: Initially, there is a decreased respiratory rate and tidal volume after tachypnea, cold-induced bronchorrhea, and depression of cough and gag reflex.

Acid-base disorder: Acid-base changes are common in hypothermia, but not only a single pattern is observed. In the blood gas analysis of the patients, it incorrectly gives a higher partial oxygen and partial carbon dioxide pressure and a lower pH value since the measurement device is sensitive to 37^0C. Therefore, a temperature correction must be made. Generally, there is severe respiratory depression and acidosis due to CO2 retention and lactic acidosis due to poor tissue perfusion.

Central Nervous System: Progressive unconsciousness and limited cooperation are observed. Gait is impaired, confusion, and lethargy and coma occur in the last period.

Renal System: The concentration ability decreases, and cold diuresis occurs. If the patient is immobile, rhabdomyolysis is observed. Acute kidney damage may develop due to myoglobinuria.

Hematological System: There is platelet dysfunction and a predisposition to secondary thromboembolism in patients. Coagulation systems are disrupted and DIC may be observed in the last stage.

Table 3. Clinical stages of hypothermia

37 °C-35 °C	Feeling cold, numbness, a slight decrease in physical performance, inability to perform complex tasks with hands. Shivering begins
35 °C-34 °C	More distinct coordination difficulties, simple confusion and insensitivity
34 °C-32 °C	Decreased coordination and frequent stumbling, falling and inability to use hands, slowed thinking and speaking, worsening memory loss
32 °C-30 °C	Cease of shivering, complete loss of coordination and muscle stiffness, inability to stand, confusion, involuntary movement
30 °C-28 °C	Severe muscle stiffness, semi-consciousness, dilated pupils, uncertain breathing and pulse
< 28 °C	Syncope, sudden cardiac death

Hypothermia Treatment

Treatment should be initiated at the site and wet, cold clothing should be exchanged for dry, warm clothing. Special blankets designed for heating should be used. Especially, if there are many patients during the disaster, priority should be given to the cure of exposure prevention. After the warming process, the patient must be protected from freezing again. For this reason, if there is a risk of freezing again during the treatment in the field, the heating process should be delayed. Direct rubbing with something hot or snow is contraindicated as it will increase the degree of injury. Alcohol or sedating agents should be avoided as they can cause vasodilation. It will be beneficial to cover the frozen areas with a warm blanket.

If the patient has chilblains or cold-affected feet, elevation, local warming, and bandaging of affected tissues should be applied to the affected limb in the treatment. The literature also recommends treatments with nifedipine, topical corticosteroids, and oral prednisone. If the patient has a deep hypothermia clinic, rapid heating with 42°C water with circulation for 10-30 minutes can warm up and soften the frozen extremities. Opioid derivative analgesics, for instance ibuprofen, are given to patients because it is a very painful process. According to some protocols, it is beneficial to use penicillin G 500,000 units four times a day for 48 hours (Zafren et al., 2014; Zafren and Danzl, 2018).

In the case of severe hypothermia, good and proper resuscitation is very important. If the patient is cardiovascularly stable, external warming is started, and heated intravenous fluid and heated O2 can be given. If the patient is cardiovascularly unstable, aggressive intervention is required. It is necessary to increase the body temperature of the patient with gastric, bladder, peritoneal, and pleural lavage routes with heated fluids. Resistant VF can develop and it is difficult to treat unless the body temperature is improved. Heating can be done via the extracorporeal circuit, but survival is low. If this is not possible, a resuscitative thoracotomy may be considered.

Severe hypothermia is associated with high mortality due to progressive systemic edema, respiratory failure and neurological complications. Today, the successful management of severe accidental hypothermia can be achieved with extracorporeal membrane oxygenation

(ECMO) using early rewarming techniques. Helicopter transport, especially from areas where transportation is difficult, provides a fast response. Central arrangements planned according to guidelines and specific protocols allow for a shorter intervention time and effective treatment. ECMO provides continuous oxygenation and hemodynamic support with rapid and safe rewarming. It also corrects cardiorespiratory instability that makes it difficult for body temperature to return to normal. Thanks to the protective effect of hypothermia, the prognosis is often good, despite prolonged hypoperfusion and cardiopulmonary resuscitation. Even prolonged cardiopulmonary resuscitation does not usually lead to hypoxic brain damage in severe hypothermia. In cases of severe hypothermia, CPR can be performed intermittently during transport if continuous CPR is not possible due to environmental conditions. However, it is recommended to minimize gaps if possible and to apply mechanical chest compressions if available. Studies have reported that survival rates in patients treated with ECMO rewarming are 37%-100% with the application of high-quality CPR following hypothermic cardiac arrest. Neurological outcomes are observed to be excellent with ECMO application for cardiorespiratory support (Darocha, 2016).

However, ECLS (Extracorporeal life support) is an invasive and resource-demanding treatment. ECMO is a critical therapeutic decision in a patient to start rewarming. It is particularly important to avoid inadequate treatment in cases of hypothermia because the neurological outcome of survivors is significantly better than that of patients after normothermic cardiac arrest. It is known that high serum potassium levels are associated with poor outcomes in the management of accidental hypothermia. Significantly elevated potassium levels, >12 mmol/L, are often incompatible with life, and levels >8 mmol/L are associated with severe brain and heart hypoxia and poor outcomes. However, in determining the patients who can benefit from extracorporeal life support, it is important not only to evaluate the serum potassium level, but also to evaluate parameters such as age, gender, body temperature at admission, hypothermia mechanism and cardiopulmonary resuscitation time (Mathieu Pasquier, 2018).

In addition, the direct transfer of hypothermic patients with risk factors for cardiac arrest (temperature < 28°C, ventricular arrhythmia, systolic blood pressure <90 mmHg) to a center where ECLS can be applied improves patient outcomes. The important factor determining the outcome in all cases of hypothermia is whether critical brain hypoxia occurs before protective brain cooling.

In a hypothermic patient with cardiac arrest, non-ECLS rewarming is only indicated if ECLS is not present for any reason. The effectiveness of non-ECLS rewarming depends on the presence of the circulation, so rewarming is extremely slow until the heart starts to work again, requiring prolonged and sustained CPR (Paal et al., 2016).

Prepare for a Winter Storm

Public education and preparation before a storm will always be the most effective treatment. Especially, the most effective method in reducing mortality cases in the winter months will be training on this subject in the eastern regions of our country. According to foreign sources, and local news and media organizations, the plan starts to work when the possibility of a storm arises within 24 hours. The civilian population begins to be warned by news channels and the media. Every family should have an emergency plan and a communication tool. When disaster strikes, family members should have a plan to keep in touch when they are not together. In the event of a disaster, it is especially desirable for people to stay in a warm indoor environment. If this opportunity cannot be provided individually, sheltered areas are reported by the state authorities.

The first sign of exposure to hypothermia is uncontrolled shivering. If there are many patients at the same time, patients with neurological findings such as memory loss, disorientation, and speech disorder should be given priority and taken to a warm and safe environment. As described above in the treatment of general hypothermia, the wet, cold clothes of the patients should be removed and they should be warmed with warm clothes or blankets. If these people are awake, non-alcoholic hot drinks can be given. Signs of hypothermia require quick treatment.

Recommendations have also been determined for those who travel individually by car. An emergency bag should be ready in the vehicles belonging to individuals who are likely to be exposed to winter storms during travel. The technical equipment of the car must be made ready for winter. If possible, do not travel alone, inform others of your travel route, travel on main roads, and provide an estimated time of arrival. There are also rules that must be followed when the car is stranded on the road while traveling. The car must be pulled aside so that it does not pose a danger to the traffic, a colored warning must be attached to the radio antenna or the window, and the warning lights of the car must be turned on. Especially staying inside the car increases the chances of being rescued. Starting the engine of the car every 10 minutes can keep the car warm enough. If possible, it is recommended to drink and eat fluids to prevent dehydration. However, alcohol or caffeine is not recommended in hypothermia.

Patient Evaluation

The most important medical condition for people who have been exposed to a winter storm or freezing cold is hypothermia. This is followed by frostbite, carbon monoxide poisoning and soft tissue traumas. Along with the vital signs of the patients, their core temperature should also be monitored. Management in accordance with the disaster plan should be started in the nearest health center. Laboratory tests, blood gases, tests for rhabdomyolysis, bleeding and coagulation tests should definitely be requested. Additionally, anomalies such as dysrhythmias or the Osborne wave should be detected early by taking an ECG. Investigations for a general trauma process should be completed. In the case of mild hypothermia, the core temperature is 32-35°C, and tachypnea, tachycardia, shivering, and changes in mental status are observed. Wet and cold clothing must be removed before passive external heating begins.

If present, special insulated blankets, metallic foil insulators, chemical heating blankets and chemical heat packs can be used in the external environment. An external heater should be applied to the anatomical areas that provide the most efficient heat transfer: the armpit, chest and back area (Frederike, 2018).

In the case of moderate hypothermia, the core temperature is 28-32°C, and cardiac, respiratory and central nervous system parameters begin to be suppressed in these patients. Fatal rhythms such as heart failure, atrial fibrillation, bradycardia or asystole may be observed. Warm blankets, heating pads and a warm environment should be provided to the patients. In the treatment of the patient, heating should be applied especially to the dorsum of the patient. The objective is to prevent further peripheral vasodilation.

In severe hypothermia, the core temperature drops below 28°C. Hypotension, bradycardia, ventricular fibrillation, pulmonary edema and coma are observed at this stage. These patients should be protected from ventricular fibrillation by careful intervention.

Internal warming can be applied in addition to the simple external warming techniques described above. The patient is treated with humidified oxygen and warm intravenous fluids. The peritoneal space, pleural space and bladder can be washed with fluids at approximately 45°C. Pleural lavage is not performed in all patients because ventricular arrhythmias may occur in patients with no cardiac rhythm. The most appropriate extracorporeal treatments may be warm hemodialysis or cardiopulmonary bypass treatments. In cases of hypothermia, arrhythmia treatment is performed according to ACLS guidelines. The patient may not respond to resuscitation until they are at normal temperature.

Patients may often require long-time CPR. High-quality CPR is the key to the best outcome. In the literature, groups of patients who underwent CPR for 6 to 8 hours and were successfully restored to spontaneous circulation after rewarming have been described (Paal et al. 2016).

Damages as a result of freezing due to cold in winter storms are more common in some risk groups. These risk groups include conditions such as mental status change, advanced age, malnutrition, peripheral vascular disease, and coronary artery disease. The frost defined as frostnip starts at -2°C. The first thing is the disruption of the extracellular matrix by freezing of the cells. The second is necrosis, which is the occurrence of reperfusion injury during the warming of the patient. Do not rub the frozen part and do not manipulate excessively. Do not take a bath over 40-42°C during treatment. The affected limb should remain in the bath for 15 to 30 minutes. If there are bullae, they should not be opened and if there are opened bullae, they should be covered and sterile. Aloe vera can be used in the dressing. Pain control with nonsteroidal anti-inflammatory and tetanus vaccination should be done.

Management of Hypothermic Trauma Patients

Hypothermia is common in severe trauma patients; it is multifactorial and increases morbidity in these patients. It is an extremely important part of the "fatal triad" with acidosis and coagulopathy, often neglected in management, worsening the prognosis. It has been reported that mortality rates in hypothermic trauma patients are much higher than in normothermic patients, and the mortality in patients with a core temperature below 34°C is 40%. Hypothermia is quite harmful in terms of hemodynamics in multiple trauma patients.

It increases the risk of massive bleeding and the need for transfusion by contributing to coagulopathy. It is associated with a non-negligible risk of infection as it causes suppression of the immune system. Preventive measures should be initiated as soon as the patient is admitted to the emergency room. Simple and easy-to-use methods such as passive external warming of hypothermic trauma patients using warming blankets, removing cold, wet clothing, administering heated intravenous fluids and heated humidified oxygen for inhalation, or warming the emergency room are an integral part of medical care (Vardon, 2016).

Hypothermia is associated with higher mortality, both in trauma patients in general and in patients with traumatic brain injury in particular. All precautions should be taken to prevent hypothermia in the prehospital care of trauma patients and in the emergency department (Rösli D, 2020).

Conclusion

There are some points to be considered when applying CPR in hypothermia patients. Cardiopulmonary resuscitation should be performed in the absence of vital signs.

1) Cardiac and ETCO2 monitoring are required.
2) The application rate and depth of chest compressions are not different from normothermic patients.
3) If the body temperature is below 30°C, "Single Shock and Maximum Power" should be applied in patients with VF.
4) Before additional shocks, it is necessary to warm the body 1-2°C.
5) Vasoactive drugs are not started until the body temperature rises above 30°C.
6) If the body temperature is between 30 and 35 °C, it is recommended to apply the vasoactive drug at twice the normal dose.
7) There are no temperature thresholds and limits for initiating or performing CPR.
8) If there are no vital signs, if there is no rhythm improvement in the ECG, if cardiac activity cannot be detected by USG, if the K+ level is >12 meq, CPR is terminated in the patient.

References

Danzl, D F, Pozos, R. F. (1994). Accidental hypothermia. *N. Engl. J. Med.* 331: 1756.

Darocha, T., Kosiński, S., Jarosz, A., Sobczyk, D., Gałązkowski, R., Piątek, J., Konstany-Kalandyk, J., & Drwiła, R. (2016). The chain of survival in hypothermic circulatory arrest: encouraging preliminary results when using early identification, risk stratification and extracorporeal rewarming. *Scandinavian journal of trauma, resuscitation and emergency medicine*, 24, 85.

Fanny V, Ségolène M, Thomas G, Olivier Fourcade. (2016). Accidental hypothermia in severe trauma. *Anaesthesia Critical Care & Pain Medicine.* 35, Issue 5, 355-361.

Frederike J.C. Haverkamp, Gordon G. Giesbrecht, Edward C. T. H. Tan. (2018). The prehospital management of hypothermia — An up-to-date overview. *Injury.* 49(2), 149-164.

Guyatt G, Gutterman D, Baumann M H, et al., (2006) Grading strength of recommendations and quality of evidence in clinical guidelines: report from an American College of Chest Physicians task force. *Chest.* 129:174–181.

Marx A. J., Hockberger S. R., Walls M. R. (2014) *Rosen'Emergency Medicine Concepts and Clinical Practice* 8 th. Edition, 2145-2168.

Mathieu P, Olivier H, Peter P, Tomasz D, Marc B, et al., (2018) *Hypothermia outcome prediction after extracorporeal life support for hypothermic cardiac arrest patients*: The HOPE score, Resuscitation, Volume 126, 58-64.

Paal, P., Gordon, L., Strapazzon, G. et al., (2016) Accidental hypothermia–an update. *Scand. J. Trauma Resusc. Emerg. Med.* 24, 111.

Robert W. (2020) Cardiac Arrest Secondary to Accidental Hypothermia: The Physiology Leading to Hypothermic Arrest: Air Medical Journal, 39(2), 133-136.

Rösli D, Schnüriger B, Candinas D, Haltmeier T. (2020) The Impact of Accidental Hypothermia on Mortality in Trauma Patients Overall and Patients with Traumatic Brain Injury Specifically: A Systematic Review and Meta-Analysis. World J Surg. 44:4106-4117.

Wittmers LE. (2001) Pathophysiology of cold exposure. Minn Med 84: 30.

Zafren et al., (2014) Wilderness Medical Society Practice Guidelines for the Out-of-Hospital Evaluation and Treatment of Accidental Hypothermia: 2014 Update. Wilderness Environ Med. Dec;25(4 Suppl):S66-85.

Zafren K, Danzl D. (2018) Frostbite and nonfreezing cold injuries. In: Schaider JJ, Hayden RS, Wolfe ER, Barkin MR, Rosen P, eds. Rosen's Emergency Medicine 9th ed. Philadelphia, PA: Lippincott Williams & Wilkins; Ch: 131; 1735- 1741.

Chapter 3

Cold Injuries

Serhat Koyuncu[1,*], MD and Halil İbrahim Akdogan[2], MD

[1]Emergency Medicine Clinic, Kayseri City Hospital, Kayseri, Turkey
[2]Emergency Service, Tokat State Hospital, Tokat, Turkey

Abstract

While cold injuries were seen primarily in military personnel in the past, today, they are an urgent health problem seen in the elderly living in cold climates, especially in the elderly with diabetes, homeless people, individuals using alcohol or substances, and athletes engaged in winter sports. Different names of frostbite injuries have been defined according to the affected area of the body and the type of cold exposure. Although different names define it, the basic principle in the treatment is stabilizing the affected tissue and restoring body temperature immediately. The main goal of clinicians is to prevent mortality and morbidity with different treatment methods.

Keywords: frostbite, cold, injury, environmental, emergency

Introduction

Although frostbite, hypothermia, and cold injuries are conditions that mainly affect military personnel, they have recently started to be seen frequently in adventurous people who are elderly, homeless, use alcohol or drugs and do mountain/winter sports. The degree of influence depends on individual factors and environmental factors, and exposure to the cold depends on the duration. Factors such as dry or wet exposure, chronic or short-term exposure, the humidity and wind degree of the environment, and temperatures below freezing determine the type of cold injury. Individual factors such as peripheral vascular disease, malnutrition, cardiovascular diseases, anemia, Raynaud's disease, diabetes, and smoking can worsen frostbite-related tissue damage.

---

* Corresponding Author's Email: dr_serhats@hotmail.com.

In: Environmental Emergencies and Injuries in Nature
Editors: Murat Yücel, Murat Güzel and İbrahim İkizceli
ISBN: 978-1-68507-833-1

Cold Injuries

Pernio (Chilblain)

Pernio or chilblain is characterized by mild but bothersome inflammatory skin lesions caused by prolonged and intermittent exposure to humid, nonfreezing ambient temperatures. It usually manifests as itchy red or purple lesions on the feet and hands. Lesions often appear 12 hours after exposure to cold. Single or multiple erythematous papules, nodules, and ulcerated, necrotized, vesicular, and bullous lesions can be seen. The lesions are painful and itchy, and there is often a burning sensation. Treatment is conservative. Elevation and application of moisturizing lotions are usually sufficient.

Immersion Injury - Trench Foot

This is a soft tissue injury caused by exposure to cold, humid, and freezing temperatures (0-10°C) for a long time. It is frequently seen in homeless people, drug users, and psychiatric patients (Ingram and Raymond, 2013). It is classically described in four stages. In the first stage (during exposure to cold), lethargy is the most common symptom. Due to excessive vasoconstriction, the extremities may appear bright red but soon become pale or white. At this stage, there is no pain or swelling. In the second stage, peripheral blood flow gradually returns after removal from the cold environment or during rewarming. The extremities become mottled and pale blue; there may be pain and edema. This phase can last from a few hours to a few days. In the third stage, blood flow increases markedly, and the extremity becomes hot and red. Hyperalgesia, edema, and bullae can be seen at this stage. This stage can take time ranging from weeks to months. The tissue usually appears as normal in the fourth stage, but pain may persist. This stage can last from weeks to years or be permanent.

Frostbite

Frostbite is local tissue death due to cold. Cellular damage occurs by various mechanisms. These mechanisms can be explained as ice crystal formation (intracellular and extracellular), cell dehydration, electrolyte disturbances, and denaturation of lipid-protein complexes. Secondarily, dissolution follows endothelial damage and subsequently microvascular thrombosis, resulting in continued cell damage and death. Endothelial damage, intravascular sludge, increase in inflammatory mediators and free radicals, reperfusion injury, and thrombosis contribute to progressive dermal ischemia (Mohr et al., 2009) The temperature, duration, and freezing rate of exposure determine the degree of injury. A visual determination of tissue viability is difficult during the first few weeks after injury. Viable tissue necrosis can only be determined after the demarcation boundaries of the tissue are clarified.

Cold bites are generally classified into four categories, depending on the appearance after rewarming, the depth of the injury, and the amount of tissue damage. First-degree injury is defined as frostbite or frostnip. These are superficial frostbite injuries that are not accompanied by permanent tissue loss or tissue damage. Generally, the fingers, toes, nose, ears, and penis are at risk. There is numbness, tingling, coldness, and paleness in the affected area. Afterward, swelling and peeling can be observed. It usually heals in a short time without leaving any damage after heating (Handford et al., 2017).

In second-degree cold bites, full-thickness freezing of the skin and then widespread edema and bullae formation filled with serous fluid are observed. When intervened at this stage, the bullae disappear after a few days. At first, paresthesia is seen, and in the long term, throbbing pain is seen. It has a good prognosis.

In third-degree injury, the reticular dermis and dermal vascular plexus are affected in deeper tissues. The bullae are hemorrhagic, and blue-gray skin discoloration is observed. The patient initially feels numb and painless, like a piece of wood, but burning and severe pain begin later (McIntosh et al., 2011). The prognosis is severe. The fourth-degree injury extends to the subcutaneous tissues, muscles, bones, and tendons. The affected tissue takes on a black, dry, and mummy-like appearance. Almost all result in tissue and limb losses (Table 1).

Management and Treatment

Treatment of frostbite injuries is complex and controversial. Incorrect interventions during treatment will cause increased mortality and morbidity. Therefore, it is vital to make the proper intervention quickly after the case is detected. There are several universally accepted principles in terms of treatment modalities, and in line with these principles, treatment modalities are grouped under three main headings. These titles are pre-hospital care, hospitalization, and post-dissolution rehabilitation. The post-dissolution rehabilitation phase can last for weeks (Murphy et al., 2000).

Pre-Hospital Management

After detection of the case in the field by professional health workers, first of all, the patient's vital functions should be evaluated. In cases with regression in vital functions, basic and advanced life support should be started to prevent mortality. In cases with normal vital signs, it is essential to initiate a very rapid and correct intervention to prevent mortality and morbidity that may develop due to freezing.

Table 1. Classification of frostbite

First Degree	Superficial involvement, numbness, tingling, peeling, and swelling around mild edema
Second Degree	Diffuse edema, full-thickness skin involvement, serous bullae, paresthesia, edema, and erythema
Third Degree	Involvement of the subcutaneous folds, hemorrhagic bullae, blue-gray skin color
Fourth Degree	Deep tissue involvement, resulting in tissue loss, black color

After detecting the case, the casualty should be quickly taken to a warmer environment, and re-exposure to cold should be prevented. Re-exposure to cold after warming a frozen body part causes increased tissue damage. The frozen area must be buffered and stabilized to prevent injury that may occur with movement. If the frozen areas are on the patient's foot, walking should be avoided. Wet clothing on the casualty should be removed. The frozen area should be treated with warm water or body temperature water during the pre-hospital warming stages. Physical interventions should be avoided to warm the frozen area.

It should be noted that heating the frozen area by rubbing may cause tissue damage, and high heat contact with hot compresses or heaters may cause hot burns. Another important issue in patients who need to be heated is the pain sensation that occurs with warming up. With the effect of warming, severe pain can occur in patients. In order to prevent this, the use of pre-hospital analgesia is essential (Biem et al., 2003, Murphy et al., 2000).

Emergency Service and Hospital Management

As a continuation of the pre-hospital management done quickly and accurately, tissue damage can be minimized with appropriate treatment models to be made in the emergency services and hospitals. The main goal of the treatment in the hospital is to quickly warm the frozen areas of the injured before tissue damage occurs. Studies have shown that the most appropriate method during the heating process is a water bath with an antibacterial agent such as povidone-iodine or hexachlorophene. Another critical parameter here is the optimal temperature of the water. In the studies carried out, it has been determined that the most suitable temperature range is between 40 and 42°C (Britt et al., 1991, McCauley et al., 1983). It has also been reported that the temperature value of water can be 37-39°C from different sources (Hallam et al., 2010, McIntosh et al., 2014). While the chance of tissue survival is less at lower temperatures, burn cases have been reported at higher temperatures, which will increase the level of injury. Active movement is beneficial during the warm-up process. However, physical contact and force such as massaging the wound area should be avoided. Reheating should be continued until thawing is complete. A red-purple coloration of the wound area and a regaining of flexibility are signs of resolution and a marker for ending the heating process. Analgesic agents are recommended to treat pain that will occur during heating. Intravenous fluid therapy is not routinely recommended in frostbite cases. However, cases of renal failure due to rhabdomyolysis due to freezing have been reported in the literature. In addition, intravenous fluid therapy should be applied in necessary cases since diuresis may develop due to hypothermia suppressing the release of antidiuretic hormone (Murphy et al., 2000).

Freezing treatment protocols were defined by McCauley et al. to provide better pathophysiological healing of the wound after thawing. According to these treatment protocols, the steps in Table 2 should be followed in the cases (McCauley et al., 1983).

In bullous lesions containing serous fluid after dissolution, the amount of damage is considered to be superficial, and these lesions are debrided. However, the damage is deeper in bullous lesions containing hemorrhagic fluid, and in studies it has been argued that it would be better to leave these lesions without debridement. The use of topical aloe vera in wounds with both types of lesions inhibits thromboxane A2 synthesis and benefits wound healing. In the study of Heggers et al., it was shown that using ibuprofen and prophylactic penicillin together with aloe vera reduced tissue loss (Heggers et al., 1987).

Table 2. Treatment protocol for freezing

1. If hospital conditions allow, frostbite cases should be followed up in appropriate clinics.
2. Affected areas should be warmed up quickly. The optimum temperature value for heating is 40-42°C (104-108°F), and heating should be continued until the injured tissue is thawed (15-30 minutes).
3. After reheating is completed:
• Debride bullous lesions containing serous fluid and apply topical aloe vera every 6 hours.
• Do not touch bullous lesions of hemorrhagic character. Apply topical aloe vera once every 6 hours.
• Stabilize and elevate the affected body part with a splint.
• Tetanus prophylaxis.
• Pain control with strong analgesic agents such as Opiad.
• Apply ibuprofen 400 mg once every 12 hours.
• Antibiotic prophylaxis for secondary infections.
• Apply hydrotherapy daily for 30-45 minutes with water at 40°C.
• Documentation: Record the lesion with a photograph at the entrance, at the 24th hour, and once every 2-3 days until discharge.
• Do not allow smoking.

Edited and excerpted from McCauley et al., 1983.

Studies suggest the use of anticoagulant treatments to prevent thrombosis in the first days of freezing. However, there is no evidence that heparin or other anticoagulants contribute positively to the course of frostbite (McCauley et al., 1983). Studies with the intra-arterial use of vasodilator agents have been shown to reduce vasospasm. However, no superiority could be demonstrated in reducing vasospasm compared to rapidly warming patients. Although it is thought that the heating process may be beneficial in cases where it is delayed, there is no evidence of this (Murphy et al., 2000).

Thrombolytic Therapy

The use of thrombolytic agents in patients to prevent tissue loss has been suggested in many studies. The main goal of thrombolytic therapy is to prevent microvascular thrombosis and tissue loss. Tissue plasminogen activator (tPA) is often used for this purpose. After the 0.15 mg/kg bolus dose, 0.15 mg/kg (not to exceed a total of 100 mg) should be given over 6 hours. Heparin therapy is recommended for 24-72 hours after thrombolytic therapy (Hickey et al., 2020, Jones et al., 2017).

Surgical Treatment

In frostbite cases, compartment syndrome may develop due to reperfusion and increased tissue edema due to rewarming or treatments. It is vital to remove the compartment quickly with fasciotomy in these cases. Amputation is life-saving in the early period in tissue necrosis and sepsis due to infection. Clinicians need to be mindful of the timing of amputation. If amputation is indicated in delayed cases, it is essential to wait for the demarcation line in terms of the functionality of the remaining tissue to minimize morbidity (Handford C et al., 2017).

In addition to the known treatment modalities, there are many studies on auxiliary treatment methods such as hyperbaric oxygen and sympathectomy. However, there is currently no scientific evidence value for the benefit of these treatments (McIntosh et al., 2014).

Conclusion

As a result, frostbite injuries are an important health problem leading to death or permanent damage. First, the necessary social measures should be taken to prevent its formation. It is very important to start the treatment very early in injured individuals to prevent mortality and morbidity. Sequela-free survival should be aimed for with transportation and correct interventions in the early pre-hospital period and with appropriate treatment approaches by clinicians specialized in this field in hospitals.

References

Biem, J., Koehncke, N., Classen, D., & Dosman, J. (2003). Out of the cold: management of hypothermia and frostbite. *Cmaj*, 168(3), 305-311.

Britt, L. D., Dascombe, W. H., & Rodriguez, A. (1991). New horizons in management of hypothermia and frostbite injury. *Surgical Clinics of North America*, 71(2), 345-370.

Hallam, M. J., Cubison, T., Dheansa, B., & Imray, C. (2010). Managing frostbite. *Bmj*, 341, Tintinalli.

Handford, C., Thomas, O., & Imray, C. H. (2017). Frostbite. *Emergency Medicine Clinics*, 35(2), 281-299.

Heggers, J. P., Robson, M. C., Manavalen, K., Weingarten, M. D., Carethers, J. M., Boertman, J. A., & Sachs, R. J. (1987). Experimental and clinical observations on frostbite. *Annals of Emergency Medicine*, 16(9), 1056-1062.

Hickey, S., Whitson, A., Jones, L., et al. (2020). Guidelines for thrombolytic therapy for frostbite. *Journal of Burn Care & Research*, 41(1), 176-183.

Ingram, B. J., & Raymond, T. J. (2013). Recognition and treatment of freezing and nonfreezing cold injuries. *Current Sports Medicine Reports*, 12(2), 125-130.

Jones, L. M., Coffey, R. A., et al. (2017). The use of intravenous tPA for the treatment of severe frostbite. *Burns*, 43(5), 1088-1096.

McCauley, R. L., Hing, D. N., Robson, et al. (1983). Frostbite injuries: a rational approach based on the pathophysiology. *The Journal of Trauma*, 23(2), 143-147.

McIntosh, S. E., Hamonko, M., Freer, L., et al. (2011). Wilderness Medical Society practice guidelines for the prevention and treatment of frostbite. *Wilderness & Environmental Medicine*, 22(2), 156-166.

McIntosh, S. E., Opacic, M., Freer, L., et al. (2014). Wilderness Medical Society practice guidelines for the prevention and treatment of frostbite: 2014 update. *Wilderness & Environmental Medicine*, 25(4), S43-S54.

Mohr, W. J., Jenabzadeh, K., & Ahrenholz, D. H. (2009). Cold injury. *Hand Clinics*, 25(4), 481-496.

Murphy, J. V., Banwell, P. E., Roberts, A. H., & McGrouther, D. A. (2000). Frostbite: pathogenesis and treatment. *Journal of Trauma and Acute Care Surgery*, 48(1), 171.

Chapter 4

Heat Emergencies

İlker Şallı[1,*] and Başak Bayram[2]

[1]Department of Emergency Medicine, University of Health Sciences Tepecik Research and Education Hospital Izmir, Turkey
[2]Department of Emergency Medicine, School of Medicine, Dokuz Eylul University, Izmir, Turkey

Abstract

Recently, with climate changes and global temperature increases, heat waves have been more common. The number of emergency department visits and mortality rates has increased due to heat emergencies during extreme heatwaves. Heat-related illnesses can occur in a wide spectrum of clinical disorders that can be corrected with simple measures such as heat edema or heat cramps to life-threatening heatstroke. In addition to individuals who are dependent on others, such as the elderly or bedridden people who cannot take the necessary precautions, healthy individuals such as young athletes and workers who must stay in a hot environment for a long time can also be affected. For this reason, healthcare professionals who care for patients from all age groups should be aware of heat illnesses, especially during heat waves, and be familiar with risk factors and emergency treatment. In this section, the pathophysiology, epidemiology and risk factors, characteristics, and management of heat illnesses are reviewed.

Keywords: heat, emergencies, emergency room, emergency service, heat stroke, heat edema

Introduction

Owing to climate changes and global temperature increases, the frequency of exposure of the population to heat waves is increasing, and this affects public health. Heat emergencies occur when body heat is not sufficiently removed and temperature cannot be regulated. Environmental factors such as air temperature, atmospheric pressure due to altitude, and weather may affect the disruption of the body's normal thermoregulation. Heat illnesses can range from benign conditions such as heat edema, heat cramps, heat exhaustion, and prickly heat to life-threatening hyperthermia, also known as heatstroke (Kenny et al., 2018). Especially

* Corresponding Author's Email: ilkersalli@hotmail.com.

In: Environmental Emergencies and Injuries in Nature
Editors: Murat Yücel, Murat Güzel and İbrahim İkizceli
ISBN: 978-1-68507-833-1

during sudden heat waves, serious health problems may occur in fragile people such as the elderly and children, and there is an increase in emergency department (ED) admissions and deaths from all causes (Schaffer et al., 2011; Oray et al., 2018; Williams et al., 2012; Zhang et al., 2015). It is thought that annual heat-related deaths will increase substantially in the next decades (Li et al., 2015; Hajat et al., 2014).

Although it is thought that elderly people experience heat-related illnesses most frequently, sudden temperature changes can affect any age group. It was reported that there was an increase in deaths from the age of 35 in the 2003 heat wave in France (Fouillet et al., 2006). Temperature changes can affect individuals working outdoors and young people doing sports. Heatstroke is one of the leading causes of sudden death in young athletes (Maron et al., 2007). It has been reported that there is a 1% increase in occupational accidents for every 1°C increase in temperature (Fatima et al., 2021). As a result, individuals from all age groups can apply to health institutions with heat emergencies. Therefore, physicians who care for the elderly, children, athletes and outdoor workers need to be aware of heat emergencies, especially in areas with sudden temperature rises. In this section, the pathophysiology, characteristics and management of heat illness are reviewed.

Pathophysiology

Living beings are divided into two according to their body temperature; ectotherm and endotherm. Ectotherm creatures do not have thermoregulation systems and their temperature depends on the external environment. Endotherm creatures have thermoregulation systems, that is, they maintain the appropriate internal temperature for themselves even if the outside temperature changes. Humans are an example of endotherm creatures. The basic human body temperature is between 36.5 and 37.5°C.

Temperatures between 35 and 41°C can be tolerated by thermoregulation systems, but the body cannot compensate for thermal loads greater than this range. Thermoregulation is a type of homeostasis for humans and necessary for survival. It also plays an adaptive role in fighting infections (Sessler, 2009). The core temperature of the body is the sum of the external environment, and heat and mechanical work originating from metabolism. The balance between environmental factors such as external temperature and humidity, and internal factors such as active metabolic hormones, causes heat loss from or increase in the body. Heat exchange with the external environment occurs by radiation, evaporation, conduction, and convection (Leiva and Church, 2021). Increasing blood flow to the skin (i.e., convection) and loss of sweat (i.e., evaporation) are the primary responses of the body to thermal stress.

Radiation is the release of heat from the body surface into the surrounding air. Conduction is the transfer of heat by contact with cold objects. Measures such as air conditioners indoors, and wearing hats and quick-drying clothing outdoors help in maintaining body temperature. However, people without a chance to relocate or who are dependent are not able to change these factors (Miyake, 2013). Sweating is a powerful process that accounts for about 70% of body heat loss and this is the main route as radiation and conduction will be ineffective when outdoor temperature and humidity increase (Leiva and Church, 2021; Gomez, 2014).

The acclimatized person can produce twice as much sweat as non-acclimatized individuals. With heat acclimatization, the body temperature threshold for sweating decreases, and the sodium concentration in the sweat component is reduced (Tansey and Johnson, 2015).

Electrolyte disturbances may develop with excessive sweating. This is the cause of painful skeletal muscle contractions due to prolonged activity in the heat. In patients with severe hypovolemia, heat exhaustion is seen due to water and salt depletion (Székely, et al., 2015).

Intravascular volume and cardiac function are two other variables in the regulation of body temperature. Severe dehydration increases blood viscosity, putting more strain on the heart. In patients with heart failure or in those who use drugs that suppress cardiac function for reasons such as hypertension, the heart cannot pump enough blood to the body's surface and this finally leads to the accumulation of heat in the body. For these reasons, cardiovascular diseases are risk factors for heat illnesses (Leiva and Church, 2021).

Core body temperature is maintained as long as the increase in body temperature is compensated by adequate heat loss. The non-compensable stage starts with decreasing central venous pressure and an increase in core body temperature occurs. The inflammatory response causes life-threatening heatstroke with cardiovascular collapse and multiple organ failure. The inflammatory response associated with heatstroke is similar to the systemic inflammatory response syndrome. Pathogens and endotoxins enter the systemic circulation because of ischemia due to decreased intestinal blood flow (Epstein and Yanovich, 2019). Finally, a life-threatening clinical situation may arise with ongoing multiorgan failure.

While classical non-exertional heat illness affects the elderly and people with comorbidities, exertional heat illness affects healthy individuals at a younger age who have to work in a heated environment or endure strenuous exercise such as sport activities (Gomez, 2014). A significant amount of heat is generated from the muscles during exercise and by metabolic activities to maintain hemostasis. If the excessive heat generation cannot be eliminated by physiological mechanisms, it causes serious life-threatening disorders. It is thought that many factors such as high ambient temperature and intensity of exercise, physical fatigue, sleep deprivation, dehydration, hot incompatible clothes and the use of drugs that affect thermoregulation (such as anticholinergics that reduce sweating, calcium channel blockers that affect skin blood supply or hormones) increase the risk of exertional heatstroke (Casa et al., 2012).

Epidemiology

Heat illnesses are a global problem that is increasing with the effect of global warming. The United States Centers for Disease Control and Prevention (CDC) reported that 7,233 heat-related deaths occurred between 1999 and 2009, an average of 658 per year in the United States (Fowler et al., 2013). However, a later study reported that an average of 5608 deaths per year between 1997 and 2006 in 297 counties of the USA were attributable to heat (Weinberger et al., 2020). Between June and September 2003, more than 70,000 deaths were reported in 12 European countries (Robine et al., 2008). Heat-related deaths are expected to increase in the next years with the aging population (Li et al., 2015). Heat-related deaths in the UK are expected to increase by 257% after 30 years (Hajat et al., 2014).

In the case of sudden temperature changes during heat waves, acute heat illness ED visits are increasing. It has been reported that during the 2006 heat wave in California, USA, ED admissions with heat illnesses increased 6 times and hospitalizations increased 10 times. Hospitalizations and deaths are higher in older age, male, urban and low-income people and those with chronic diseases (Knowlton et al., 2009). The most common reason for admission to EDs due to heat illnesses is heat exhaustion, and heatstrokes are the most common cause of hospitalization and mortality (Hess et al., 2014).

Temperature changes can affect individuals from all age groups, however, older people are more vulnerable to the health effects of heat waves. Sweating capacity reduces with aging and skin blood flow is approximately 2-3 times lower than in younger people. With reducing sweating and cardiovascular functions in the elderly heat dissipation decreases (Millyard et al., 2020). Larose et al., reported that, impairment in heat dissipation begins after the age of 40, and therefore, the risk of heat-related illness increases from middle age when doing physical activity in the heat (Larose et al., 2013). Most deaths due to heat illnesses are seen in elderly patients over 65 years of age and those of the male gender. Alcohol and drug users and people using psychiatric medications are at risk of classic heatstroke.

The increase in temperature also negatively affects the health of children. It has been reported that there is an increase in ED admissions of children with the increase in temperature and humidity. Children aged 0-4 years are the most affected group (Sheffield et al., 2018; Niu et al., 2021). Children are at risk of heat illness, since they have a larger surface area than their body mass, sweat less and have a low acclimation rate. Additionally, their tendency to consume water during intense exercise is more blunted than in adults (Bytomski and Squire, 2003).

Risk factors associated with heat illness can be classified as individual and environmental factors. Individual factors include the specific characteristics as well as medical history and medication use. Individual predisposing factors associated with heat illness include; (Pryor et al., 2015; Westwood et al., 2020; Kenny et al., 2010; Leiva and Church, 2021; Nelson et al., 201; Epstein and Yanovich, 2019; Gauer and Meyers, 2019):

- Age (i.e., older adults, infants and children)
- Obesity
- Malnutrition
- Lack of acclimatization
- Lack of physical fitness
- Physical fatigue
- Sleep deprivation
- Strenuous exercise in hot temperatures (e.g., athletes, outdoor laborers, military personnel)
- Comorbidities
  - Cardiovascular diseases
  - Hypertension
  - Hypohidrosis
  - Diabetes mellitus
  - Respiratory disease
  - Psychiatric illness
  - Malignant hyperthermia
  - Sickle cell disease
- Medications
  - Those that decrease sweating capacity and interfere with central thermoregulation: Anticholinergics, antihistamines, tricyclic antidepressants, benzotropine; phenothiazines.

- Those that increase heat production: Amphetamines, LSD, cocaine, phencyclidine; MAO inhibitors (↑ muscle activity)
- Those that cause dehydration and electrolyte imbalances: Lithium, Haldol, Navane, prolixin; diuretics, alcohol.

Environmental predisposing factors associated with heat illness include; Increased endogenous heat load (e.g., heat, temperature and/or high ambient humidity), lack of adequate cooling and shading, and lack of access to water (Gauer and Meyers, 2019). Exertional heatstroke is common in young athletes, outdoor laborers and soldiers (Gomez, 2014). In environments with high humidity, the heat loss capacity decreases with high ambient humidity regardless of age, and therefore the risk increases (Larose et al., 2014).

Behavioral thermoregulation is an important response for maintaining body temperature in a hot environment and avoiding heat illnesses (Flouris and Schlader, 2015). Recognizing the increase in temperature and moving to a cooler environment, using air conditioning or a fan, limiting exercises and increasing fluid intake are examples of behavioral responses. Older people, those who are bedridden, mentally ill people, individuals under the influence of drugs or alcohol and those with limited mobility cannot make such behavioral changes (Miyake, 2013; Flouris and Schlader, 2015). Individuals who depend on others, lack social support and are alone are particularly at risk during heat waves. A meta-analysis evaluating risk factors for death in a heatwave reported that, air conditioning at home, visiting a cool environment, and increased social contact reduced heat-related deaths during a heatwave, while being bedridden and living alone increased the risk (Westwood et al., 2020).

Heat-Related Illnesses

Heat Edema
This can be described as swelling in the distal extremities with the effect of gravity, venous stasis and vasodilation after exposure to heat. It is more common in older individuals. Pitting edema may occur due to heat-induced hyperaldosteronism. Elevation of the extremities and compression garments such as compression stockings are used for treating heat edema Diuretics should be avoided as they increase the volume deficit (Lipman et al., 2019).

Heat Rash (Miliaria or Prickly Heat)
This is a condition that occurs because of the blockage of the eccrine sweat glands, after exposure to hot climates. Heat rash generally occurs on parts of the body where clothing is sticking or rubbing.

There are 3 types of heat rash (Leiva and Church, 2021);

- Miliaria crystallina: This is the mildest and fortunately the most common form. It occurs in the stratum corneum, the outermost layer of the epidermis. It is usually seen in childhood with small clear vesicles on the face and trunk.
- Miliaria rubra: This occurs in the deep epidermis. Rashes are macular and papular, and covered with vesicles. Patients may feel itching or burning in the areas of the rash.

- Miliaria profunda: This is a more severe form, occurring at the dermal-epidermal junction. Rashes appear as large, white vesicles.

In treatment, clothing should be removed, the person placed in a cool environment, and topical emollients should be avoided (Gauer and Meyers, 2019). Miliaria crystallina is self-limiting and resolves within 24 hours. In miliaria rubra, a low-potency topical steroid can be used to limit inflammation. To protect against secondary infections, topical antibiotics should be added to the prescription in patients with miliaria profunda (Guerra et al., 2021).

Heat Cramps

These can be defined as spasmodic and painful contractions of large muscle groups that develop after exercise in a hot environment (Lipman et al., 2019). The mechanism of focal exercise-associated muscle was first described by the theory of dehydration and electrolyte imbalance. According to the theory, severe sweating can lead to dehydration and electrolyte deficits (sodium, potassium, magnesium and chloride). The osmolality of the extracellular fluid increases due to fluid loss and the intracellular fluid is displaced into the extracellular space. The interstitial space expands and causes mechanical deformation in the nerve endings. This causes excessive excitation in the motor nerve terminals. According to the neuromuscular theory, repetitive exercises cause muscle fatigue, and an increasing excitatory drive to the alpha motor neuron activity produces localized muscle cramps (Nelson and Churilla, 2016; Giuriato et al., 2018). Although the neuromuscular theory is more supported with new evidence, it is thought that dehydration and electrolyte disorders may affect the etiology, especially in sensitive individuals (Nelson and Churilla, 2016).

Heat-related cramps are probably different from the local muscle cramps associated with repetitive exercise seen in athletes. Exercise-related cramps can occur in a warm or cool environment and without passive warming. Oral salt solutions or electrolyte replacement may relieve heat cramps (Lipman et al., 2019).

Generally, there is no abnormality in the patient's consciousness and vital signs. Evaluation should be done for more serious medical conditions such as heat exhaustion. Physical activity should be terminated and resting should occur. Oral isotonic or hypertonic solution should be given to patients who can tolerate fluid intake. Intravenous fluid administration should be considered in patients whose oral intake is not tolerated (Casa et al., 2015).

Heat Syncope

Heat syncope and exercise-related syncope are two confusing definitions. Heat syncope refers to transient loss or near-loss of consciousness, which occurs in a few days of exposure when high ambient temperature without acclimatization is completed (O'Connor and Casa, 2021). The risk factors involve advanced age, having comorbid conditions that decrease cardiac output, prolonged standing and dehydration (Lipman et al., 2019). Exercise-related syncope describes an athlete's inability to stand or syncope without hyperthermia because of an impaired baroreceptor reflex or lower extremity venous pooling (Lipman et al., 2019; O'Connor and Casa, 2021).

The victim should be taken to a shaded area or air-conditioned area and placed in a supine position with their feet elevated above the level of the heart. Oral fluids should be given to patients who can tolerate oral intake. With this intervention, the person is expected to recover in 15-20 minutes. Other causes of syncope should be considered in patients who do not improve within this period (O'Connor and Casa, 2021). A careful examination should be made for fall-related injuries. Patients with risk factors for significant causes of syncope or with prolonged symptoms should be evaluated like other syncope patients presenting to the ED (Lugo-Amador et al., 2004; O'Connor and Casa, 2021; Gauer and Meyers, 2019).

Heat Stress or Heat Exhaustion

Heat exhaustion is a more severe and the most common form of heat illness among patients admitted to EDs (Hess et al., 2014). It may occur as a result of exposure to high environmental heat or strenuous physical activity. Skin blood supply increases during heat stress, stroke volume reduces due to impaired end-diastolic filling, and presyncope symptoms occur due to insufficient cardiac output (Lipman et al., 2019; Nybo et al., 2011). Most of the patients present with volume depletion and/or fluid depletion (Atha, 2013). Core body temperature may be normal or slightly elevated (>37°C but <40°C). The patient can present with syncope, fatigue, tachycardia, excessive sweating, nausea/vomiting, and weakness without neurological symptoms.

The patient should be taken to a shaded or air-conditioned area and placed in a supine position with their feet elevated above the level of the heart. Then, the patient should be strictly monitored including mental status, heart rate, respiratory rate, blood pressure, and core body temperature. The patient should be peeled as much as possible and start cooling until the rectal temperature is lower than 38.3°C (O'Connor and Casa, 2021). Any technique may be used for cooling such as evaporative, convective, or conductive cooling (Lipman et al., 2019). Peroral chilled water or sports drinks can be given to patients who can tolerate oral intake. In patients who develop symptoms such as nausea and vomiting, care should be taken in terms of aspiration and giving antiemetics should be considered. Intravenous fluids should be started immediately in patients with impaired consciousness or nausea/vomiting. One recommended approach for fluid resuscitation is to give 1 liter of normal saline followed by an infusion according to the patient's response (O'Connor and Casa, 2021). It should be considered that especially dehydrated patients may need more fluids.

If rapid improvement does not occur after the first interventions or patients have high-risk comorbidities, older people should be transferred to the hospital. Electrolyte abnormalities (sodium, potassium, glucose, magnesium, calcium, and phosphorus), complete blood count, kidney and liver functions, coagulation studies, and studies for rhabdomyolysis (e.g., creatine kinase and myoglobin level) should be evaluated in the ED. Younger patients who are adequately responsive to treatment and without comorbidities can be discharged home from the ED after observation. Elderly or other patients with comorbidities or patients with significant electrolyte abnormalities should be admitted to the hospital (Lugo-Amador et al., 2004).

Heatstroke

Heatstroke is a condition in which the body cannot tolerate high temperatures due to impaired thermoregulation. With the loss of hypothalamic regulation, body temperature rises inexorably and may rise above 40.5°C. Rapidly increasing body temperature causes dysfunction in the central nervous system and multiorgan failure (Epstein and Yanovich, 2019). Heatstroke is the most common cause of death due to heat illness in the EDs (Hess et al., 2014). Excess water and salt are lost through sweating despite a hot environment. Significant cardiac stress occurs because of dehydration, hypovolemia, and vasodilation. Since vasodilation will return with cooling, which is the first step in heatstroke treatment, the blood pressure of the patient recovers without the need for excessive fluid loading.

There are two types of heatstroke. Classical (passive) heatstroke (CHS) is more common in vulnerable (elderly, young, or chronically ill) people. For example, children who are left in a car with closed windows in hot weather, the elderly living in care homes without air conditioning, and people with neuropsychiatric issues are at risk of CHS. Although mortality decreases with early diagnosis and treatment, it varies from 17% to 63.6% (Rublee et al., 2021). There is a prodromal period similar to heat exhaustion, but patients admitted to the hospital have severe clinical symptoms such as altered mental status, coma, seizure, and hypotension.

Exertional heatstroke (EHS): Unlike CHS, this occurs in young and athletic people. It develops within hours in people who are not accustomed to the climate after intense exercise in hot and humid weather. Patients suffer from high-output heart failure. The mortality rate is lower than 5% (Epstein and Yanovich, 2019). Patients usually present to the ED with complaints such as tremors in the trunk and upper extremities, feeling dizzy, throbbing headache, nausea, and dizziness.

Myocardial oxygen consumption increases after cardiac stress in both types. If there is an underlying disease such as coronary artery disease, heart failure, atherosclerosis, myocardial infarction and malignant dysrhythmia may occur. Above 41.5°C, protein denaturation develops and neurons begin to die rapidly (Ye et al., 2019). Confusion, lethargy, disorientation, and coma may occur. A fixed dilated pupil is seen in patients with severe neurological involvement (Epstein and Yanovich, 2019).

The respiratory rate of patients was increased to remove the increased body temperature and to compensate for the lactic acidosis that occurred. Pulmonary edema may develop due to heart failure after cardiac stress. A breath sounds examination is critical in this respect. The cardiovascular system enters the hyperdynamic phase primarily to remove heat. Tachycardia and hypertension are seen. However, because of increased stress, pulmonary edema and malignant dysrhythmias develop together with pump failure. The second phase is hypotension (Lugo-Amador et al., 2004). If the patient has developed hypotension, This indicates a poor prognosis.

The skin is hot and reddened due to vasodilation. Sweating varies according to the type of heatstroke. Sweating is not usually seen in CHS due to the affected population because the sweat glands are tired or not yet functioning adequately. However, the cause of heatstroke is not, of course, the absence of sweating. In EHS, on the other hand, some patients are sweating due to the increased catecholamine discharge. If liver involvement is developed, the production of coagulation factors is disrupted. DIC may develop due to platelet disruption and increased permeability of vessels (Leon and Helwig, 1980; al-Mashhadani et al., 1994). In the presence of petechiae and purpura on the skin, internal organ bleeding should be investigated. Electrolyte disturbances play an important role in clinical worsening. Sudden cardiac collapse may develop, especially due to the development of hypokalemia. Acute tubular necrosis may develop due to renal hypoperfusion, and rhabdomyolysis may develop due to tissue hypoperfusion.

Treatment

Treatment should be started on first contact with the patient. In the out-hospital setting the initial resuscitation should be focused on evaluation and stabilization of the airway, breathing, and circulation using standard advanced life support protocols. The rectal body temperature is evaluated, and classical heatstroke patients are immediately transported to the ED. In patients with exertional heat, stroke cooling should be initiated with cold-water immersion before the transport. Measurement methods other than rectal body temperature (such as oral, tympanic, axillary) are not recommended. Instead, it is recommended to cool the patient until the patient begins to shiver (O'Connor and Casa, 2021). The health care providers should give 1-2 L of isotonic saline. The seizures should be treated with benzodiazepines (Epstein and Yanovich, 2019).

The core temperature should be monitored by rectal or intravesical measurement in the hospital. Rapid cooling is the first-line treatment for the preservation of the central nervous system and should not be delayed for any reason other than cardiopulmonary resuscitation. The rate of cooling the patient should be faster than 0.2°C/minute. In general, below 39°C is targeted (Epstein and Yanovich, 2019). Conductive cooling with cold water immersion and evaporative and convective cooling with sprayed water and forced air are the most common cooling methods in hospitals. The Wilderness Medical Society Clinical Practice Guidelines recommend cold water immersion over evaporative and convective cooling in the hospital setting (Lipman et al., 2019). Antipyretics such as aspirin or acetaminophen have no place in treating heatstroke because there is no problem in the hypothalamic set point in the pathogenesis of heatstroke. Complications such as liver damage and DIC may be exacerbated by the use of these drugs (Lugo-Amador et al., 2004).

Patients should be evaluated for airway, respiration, and circulation in the ED. Patients may develop seizures and there is a risk of aspiration due to acute changes in mental status. Most of the patients with heatstroke have impaired consciousness and seizures can develop. Patients should be assessed for the necessity of advanced airway interventions. Benzodiazepines (5 mg, repeatable) and phenytoin (loading dose 15-20 mg/kg) can be used to treat seizures (Epstein and Yanovich, 2019). Two large vascular accesses should be obtained for fluid needs, and oxygen support should be provided if necessary. Fluid replacement with 30 mL/kg of isotonic saline should be performed in the presence of circulatory failure. The goal of resuscitation in the ED is to maintain mean arterial pressure >65 mmHg and urine output >50 mL/kg/h, and to achieve normal lactate levels. Vasopressors should be considered in patients who do not respond adequately to fluid therapy (Epstein and Yanovich, 2019). Fluid replacement should be done carefully because with cooling, peripheral vasodilation will regress and additional volume will be added to the central circulation. The excessive volume load will accelerate the development of pulmonary edema in the patient (Seraj et al., 1991). Chinese guidelines recommend evaluating cardiac functions with a bedside USG and a dynamic response to fluid (e.g., passive leg raise) in the presence of circulatory dysfunction and hypoperfusion (Liu et al., 2020).

Serum electrolytes (sodium, potassium, glucose, magnesium, calcium, and phosphorus), complete blood count, kidney and liver functions, urinalysis, coagulation studies, and studies for rhabdomyolysis (e.g., creatine kinase and myoglobin level) should be evaluated in the ED. Metabolic and electrolyte disturbances should be corrected appropriately.

Conclusion

Heat emergencies can be seen in a wide spectrum of illnesses from mild cases with heat edema or heat cramps to life-threatening heatstroke. Although mortality due to heat illnesses is more common among people of older age with comorbidities, heat-associated illnesses can affect people of all age groups especially considering exertional heatstroke, which is common among younger people. Risk factors include individual factors such as obesity and age, as well as environmental factors such as heatwaves and lack of adequate cooling, shading, and access to water. People can prevent most of the heat-related illnesses with simple precautions, and basic behavioral changes such as air conditioning at home and visiting a cool environment, and social contact may protect people from death during heat waves.

Most heat illnesses can be treated with simple medical interventions, the interruption of exercise, and removal of the patient from the hot environment. Early recognition of more serious conditions such as heat exhaustion and heatstroke is crucial. Monitoring core temperature by rectal or intravesical measurement is the safest method of evaluating a suspected patient in the ED. Rapid recognition of patients with heatstroke and prompt initiation of cooling improve outcomes. Coldwater immersion should be considered for cooling in the hospital. Antipyretics should not be used for temperature control. Fluid replacement should be performed by evaluating circulatory status and the presence of hypoperfusion. Cardiac functions can be evaluated with bedside ultrasound to avoid volume overload. Heatstroke treatment requires special equipment, from body temperature monitoring to cooling methods. Standard algorithms should be established for the management of patients in EDs and adequate equipment should be available.

Recent studies have drawn attention to a significant increase in ED admissions and mortality during heatwaves. Considering the temperature increases due to climate changes, it is clear that more important health problems will be seen, especially with the aging of the population. Prevention of heat-related illnesses is more effective than treatment and certainly easier. Studies need to be carried out to identify effective prevention methods and health care providers and policymakers need to work effectively for their wider acceptance.

References

Atha, W. F. (2013). Heat-related illness. *Emergency Medicine Clinics*, 31(4), 1097-1108.

Al-Mashhadani, S. A., Gader, A. G., Al Harthi, S. S., Kangav, D., Shaheen, F. A., & Bogus, F. (1994). The coagulopathy of heat stroke: alterations in coagulation and fibrinolysis in heat stroke patients during the pilgrimage (Haj) to Makkah. *Blood coagulation & fibrinolysis: an international journal in haemostasis and thrombosis*, 5(5), 731-736.

Bytomski, J. R., & Squire, D. L. (2003). Heat illness in children. *Current sports medicine reports*, 2(6), 320-324.

Casa, D. J., Armstrong, L. E., Kenny, G. P., O'Connor, F. G., & Huggins, R. A. (2012). Exertional heat stroke: new concepts regarding cause and care. *Current sports medicine reports*, 11(3), 115-123.

Casa, D. J., DeMartini, J. K., Bergeron, M. F., Csillan, D., Eichner, E. R., Lopez, R. M., ... & Yeargin, S. W. (2015). National Athletic Trainers' Association position statement: exertional heat illnesses. *Journal of athletic training*, 50(9), 986-1000.

Epstein, Y., & Yanovich, R. (2019). Heatstroke. *New England Journal of Medicine*, 380(25), 2449-2459.

Fatima, S. H., Rothmore, P., Giles, L. C., Varghese, B. M., & Bi, P. (2021). Extreme heat and occupational injuries in different climate zones: A systematic review and meta-analysis of epidemiological evidence. *Environment international*, *148*, 106384.

Flouris, A. D., & Schlader, Z. J. (2015). Human behavioral thermoregulation during exercise in the heat. *Scandinavian journal of medicine & science in sports*, *25*, 52-64.

Fowler, D. R., Mitchell, C. S., Brown, A., Pollock, T., Bratka, L. A., Paulson, J., ... & Radcliffe, R. (2013). Heat-related deaths after an extreme heat event—four states, 2012, and United States, 1999–2009. *MMWR. Morbidity and mortality weekly report*, *62*(22), 433.

Fouillet, A., Rey, G., Laurent, F., Pavillon, G., Bellec, S., Guihenneuc-Jouyaux, C., ... & Hémon, D. (2006). Excess mortality related to the August 2003 heat wave in France. *International archives of occupational and environmental health*, *80*(1), 16-24.

Gauer, R., & Meyers, B. K. (2019). Heat-related illnesses. *American family physician*, 99(8), 482-489.

Giuriato, G., Pedrinolla, A., Schena, F., & Venturelli, M. (2018). Muscle cramps: a comparison of the two-leading hypothesis. *Journal of electromyography and kinesiology*, *41*, 89-95.

Gomez, C. R. (2014). Disorders of body temperature. *Handbook of clinical neurology*, *120*, 947-957.

Guerra, K. C., Toncar, A. & Krishnamurthy K. Miliaria. (2021). In: *StatPearls* [Internet]. Treasure Island (FL): StatPearls Publishing; 2021 Jan–. PMID: 30725861.

Hajat, S., Vardoulakis, S., Heaviside, C., & Eggen, B. (2014). Climate change effects on human health: projections of temperature-related mortality for the UK during the 2020s, 2050s and 2080s. *J Epidemiol Community Health*, *68*(7), 641-648.

Hess, J. J., Saha, S., & Luber, G. (2014). Summertime acute heat illness in US emergency departments from 2006 through 2010: analysis of a nationally representative sample. *Environmental health perspectives*, *122*(11), 1209-1215.

Kenny, G. P., Yardley, J., Brown, C., Sigal, R. J., & Jay, O. (2010). Heat stress in older individuals and patients with common chronic diseases. *Cmaj*, *182*(10), 1053-1060.

Kenny, G. P., Wilson, T. E., Flouris, A. D., & Fujii, N. (2018). Heat exhaustion. *Handbook of clinical neurology*, *157*, 505-529.

Knowlton, K., Rotkin-Ellman, M., King, G., Margolis, H. G., Smith, D., Solomon, G., ... & English, P. (2009). The 2006 California heat wave: impacts on hospitalizations and emergency department visits. *Environmental health perspectives*, *117*(1), 61-67.

Larose, J., Boulay, P., Wright-Beatty, H. E., Sigal, R. J., Hardcastle, S., & Kenny, G. P. (2014). Age-related differences in heat loss capacity occur under both dry and humid heat stress conditions. *Journal of Applied Physiology*, *117*(1), 69-79.

Larose, J., Boulay, P., Sigal, R. J., Wright, H. E., & Kenny, G. P. (2013). Age-related decrements in heat dissipation during physical activity occur as early as the age of 40. *PLoS One*, *8*(12), e83148.

Leiva, D. F., & Church, B. (2020). Heat Illness. In: *StatPearls* [Internet]. Treasure Island (FL): StatPearls Publishing; 2021 Jan–. PMID: 31971756.

Leon, L. R., & Helwig, B. G. (2010). Heat stroke: role of the systemic inflammatory response. *Journal of applied physiology*, 109(6), 1980-1988.

Li, T., Ban, J., Horton, R. M., Bader, D. A., Huang, G., Sun, Q., & Kinney, P. L. (2015). Heat-related mortality projections for cardiovascular and respiratory disease under the changing climate in Beijing, China. *Scientific reports*, *5*(1), 1-8.

Liu, S. Y., Song, J. C., Mao, H. D., Zhao, J. B., & Song, Q. (2020). Expert consensus on the diagnosis and treatment of heat stroke in China. *Military Medical Research*, *7*(1), 1-20.

Lugo-Amador, N. M., Rothenhaus, T., & Moyer, P. (2004). Heat-related illness. Emergency Medicine Clinics, 22(2), 315-327.

Maron, B. J., Doerer, J. J., Haas, T. S., Tierney, D. M., & Mueller, F. O. (2009). Sudden deaths in young competitive athletes: analysis of 1866 deaths in the United States, 1980–2006. *Circulation*, *119*(8), 1085-1092.

Millyard, A., Layden, J. D., Pyne, D. B., Edwards, A. M., & Bloxham, S. R. (2020). Impairments to Thermoregulation in the Elderly During Heat Exposure Events. *Gerontology and Geriatric Medicine*, *6*, 2333721420932432.

Miyake, Y. (2013). Pathophysiology of heat illness: Thermoregulation, risk factors, and indicators of aggravation. *Japan Med Assoc J, 56*(3), 167-73.

Nelson, N. G., Collins, C. L., Comstock, R. D., & McKenzie, L. B. (2011). Exertional heat-related injuries treated in emergency departments in the US, 1997–2006. *American journal of preventive medicine, 40*(1), 54-60.

Nelson, N. L., & Churilla, J. R. (2016). A narrative review of exercise-associated muscle cramps: Factors that contribute to neuromuscular fatigue and management implications. *Muscle & nerve, 54*(2), 177-185.

Niu, L., Herrera, M. T., Girma, B., Liu, B., Schinasi, L. H., Clougherty, J. E., & Sheffield, P. (2021, August). Associations between Heat Index and Child Emergency and Hospital Visits in New York City. In *ISEE Conference Abstracts* (Vol. 2021, No. 1).

Nybo, L., Rasmussen, P., & Sawka, M. N. (2011). Performance in the heat—physiological factors of importance for hyperthermia-induced fatigue. *Comprehensive Physiology, 4*(2), 657-689.

O'Connor, F. G., Casa, D., & Fields, K. B. (2015). *Exertional heat illness in adolescents and adults: Management and prevention.* Uptodate [Internet]. Availabe at: https://www.uptodate.com/contents/exertional-heat-illness-in-adolescents-and-adults-management-andprevention?sectionName=Heat%20syncope%20and%20exercise%20associated%20collapse&search=exertional%20heat%20illness&topicRef=13788&anchor=H12884550&source=see_link#H12884550 (Last Accessed: 01 Jan 2022).

Oray, N. C., Oray, D., Aksay, E., Atilla, R., & Bayram, B. (2018). The impact of a heat wave on mortality in the emergency department. *Medicine, 97*(52).

Pryor, R. R., Bennett, B. L., O'Connor, F. G., Young, J. M., & Asplund, C. A. (2015). Medical evaluation for exposure extremes: heat. *Wilderness & environmental medicine, 26*(4), 69-75.

Robine, J. M., Cheung, S. L. K., Le Roy, S., Van Oyen, H., Griffiths, C., Michel, J. P., & Herrmann, F. R. (2008). Death toll exceeded 70,000 in Europe during the summer of 2003. *Comptes rendus biologies, 331*(2), 171-178.

Rublee, C., Dresser, C., Giudice, C., Lemery, J., & Sorensen, C. (2021). Evidence-Based Heatstroke Management in the Emergency Department. *Western Journal of Emergency Medicine, 22*(2), 186.

Schaffer, A., Muscatello, D., Broome, R., Corbett, S., & Smith, W. (2012). Emergency department visits, ambulance calls, and mortality associated with an exceptional heat wave in Sydney, Australia, 2011: a time-series analysis. *Environmental Health, 11*(1), 1-8.

Seraj, M. A., Channa, A. B., Al Harthi, S. S., Khan, F. M., Zafrullah, A., & Samarkandi, A. H. (1991). Are heat stroke patients fluid depleted? Importance of monitoring central venous pressure as a simple guideline for fluid therapy. *Resuscitation, 21*(1), 33-39.

Sheffield, P. E., Herrera, M. T., Kinnee, E. J., & Clougherty, J. E. (2018). Not so little differences: Variation in hot weather risk to young children in New York City. *Public health, 161*, 119-126.

Székely, M., Carletto, L., & Garami, A. (2015). The pathophysiology of heat exposure. *Temperature, 2*(4), 452-452.

Tansey, E. A., & Johnson, C. D. (2015). Recent advances in thermoregulation. *Advances in physiology education.* 2015 Sep;39(3):139-48.

Weinberger, K. R., Harris, D., Spangler, K. R., Zanobetti, A., & Wellenius, G. A. (2020). Estimating the number of excess deaths attributable to heat in 297 United States counties. *Environmental Epidemiology (Philadelphia, Pa.), 4*(3).

Williams, S., Nitschke, M., Weinstein, P., Pisaniello, D. L., Parton, K. A., & Bi, P. (2012). The impact of summer temperatures and heatwaves on mortality and morbidity in Perth, Australia 1994–2008. *Environment international, 40*, 33-38.

Ye N., Yu T., Guo H., Li J. (2019). Intestinal Injury in Heat Stroke. *J Emerg Med*, 57:791.

Zhang, K., Chen, T. H., & Begley, C. E. (2015). Impact of the 2011 heat wave on mortality and emergency department visits in Houston, Texas. Environmental Health, 14(1), 1-7.

Westwood, C. S., Fallowfield, J. L., Delves, S. K., Nunns, M., Ogden, H. B., & Layden, J. D. (2021). Individual risk factors associated with exertional heat illness: A systematic review. *Experimental physiology, 106*(1), 191-199.

Chapter 5

Thermal Burns

Ali Kemal Erenler[*]

Department of Emergency Medicine, Hitit University, Çorum, Turkey

Abstract

According to the reports of the World Health Organization, 11 million thermally injured patients present annually, requiring dedicated specialist services worldwide. Although the risk factors, mechanism of injury, and pathophysiology of thermal burns (TB) are well-defined in the literature, they remain a significant cause of morbidity and mortality. They also have psychological and economic impacts that can last for a lifetime.

The impact of thermal injuries on the human body may be divided into two categories as local and systemic responses. Locally, they cause coagulation necrosis and protein denaturation, stasis, and hyperemia due to damage to the circulation. Their systemic consequences are hypotension, pulmonary edema, and decreased circulation to end organs due to the release of systemic inflammatory mediators and cytokines. Death results from multi-organ failure, and the presence of an inhalation injury increases the risk of death.

The current standard for any burn treatment was first described in the 1960s. It can be summarized as removing clothing and jewelry from the affected site, applying cool running water, covering the wound, and seeking medical help. Despite this fact, there is still a lack of consensus on an ideal initial treatment for thermal burn injuries. Since management requires a multidisciplinary approach, numerous rehabilitation programs are proposed in the literature. This chapter summarizes the pathophysiology and novel treatment approaches in TB injuries.

Keywords: thermal injury, heat, trauma

Introduction

TBs are the most common type of burn injury. Up to 86% of the burned patients require burn center admission. The most common causes of TBs are hot liquids, steam, flame or flash, and electrical injury (Shaefer et al., 2021).

---

[*] Corresponding Author's Email: akerenler@hotmail.com.

In: Environmental Emergencies and Injuries in Nature
Editors: Murat Yücel, Murat Güzel and İbrahim İkizceli
ISBN: 978-1-68507-833-1

Thermal burns are a significant cause of worldwide morbidity and mortality. They can lead to debilitating, lifelong injuries and have serious psychological and economic impacts (Walker et al., 2021). The well-known risk factors for TBs are young age (children tend to have contact with hot liquids and surfaces), male gender (occupation-related TB injuries are commonly seen in the male population), summer months, lack of smoke detectors at home, and alcohol abuse. In addition, when an immersion scald burn is present in a child, abuse by a parent or caregiver should be kept in mind (Shaefer et al., 2021).

The depth of the tissue injury classifies thermal burns. The American Burn Association sets four classifications:

1. Superficial: Only the epidermal layer is involved and does not blister. It is painful and usually resolves by itself in a week.
2. Partial Thickness: This is also called a second-degree burn. Besides the epidermal layer, some parts of the dermal layer are involved. Superficial partial-thickness burns blister and are painful but resolve within 21 days, usually without scarring. Patients are at risk for infection, so that grafting may be required depending on the surface width of the injury. These injuries take up to 9 weeks to heal, usually with hypertrophic scarring.
3. Full Thickness (third-degree): These burns go through the entire dermal layer and frequently injure the subcutaneous tissue. In the acute phase, the denatured dermal layer remains intact. The necrotic nature of the burn usually causes anesthesia. The appearance of the injury site is waxy with a color of grey to black. The eschar of the burn falls off in time, and a bed of granulation tissue becomes visible. Contracture may develop if surgical treatment is not performed. These burns do not heal spontaneously.
4. Extension into deep tissues (fourth-degree): The burn affects underlying tissue such as muscle or bone. This situation is a major reason for mortality and needs immediate treatment (Edwards et al., 2021). There is strong agreement that the rehabilitation of patients after burn injuries requires a multidisciplinary team (Neubauer et al., 2019).

We searched the MEDLINE/PubMed database for this narrative review by entering the keywords "burn" and "thermal injury." The relevant articles (original articles, reviews, case reports, case series, etc.) published in the last five years were involved in the study. Those without full texts, with non-explanatory abstracts, or written in a language other than English were excluded.

Approach to Thermal Burn Patients

Thermal burn injuries are a significant public health problem, particularly in low- and middle-income countries with socio-economic consequences. The incidence of TBs is reported as 1.3 per 100,000 population in these countries. On the other hand, in high-income countries, the incidence of TBs is ten times lower (0.14 per 100,000 population). Although a reduction in deaths related to TBs has been determined in recent years, 90% of these deaths occur in low- and middle-income countries (Holley et al., 2020).

The reduction as mentioned above in mortality rates in TB patients is linked to improvements in care protocols, injury evaluation, resuscitation, management of inhalation injury, nutrition, and early excision/grafting therapy (Holley et al., 2020).

In TB patients, outcome prediction is another challenge. The questions, "who gets sick and why?" arise as a problem to be solved. The comorbidities of the patients may complicate thermal burns. Advanced age, inactivity, diabetes mellitus, hypertension, obesity, substance abuse, and polytrauma are associated with bad outcomes (Moffat et al., 2020).

In a 2-year retrospective study by Smith et al., it was reported that acute kidney injury, infection and received vasopressor(s), the percentage TBSA injured, admission serum ethanol level, maximum C-reactive protein, and maximum total bilirubin were significantly associated with the length of hospital stay in patients with thermal injury (Smith et al., 2020).

Cell membrane potential alterations are the reason for the fluid and electrolyte abnormalities in burn shock. These alterations result in an intracellular influx of water and sodium and extracellular migration of potassium due to sodium pump dysfunction (DeKoning et al., 2019).

Multisystem organ failure (MOF) is the most common reason for death in TB patients. A study revealed that inhalation injury requiring mechanical ventilation significantly increases the death rate. In the study, advanced age was also related to increased mortality. The total body surface area and the APACHE III score in survivors were significantly higher in non-survivors when compared to survivors. The APACHE III score is proposed as a useful prognostic tool in patients with TB (Shalaby et al., 2019).

Criteria for Burn Center Transport

Patients with the injuries below should be treated in an advanced burn center:

a) Full-thickness/third-degree burns in any age group
b) Partial-thickness burns > 10% of total body surface area
c) Burns involving the face, hands, feet, genitalia, perineum, or major joints
d) Electrical burns, including lightning injury
e) Chemical burns
f) Inhalation injury
g) Burn injury in patients with preexisting medical disorders that could complicate management, prolong recovery or affect mortality
h) Burn injury in any patients with concomitant trauma (e.g., fractures) in whom the burn injury poses the most significant risk of morbidity or mortality
i) Burn injury in children in hospitals without qualified personnel or equipment to care for children
j) Burn injury in patients who will require special social, emotional, or long-term rehabilitation
k) Burn injury in children < 10 years and adults > 50 years of age (DeKoning et al., 2019).

Treatment

As in all trauma patients, ABC is the mainstay of treatment. Early fluid resuscitation also plays an important role. The Rule of Nines is the most common and simplest method for burn size calculation (See Figure 1) (DeKoning et al., 2019).

The Parkland Formula is widely used for fluid resuscitation. For adults the dosage is: 4 mL LR × weight (kg) × % BSA burned over the initial 24 hours; half over the first eight hours from the time of the burn and another half over the next 16 hours. For children, 3 mL LR × weight (kg) × % BSA burned over an initial 24 hours plus maintenance; half over the first eight hours from the time of the burn, and another half over the next 16 hours (DeKoning et al., 2019).

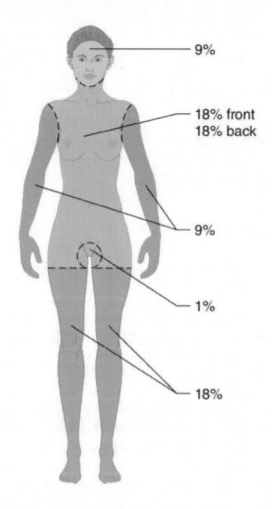

DeKoning et al., 2019.

Figure 1. The Rule of Nines for body surface area calculation.

Following inhalation injury, carbon monoxide poisoning may occur. Carbon monoxide poisoning may result in brain hypoxia and coma. In these patients, airway protective mechanisms deteriorate. Subsequently, aspiration and pulmonary damage may emerge. Patients with carbon monoxide poisoning must be treated with 100% oxygen therapy by a non-breather mask and evaluated in detail for hyperbaric oxygen therapy. Cyanide formed by the combustion of nitrogen-containing polymers binds to mitochondrial oxidative phosphorylation, which is another reason for tissue hypoxia (DeKoning et al., 2019).

In a review of 42 studies, mesenchymal stem cell therapy was revealed to significantly reduce inflammation. The therapy also provided burn wound progression and healing rate acceleration. In this complex and not-fully-understood process, the paracrine modulators, such as immunomodulatory, antioxidative, and trophic factors, are anticipated to play a role. Allogenic mesenchymal stem cell therapy may be used in the prompt treatment of TBs in humans (Rangatchew et al., 2020).

In order to design new treatment strategies, researchers should focus on the early identification of patients at risk for the development of laryngotracheal stenosis (Lowery et al., 2019).

For the rehabilitation of TB patients, a multidisciplinary team should be gathered. This team may consist of psychologists, physiotherapists, occupational therapists, burn specialists, and rehabilitation physicians (DeKoning et al., 2019).

Special Considerations

For children, rapid assessment, admission to specialized burn centers, and telemedicine are the essentials in management. Hemodynamic management, airway management, management of inhalation injury, anesthesia and analgesia, burn wound treatments, and other treatments must be considered in pediatric and adult patients (Holley et al., 2020).

Another critical form of TBs is ocular burn injuries (OBIs). The incidence of eye traumas in the ED is 3%, and of these, only 7% comprises OBIs. Even though their incidence is relatively low, emergency physicians should be aware of this entity to reduce morbidity. Thanks to blinking reflexes and Bell's phenomenon characterized by the movement of the eyeballs up and outward when the eye is opened (also known as an oculogyric reflex), OBIs are a rare condition. The majority of the complaints related to the eye are corneal abrasions and foreign bodies. Following a complete physical examination for TB, OBIs should be evaluated in terms of visual acuity, extraocular motion, intraocular pressure, and fluorescein staining. Also, a detailed examination of the eyes for the presence of a foreign body should be performed. Normal saline is commonly used for irrigation due to its availability; however, a physician must keep in mind that it is a hypotonic solution compared to aqueous humor, leading to increased corneal uptake. Due to the similar osmolarity of aqueous humor and lactated ringer, lactated ringer may prevent the cornea from swelling. Irrigation must not be performed with less than 1 L of fluid (Bawany et al., 2020).

As discussed earlier, inhalation injury is a strong predictor of morbidity and mortality. Following injury, airway epithelial cells secrete tissue factor, and its inhibition can decrease cellular proliferation by up to 60%. Reactive nitrogen species may cause the growth of facultative anaerobes following injury. Also, iatrogenic interventions, particularly intubation, may cause upper respiratory flora to spread through the infraglottic airway. Bronchoalveolar lavage fluid analyses revealed that inflammatory marker release correlates with inhalation injury severity. Plasma interleukin-1 receptor antagonist levels mediate the blunted immune response observed in non-survivors. The levels of IL-10, IL-6, and IL-7 were also correlated with mortality. In bronchoalveolar lavage fluid analyses, 26S proteasome activity and concentration were lower in patients with inhalation injury and even lower in patients who developed ventilator-associated pneumonia. The ubiquitin level decreases as the severity of the inhalation injury increases. It is known that an α-2-macroglobulin increase is associated with mortality in patients with an extensive cutaneous burn. Bronchoalveolar lavage fluid proteins are being widely investigated to identify inhalation injury, ventilation duration, length of stay in the intensive care unit, and bacterial respiratory infection prediction (Moffatt et al., 2020).

When hand burns are considered, conservative treatment is adequate for superficial burns. The devitalized epidermis should be removed, and a protective absorbent dressing should cover the wound. Surgical treatment is required for deep burns. Primary tangential necrectomy performed using an Esmarch bandage, followed by coverage with skin grafts or skin flaps, may be effective if deeper tissues are exposed (Stritar et al., 2020).

Hypermetabolism and hypercatabolism are correlated with the degree of catecholamine production. At the molecular level, metabolic dysfunction due to the burn persists for months to years (Moffatt et al., 2020).

In a study with 114 randomized pediatric patients, it was reported that negative pressure wound therapy (NPWT) might also be performed in small-area burns. This technique has the potential to hasten re-epithelialization; however, it also has a greater treatment burden when compared to a single dressing. It was also reported that NPWT decreased the expected time to wound closure by 22%, and the risk of referral to scar management was reduced by 60% (Frear et al., 2020).

Conclusion

Children ≤ 4 years of age, adults ≥ 65 years of age, persons living in rural areas, persons living in manufactured homes or substandard housing, and persons living in poverty are at greater risk for TB injuries.

Thermal injury is a progressive disease. It has local effects like the liberation of vasoactive substances, the disruption of cellular function, and edema formation. The subsequent systemic response alters the neurohormonal axis and further extends the injury. Implicated in these events are histamine, kinin, serotonin, arachidonic acid metabolites, and free oxygen radicals. The effects of these substances begin as local and subsequently result in the progression of the burn wound. Following a TB, cardiac dysfunction, cachexia, hyperglycemia, and hyperinsulinemia may occur due to an elevated innate immune response, apoptotic activity, and systemic inflammation. When accompanied by inhalation injury, a TB may be more lethal. The analysis of the release patterns of cytokines and other protein or RNA markers and how these patterns differ between the pulmonary and systemic responses may allow the differentiation of inhalation injury severity or even predict the development of complications or mortality.

Thermal injury results in massive and sustained catecholamine discharge. Catecholamine control is the cornerstone of further management of TBs. Following an injury, catecholamine production is correlated with the degree of hypermetabolism and hypercatabolism. In addition, neuroinflammatory processes are also correlated with postburn life quality. Systemic inflammatory response syndrome is responsible for the damage to the tissues. The central nervous system is also affected. The blood-brain barrier may deteriorate even in the absence of brain trauma. Deterioration of the blood-brain barrier results in increased intracranial pressure during the resuscitation period.

References

Bawany, S., Macintosh, T., & Ganti, L. (2020). Ocular Thermal Burn Injury in the Emergency Department. *Cureus*, 12(2), e7137. https://doi.org/10.7759/cureus.7137.

DeKoning E. P. (2019) Chapter 217: Thermal Burns. In *Emergency Medicine: A Comprehensive Study Guide*. Judith E. Tintinalli. 9th Edition. 1396-1402.

Edwards, M., Singh, M., Selesny, S., & Cooper, J. S. (2021). Hyperbaric Treatment Of Thermal Burns. In *StatPearls*. StatPearls Publishing.

Frear, C. C., Cuttle, L., McPhail, S. M., Chatfield, M. D., Kimble, R. M., & Griffin, B. R. (2020). Randomized clinical trial of negative pressure wound therapy as an adjunctive treatment for small-area thermal burns in children. *The British journal of surgery*, 107(13), 1741–1750. https://doi.org/10.1002/bjs.11993.

Holley, A., Cohen, J., Reade, M., Laupland, K. B., & Lipman, J. (2020). New guidelines for the management of severe thermal burns in the acute phase in adults and children: Is it time for a global surviving burn injury campaign (SBIC)?. *Anaesthesia, critical care & pain medicine*, 39(2), 195–196. https://doi.org/10.1016/j.accpm.2020.03.009.

Lowery, A. S., Dion, G., Thompson, C., Weavind, L., Shinn, J., McGrane, S., Summitt, B., & Gelbard, A. (2019). Incidence of Laryngotracheal Stenosis after Thermal Inhalation Airway Injury. *Journal of burn care & research: official publication of the American Burn Association*, 40(6), 961–965. https://doi.org/10.1093/jbcr/irz133.

Moffatt, L. T., Madrzykowski, D., Gibson, A., Powell, H. M., Cancio, L. C., Wade, C. E., Choudhry, M. A., Kovacs, E. J., Finnerty, C. C., Majetschak, M., Shupp, J. W., & Standards in Biologic Lesions Working Group (2020). Standards in Biologic Lesions: Cutaneous Thermal Injury and Inhalation Injury Working Group 2018 Meeting Proceedings. *Journal of burn care & research : official publication of the American Burn Association*, 41(3), 604–611. https://doi.org/10.1093/jbcr/irz207.

Neubauer, H., Stolle, A., Ripper, S., Klimitz, F., Ziegenthaler, H., Strupat, M., Kneser, U., & Harhaus, L. (2019). Evaluation of an International Classification of Functioning, Disability and Health-based rehabilitation for thermal burn injuries: a prospective non-randomized design. *Trials*, 20(1), 752. https://doi.org/10.1186/s13063-019-3910-6.

Rangatchew, F., Vester-Glowinski, P., Rasmussen, B. S., Haastrup, E., Munthe-Fog, L., Talman, M. L., Bonde, C., Drzewiecki, K. T., Fischer-Nielsen, A., & Holmgaard, R. (2021). Mesenchymal stem cell therapy of acute thermal burns: A systematic review of the effect on inflammation and wound healing. *Burns : journal of the International Society for Burn Injuries*, 47(2), 270–294. https://doi.org/10.1016/j.burns.2020.04.012.

Schaefer, T. J., & Tannan, S. C. (2021). Thermal Burns. In *StatPearls*. StatPearls Publishing.

Shalaby, S. A., Fouad, Y., Azab, S., Nabil, D. M., & Abd El-Aziz, Y. A. (2019). Predictors of mortality in cases of thermal burns admitted to Burn Unit, Ain Shams University Hospitals, Cairo. *Journal of forensic and legal medicine*, 67, 19–23. https://doi.org/10.1016/j.jflm.2019.07.011.

Smith, R. R., Hill, D. M., Hickerson, W. L., & Velamuri, S. R. (2019). Analysis of factors impacting length of stay in thermal and inhalation injury. *Burns : journal of the International Society for Burn Injuries*, 45(7), 1593–1599. https://doi.org/10.1016/j.burns.2019.04.016.

Stritar, A., & Mikša, M. (2020). Reconstructive surgery of upper extremity after thermal burns: guidelines or experience?. *Annals of burns and fire disasters*, 33(1), 47–52.

Walker, N. J., & King, K. C. (2021). Acute and Chronic Thermal Burn Evaluation and Management. In *StatPearls*. StatPearls Publishing.

Chapter 6

Chemical Burns

Hizir Ufuk Akdemir and Fatih Çalişkan*

Department of Emergency Medicine, Ondokuz Mayıs University, Samsun, Turkey

Abstract

Chemical burns are caused mainly by contact with strong acid and alkali agents, and industrial accidents, assaults, intentional/unintentional ingestion, and careless use of cleaners in the home are responsible for the exposure. Compared to a thermal burn, chemical burns cause progressive tissue damage until the agent is diluted and removed from the contaminated skin. The fundamental steps are removing dirty clothes immediately and cleaning the exposed area with water, at least 30 minutes for acid agents, and one hour for alkali agents. The use of neutralizing agents frequently generates heat, while balancing the chemical agent may cause thermal burns. The proper management of patients with chemical burns in the emergency room includes appropriate fluid resuscitation and wound management.

Keywords: burns, chemical, acids, alkalis

Introduction

Due to careless/inappropriate use of cleaning agents, occupational accidents, and intentional ingestions/assaults, chemical burns often occur as a result of contact with strong acid (pH <7) and alkaline (pH >7) substances. Petroleum products, phenol, and phosphorus compounds rarely cause chemical burns. Burns, dermatitis, allergic reactions, and systemic toxicity may develop due to chemical substances. The burn may be associated with a contact after a direct spill or another exposure, and a covert or open exposure, especially in the pediatric age group. Tissue damage continues until the responsible agent is diluted or removed from the contaminated skin.

The recommended initial intervention consists of removing the dirty clothes and washing with water for at least 30 minutes for acidic agents and at least one hour for alkaline agents.

---

* Corresponding Author's Email: mdfcaliskan@gmail.com.

In: Environmental Emergencies and Injuries in Nature
Editors: Murat Yücel, Murat Güzel and İbrahim İkizceli
ISBN: 978-1-68507-833-1

Neutralization should not be applied as it causes thermal burns due to heat generation. Inhalation or ingestion of the chemical agent through the skin may cause systemic effects. The other management contents are stabilization of the patient, appropriate fluid therapy, and wound care in those injuries (Demir and Mihmanlı, 2007). In inadequate treatment, chemical burns can lead to short-term, long-term, and life-long health problems. Suicidal oral ingestions can cause death in the early period. Considerable attention is required to treat chemical burns due to the accompanying tissue damage and the course of chemical exposure (Palao et al., 2010).

Epidemiology

A wide variety of products cause chemical burns, and these are commonly used products at home, in the workplace, and various environments. Although domestic exposures are frequent, the majority are occupational. 10.7% of all burns and approximately 6-10% of the admissions to the burn center are due to chemical burns. Morbidity and mortality rates are high, and chemical burns are responsible for approximately 30% of total deaths associated with burning (Palao et al., 2010; Hardwicke et al., 2012).

Pathophysiology

Chemical agents lead to damage according to some properties such as irritancy, acidity/alkalinity properties, strength, concentration, form (solid-liquid), area of contact, exposure time, contact site, and degree of penetration. Contact with a soft mucosal surface such as the eye, which does not have any barrier protection, leads to more extensive damage in the early stage than contact with intact skin. Immediate contact with the mucosal surface after an unintentional or intentional ingestion of a chemical agent will result in both direct and absorptive toxicity (Vanzi and Pitaro 2018). Acidic chemicals, except hydrofluoric acid, typically cause coagulation necrosis. Burns are not limited to the skin but may also be accompanied by respiratory tract and mucosal damage. Acidic chemicals that produce scar tissue have the potential to cause severe toxicity.

On the other hand, alkalis characteristically cause liquefaction necrosis. Chemical burns from alkalis tend to be more comprehensive and penetrate deeper. Alkalis combine with protein and lipids to form complexes and soaps that can dissolve and affect the depth of the tissue, and then alkalis create soft, gelatinous, brittle, and brownish eschars.

Damage in chemical burns occurs as a result of different pathophysiological mechanisms. The pathophysiological processes are briefly oxidation, reduction, corrosion, protoplasmic poisoning, and ischemia. Substances in these groups are: Oxidation: Potassium permanganate, chromic acid, and sodium hypochlorite. Reduction: Substances such as nitric acid, hydrochloric acid, and some mercury compounds. Corrosion: Strong alkalis (sodium hydroxide, potassium hydroxide, calcium hydroxide, etc.), white phosphorus, and phenols. Protoplasmic poisoning: Acetic acid, formic acid, oxalic acid, and hydrofluoric acid. Ischemia: Mustard gas used in chemical weapons, dimethyl sulfoxide, and sulfuric acid (Palao et al., 2010).

All chemical burns are pathophysiologically similar due to the limited variety of lesions caused by the skin's response to toxic effects. Chemical-induced skin lesions may present the classic signs of thermal injuries, such as erythema, bullae, or full-thickness skin necrosis. In the early period, injuries may show mild symptoms, while excessive skin damage and systemic toxicity may develop (Palao et al., 2010; Kearns et al., 2014).

Toxicokinetics

Alkaline chemical agents often cause irreversible changes in the protein matrix due to liquefaction necrosis, for which their hydroxyl group is responsible. In addition, local or systemic vascular damage may develop. Acidic chemical agents cause coagulation necrosis resulting in cytotoxicity. On the other hand, mucosal or skin alterations may prevent further toxicity and limit absorption. Alkaline agents are more toxic than acidic agents due to irreversible protein and tissue damage (Schaefer 2020).

General Approach to Chemical Burns

The goals in the approach to chemical burns are preventing irreversible damage, terminating contact with the corrosive substance, and washing the burn area with plenty of liquid. In some exceptional cases, the responsible agent (lime, Na metal, phenol, etc.) should be taken off before washing. For chemical burns due to alkaline agents, it is recommended that the washing time be more extensive than hours (Palao et al., 2010). As in all emergencies and diseases, stabilization attempts should be carried out with priority and speed. The patient should be stabilized by establishing/maintaining airway patency (A), providing/maintaining oxygenation (B), and controlling/supporting circulation (C).

Direct examination of external body areas exposed to the chemical agent is mandatory. Endoscopic evaluation is essential in oral intake/ingestion of the chemical agent. In the case of exposure to hydrofluoric (HF) acid, monitoring serum calcium and magnesium levels is critical to prevent fluoride ion chelation and cytotoxicity. Serial observation of lesions occurring in a large number of other local exposures is sufficient (Friedstat et al., 2017). Endoscopic follow-up should be performed by an experienced physician to objectively evaluate and document the improvement/worsening of gastrointestinal (GI) exposures resulting from oral intake/ingestion of the chemical agent. Similarly, in ocular chemical burns, the patient should be followed regularly by an experienced ophthalmologist, and the examination findings obtained should be used to guide the treatment.

Laboratory evaluation (complete blood count [CBC], platelets, electrolytes, calcium, magnesium, arterial/venous blood gas, liver and kidney function, lactic acid level, and sometimes coagulation studies) is indicated for gastrointestinal chemical exposures, especially when systemic absorption is suspected. Radiographic examinations, including an erect chest x-ray, may help to identify the presence of free air suggestive of perforation. In the past, radiopaque contrast material has been used as a diagnostic tool in patients with suspected perforation. But now, non-contrast computed tomography (CT) is a vital imaging modality if there is a suspicion of mediastinal free air due to post-exposure perforation (Liu et al., 2017).

Acid Burns

The self-limiting tendency of burns due to acidic chemical agents is dominant. The formation of an impenetrable barrier prevents deeper penetration of the chemical agent. The chemical agents in this group are irritating to the respiratory tract and mucous membranes, so the examination of the patient should not be limited to the skin. Factors that affect the extent of tissue damage include pH, concentration, molarity, and complex affinity for hydroxyl ions. The most crucial factor is the contact time and early decontamination of the chemical agent. We know that less than 1 minute of exposure to sulfuric acid does not cause a chemical burn, but 1 minute of exposure can cause full-thickness skin damage.

Acetic Acid

This is in the group of protoplasmic poisons that show their effects by causing ester formation with proteins. Hair straightening solutions contain diluted acetic acid, the most common cause of scalp burns in women. Emergency management includes washing the contaminated skin immediately with plenty of tap water, removing the dirty clothes, and applying a mild alkaline solution such as soda or bicarbonate. Oral antibiotics are vital in extensive burns due to the risk of secondary infection (Palao et al., 2010).

Carbolic Acid (Phenol)

This corrosive chemical causes protein denaturation due to contact, defined as corrosion. It causes chemical burns characterized by a relatively painless white or brown clot. Coagulation necrosis forms in the affected area. They tend to produce a soft eschar that can form shallow ulcerated lesions. Absorption from the necrotic tissue may temporarily extend, but phenol may become trapped under the eschar. Phenol is insoluble in water, and the skin should be cleaned first with sponges dipped in solvents such as 50% polyethylene glycol. More effective decontamination can be achieved by gently washing with isopropyl alcohol (Palao et al., 2010; Saydiari et al., 1974).

Chromic Acid

This is among the chemicals that cause damage with the oxidation mechanism, defined as protein denaturation resulting from the addition of oxygen, sulfur, or halogen atoms to living body proteins (Jelenko III, 1974). Conjunctivitis, lacrimation, and nasal septal ulcers may develop in more severe cases. Due to systemic effects, hepatotoxicity, nephrotoxicity, gastrointestinal system bleeding, coagulation, and central nervous system disorders may occur. Death may occur due to systemic toxicity. After contact with the chemical agent, the patients should be followed closely in terms of systemic effects by irrigation with plenty of water. Excision may be required to prevent systemic effects (Palao et al., 2010; Jelenko III, 1974).

Formic Acid

This is in the group of protoplasmic poisons, and shows its effects by causing ester formation with proteins, similar to acetic acid. Also, absorption of formic acid can cause intravascular hemolysis, kidney failure, and necrotizing pancreatitis (Pruitt, 1990). It can occur in contact with workers engaged in acrylate adhesive work and those working in cellulosic-related production areas. Respiratory depression and metabolic acidosis with an increased anion gap are the findings of the systemic effects (Chan et al., 1995).

Hydrochloric Acids

These are some of the chemicals that cause damage with the reduction mechanism. Reducing agents act by binding free electrons in tissue proteins. Heat can also produce a chemical reaction, thus causing a complex picture. Substances defined as desiccants, including concentrated hydrochloric (muriatic) acid, cause damage by the dehydration of tissues. As these reactions are often exothermic, heat generation often exacerbates the damage. It occurs less frequently than other acid burns, such as sulfuric acid. In contact with the skin, hydrochloric acid denatures proteins into chloride salts. Treatment consists of rapid and continuous flushing of the affected skin with water to prevent severe tissue damage associated with low pH (Yano et al., 1995). It is essential to know that inhalation of vapor due to hydrochloric acid can cause lung damage (upper airway edema, lung inflammation). Dark-brown and black colorations are characteristics of the skin. Skin damage is minor unless there is prolonged contact. Hydrochloric acid is a cleaning agent used for toilet and sewage pipes, war materials, and automobile batteries (Palao et al., 2010).

Sulfuric Acids

These cause damage to the ischemia mechanism (Bond et al., 1998). They are also among the substances defined as desiccants, similar to concentrated hydrochloric (muriatic) acid, and cause damage by the dehydration of tissues. Because these reactions are often exothermic, heat generation often exacerbates the damage. It converts the skin to a dark brown and black coloration after contamination. Skin damage is minor unless there is prolonged contact with sulfuric acid. It is found in cleaning agents of toilet and sewage pipes, war materials, and automobile batteries (Palao et al., 2010). Concentrated sulfuric acid produces extreme heat when combined with water. Therefore, neutralization with soap or lime water before lavage chemical agents is most important (Jelenko III, 1974; Leonard et al., 1982).

Hydrofluoric Acid

This is one of the most potent inorganic acids known. Organic and inorganic acids function by reacting with dermal proteins due to H+ release. This pathophysiological process, which begins with contact with a chemical substance, results in coagulation necrosis of the skin. Hydrofluoric acid (HF) is widely used in the petroleum distillation industry to produce gasoline. It is also commonly used in chemical and electronic manufacturing, glass engraving, and foundries. Dilute solutions are in household rust removers and metal cleaning products. The free fluoride conjugate base ion, releasing more free H+ during dissociation, is responsible for most tissue damage. Like strong alkalis, free H+ is excreted from fatty acids, resulting in oil saponification and liquefaction necrosis.

The free fluoride ion also affects the cations and leads to hypocalcemia and hypomagnesemia. Hypokalemia may also result from the inhibition of sodium-potassium. In ATPase and Krebs cycle enzymes progressive tissue damage can last for a few days if left untreated. HF burns are characterized by unbearable pain and progressive tissue damage. Pain may occur suddenly or be delayed depending on the magnitude of the exposure. In the following period, the hardened skin in the affected area will turn into a necrotic scar. Systemic symptoms such as nausea, abdominal pain, and muscle fasciculation may occur. QT prolongation, hypotension, and ventricular arrhythmias may occur in advanced cases due to profound electrolyte disturbances. In most chemical burns, irrigation with water is the first step in the initial treatment. Acidic chemicals generally require a shorter irrigation time than alkaline chemicals. This time is around 15-30 minutes in the case of contact with HF. Debridement of blisters is recommended for ensuring the removal of the acid trapped under the spilled epithelium. In more severe HF burns, detoxification of the fluoride ion with calcium gluconate is indicated. Calcium gluconate promotes the formation of an insoluble calcium salt that can be washed off the skin surface (Friedstat et al., 2017; Wang et al., 2014).

Calcium gluconate can be administered via different ways such as intravenous, intra-arterial injection, topically by 2.5% gel, or direct subcutaneous infiltration with a 5-10% solution. Topical and parenteral calcium salts have proven to be effective therapy for both dermal and systemic manifestations. Topical treatment is sufficient for superficial burns rather than penetrant burns, but calcium's impermeability to the subcutaneous tissue limits the use in deeper burns. Subcutaneous infiltration of calcium gluconate may be used for minor and more localized burns - a 0.5 mL per cubic centimeter injection with a 27-30-gauge needle. Burns of the fingers should be treated with direct infiltration of calcium gluconate. The procedure can be started with a regional nerve block. In the risk or presence of finger ischemia, systemic administration of calcium gluconate is recommended for finger HF burns (Yuanhai et al., 2014). Intravenous or intra-arterial injection with 10% calcium gluconate usually requires hospitalization to the ICU, telemetry, and close monitoring of serum calcium levels. Although central venous cannulation is necessary for treatment, calcium chloride is also effective. Skin exposure does not need to be extensive for systemic complications to develop (Friedstat et al., 2017).

Alkali Burns

The corrosion effect is the pathophysiological mechanism responsible for the damage after exposure to strongly alkaline chemicals. Alkalis lead to liquefaction necrosis after exposure. They cause extensive tissue damage and more penetrant burns than acidic chemicals. They create complexes and soaps which are soluble by combining with protein and cutaneous lipids and affecting the depth of the tissue. The skin damage associated with the alkali burns persists until the neutralization. A soft, gelatinous, brittle, and brownish eschar formation develops after alkali burns. Anhydrous ammonia, calcium oxide/hydroxide, and sodium or potassium hydroxide are well-known examples of alkalis used in industrial applications or households. Lime or calcium oxide/hydroxide is the most common cause of alkali burns, and the main component of cement and plaster. The burn depth is limited due to the precipitation of calcium soaps in the fat tissue, and this prevents more penetrant tissue damage. Ammonia and caustic soda do not show this property. These agents penetrate the deeper subcutaneous tissue and create more severe tissue damage (Friedstat et al., 2017). Anhydrous ammonia is a pungent, colorless gas. It is a commonly used chemical to manufacture fertilizers, synthetic textiles, and methamphetamine (Davidson et al., 2013). Anhydrous ammonia is transported and stored in refrigerated containers. Also, leaks can cause both chemical and cold injuries. Tissue damage positively correlates with the ammonium hydroxide production and the concentration of the hydroxyl ions. The ensuing damage is a product of liquefaction necrosis, resulting in burns at varying degrees.

Exceptionally, anhydrous ammonia has a high affinity for mucous membranes. Mucosal injuries are specific for anhydrous ammonia exposure. Hemoptysis, pharyngitis, pulmonary edema, and bronchiectasis are the clinical manifestations of mucosal injuries associated with anhydrous ammonia. Toxicity by inhalation is more severe (Amshel et al., 2000). Anhydrous ammonia is easily soluble in water. Therefore, the first step of the treatment is irrigation with copious amounts of water at the early stage. Alkalis tend to stay in the tissue for a long time. The physicians should irrigate the contaminated area every 4-6 hours for the first 24 hours. In the presence of facial or oropharyngeal burns, the physician should keep in mind that the patient may have a difficult airway and need mechanical ventilation for airway stabilization. The contaminated eye should be irrigated with normal saline or water to minimize ocular damage, and the goal is to lower the conjunctival sac pH below 8.5. The irrigation should be continued until the goal is reached (White et al., 2007).

Since producing the first artificial cement in France in 1812, it has been widely used worldwide. Cement burns are relatively increased in hospitals due to its easy use and access. Cement has many components combined with high heat. Calcium oxide is around 65% of the total cement weight, acting as a desiccant and alkali. The mixture of calcium oxide and water creates calcium hydroxide, and the hydroxyl ion leads to tissue damage similar to other alkalis. Wet cement causes allergic dermatitis, abrasions, and chemical burns. Liquefaction necrosis develops. The patient may not be aware of the injury in the early stage due to the silent onset of damage.

The most commonly involved anatomical region is the lower extremities, and the wounds are usually deep. The first step in the general treatment of these injuries is the removal of all contaminated clothes, including shoes. Burned areas should be irrigated with copious amounts of sterile water, and antibacterial cream should be administered against secondary skin infection. Periodic evaluation of lesions is necessary to decide whether surgical excision and skin grafting are required. The damage can be particularly devastating when cement splashes eyes not protected by safety glasses. Damage to the respiratory tract may occur due to inhalation of calcium oxide powders in the form of aerosols. Most patients ignore the dangers of cement. It is essential to use knowledge and adequate protective materials to prevent cement-related injuries (Spoo and Elsner 2001; Pike et al., 1988; Lewis et al., 2004).

Potassium Permanganate

This is among the chemicals that cause damage with the oxidation mechanism, defined as protein denaturation resulting from the addition of oxygen, sulfur, or halogen atoms to living body proteins (Jelenko III, 1974). After skin contact, the contaminated area should be washed with plenty of water, and dirty clothes should be removed. After eye contact, it should be washed with plenty of water, with the eyelid completely open, and an ophthalmologic examination is necessary.

Ocular Burns

Chemical burns of the eye and appendices are a common cause of emergency admissions, with approximately 2 million cases annually. About 15-20% of facial burns are eye-related. Ocular injury is a cause of acquired visual impairment, and it is the second cause after cataracts, especially in the United States. In etiology, alkali chemicals are the more common cause. The fact that the agent is alkaline instead of acid causes the burns to be more penetrating and extensive, adversely affecting the prognosis. The sources include cleansers, fertilizer, hair dyes, floor strippers, lime soil treatment, cement, plaster, mortar, lye cleansers, oven or drain cleaners, swimming pool cleaners, bleach, and automatic dishwasher detergents. Blurred vision, ocular pain, red eye, blepharospasm, conjunctivitis, and photophobia may occur. In severe cases, ischemia of the conjunctiva and sclera lead to the white appearance of eyeballs (Friedstat et al., 2017; Pargament et al., 2015; Liu et al., 2011; Rao and Goldstein 2014).

Alkaline chemicals such as lime and ammonia easily penetrate the layers of the eye. Injuries due to acidic chemicals are generally less severe. This is because the sudden precipitation of epithelial proteins protects from intraocular penetration and plays the role of a barrier. Periocular injuries are commonly seen, and the severity of tissue damage is often associated with scar formation. Debridement is essential for protecting the ocular surface from keratopathy and corneal ulceration. A severe penetrant skin injury can often result in tarsorrhaphy or cicatricial ectropion. Surgical excision and grafting are included in treating extreme clinical conditions (Friedstat et al., 2017; Pargament et al., 2015; Liu et al., 2011; Rao and Goldstein, 2014). Ocular burns defined as grade IV burns are representing the most severe damage.

Four grades assess the clinical severity of ocular burns. Grade I burns are associated with hyperemia, conjunctival ecchymosis, and defects in the corneal epithelium. Grade II burns involve a blurred cornea. Grade III burns are associated with deeper penetration into the cornea and present with mydriasis, gray discoloration of the iris, early cataract formation, and ischemia of less than half of the limbus. Grade IV burns look similar to grade III, but ischemia involves more than half of the limbus. They are also associated with bulbar and tarsal conjunctival necrosis (Friedstat et al., 2017; Levine and Zane, 2014).

The first step for managing eye injuries is irrigation with plenty of water. The short time between exposure and irrigation improves the clinical outcome. An intravenous tube and a polymethylmethacrylate (Morgan) lens are the best modality for prolonged copious irrigation. Still, in the absence of such a device, it is essential to keep the eyelids pulled back to ensure adequate irrigation of the conjunctiva and cornea (Friedstat et al., 2017; Paterson et al., 1975; Rihawi et al., 2007).

Air Bag Burns

Airbag-related injuries affect the face, especially around the eyes. Ocular injuries can occur mechanically and chemically after airbag deployment. Alkaline corneal burns may develop in airbag-related eye injuries. The sodium acid propellant system triggers inflation of the airbag. Sodium acid is converted to nitrogen gas, blowing up the airbags. The inflation of the airbags creates heat and alkaline aerosols. These alkalines are sodium hydroxide, sodium carbonate, and other metallic oxides. Alkali agents may crystallize and accumulate in the fornix when exposed. Eyeglasses can protect the eyes from chemical burns (Çalışkan et al., 2013; Zador and Ciccone, 1993; Lee et al., 2001).

In the presence of ocular alkaline exposure, an ophthalmological examination is recommended to exclude the eye's mucosal damage. To minimize ocular damage, the contaminated eye should be irrigated with normal saline or water. The pH of the lacrimal fluid should be checked. If the pH is above 7.4, irrigation should be started immediately and the pH checked 30 minutes later. The eye should be examined for foreign bodies remaining in the eye, and the deposits should be removed (Çalışkan et al., 2013; Lee et al., 2001).

White Phosphorus

Another cause of chemical burns is phosphorus. There are different sources. It may be the leading cause of injury, especially in industrial accidents and chemical weapon wars. White phosphorus ignites in the presence of air and burns until all the agent is oxidized or the oxygen source is removed. Therefore, irrigation with water is essential. Irrigation removes the macroscopic phosphorus aggregates. Copper sulfate (0.5%) inhibits oxidation and turns the particles black. The color change of the materials makes it easy to recognize and clean. Follow-up and monitoring are recommended for calcium, phosphorus levels, and cardiac abnormalities. The prognosis of ocular complications is relatively poor (Palao et al., 2010; Daly et al., 2005).

Conclusion

The fundamental principles in managing chemical burns include removing the chemical agent, adequate irrigation, proper use of antidotes, correct estimation of the injury size, diagnosis of systemic toxicity, early treatment of ocular or other mucosal exposure, and management of chemical inhalation injury. Clothing should be removed and the patient should be covered after irrigation to prevent hypothermia. Treatment options should be arranged individually according to patients' clinical condition. Patients stabilized after the first intervention should be referred to specialized centers for burns.

Educational activities should be carried out to increase the knowledge level of both emergency care physicians and people in the risk group. The importance of protective equipment should be emphasized and encouraged.

References

Amshel, C. E., Fealk, M. H., Phillips, B. J., and Caruso, D. M. (2000). Anhydrous ammonia burns case report and review of the literature. *Burns*, 26(5), 493-497.

Bond, S. J., Schnier, G. C., Sundine, M. J., Maniscalco, S. P., and Groff, D. B. (1998). Cutaneous burns caused by sulfuric acid drain cleaner. *Journal of Trauma and Acute Care Surgery*, 44(3), 523-526.

Chan, T. C., Williams, S. R., and Clark, R. F. (1995). Formic acid skin burns result in systemic toxicity. *Annals of emergency medicine*, 26(3), 383-386.

Çalışkan, F., Akdemir, H., Duran, L., Katı, C., Yavuz, Y., and Çolak, Ş. (2014). Ocular injury related with airbag deployment: A case report. *Journal of Experimental and Clinical Medicine*, 30(4).

Davidson, S. B., Blostein, P. A., Walsh, J., Maltz, S. B., Elian, A., and VandenBerg, S. L. (2013). The resurgence of methamphetamine-related burns and injuries: a follow-up study. *Burns*, 39(1), 119-125.

Demir, U., and Minhanlı, M. (2007). Chemical burns. *Turkiye Klinikleri J Surg Med Sci*, 3(1), 89-91.

Friedstat, J., Brown, D. A., and Levi, B. (2017). Chemical, electrical, and radiation injuries. *Clinics in plastic surgery*, 44(3), 657-669.

Hardwicke, J., Hunter, T., Staruch, R., and Moiemen, N. (2012). Chemical burns–an historical comparison and review of the literature. *Burns*, 38(3), 383-387.

Jelenko III, C. (1974). Chemicals that "burn." *Journal of Trauma and Acute Care Surgery*, 14(1), 65-72.

Kearns, R. D., Cairns, C. B., Holmes, J. H., Rich, P. B., and Cairns, B. A. (2014). Chemical burn care: a review of best practices. *EMS World*, 43(5), 40-45.

Lee, W. B., O'Halloran, H. S., Pearson, P. A., Sen, H. A., and Reddy, S. H. (2001). Airbags and bilateral eye injury: five case reports and a literature review. *The Journal of emergency medicine*, 20(2), 129-134.

Leonard, L. G., Scheulen, J. J., and Munster, A. M. (1982). Chemical burns: effect of prompt first aid. *The Journal of Trauma*, 22(5), 420-423.

Levine, M. D., Zane, R. Chemical injuries. In: Marx, J. A., Hocksberger, R. S., Walls, R. M., editors. *Rosen's emergency medicine concepts and clinical practice*. 8th. Philadelphia: Saunders; 2014. p. 818-29.

Lewis, P. M., Ennis, O., Kashif, A., and Dickson, W. A. (2004). Wet cement remains a poorly recognized cause of full-thickness skin burns. *Injury*, 35(10), 982-985.

Liu, H., Wang, K., Wang, Q., Sun, S., and Ji, Y. (2011). A modified surgical technique in the management of eyelid burns: a case series. *Journal of medical case reports*, 5(1), 1-4.

Liu, H. F., Zhang, F., and Lineaweaver, W. C. (2017). History and advancement of burn treatments. *Annals of plastic surgery*, 78(2), S2-S8.

Palao, R., Monge, I., Ruiz, M., and Barret, J. P. (2010). Chemical burns: pathophysiology and treatment. *Burns*, 36(3), 295-304.

Pargament, J. M., Armenia, J., and Nerad, J. A. (2015). Physical and chemical injuries to eyes and eyelids. *Clinics in dermatology*, 33(2), 234-237.

Paterson, C. A., Pfister, R. R., and Levinson, R. A. (1975). Aqueous humor pH changes after experimental alkali burns. *American journal of ophthalmology*, 79(3), 414-419.

Pike, J., Patterson Jr, A., and Arons, M. S. (1988). Chemistry of cement burns: pathogenesis and treatment. *The Journal of burn care & rehabilitation*, 9(3), 258-260.

Pruitt, B. A. (1990, March). Chemical injuries: epidemiology, classification and pathophysiology. In *annual meeting of the American Burns Association*.

Rao, N. K. and Goldstein, M. H. Acid and alkali burns. In: Yanoff, M., Duker, J., editors. *Ophthalmology*. 4th. Philadelphia: Saunders; 2014. p. 296-8.

Rihawi, S., Frentz, M., Becker, J., Reim, M., and Schrage, N. F. (2007). The consequences of delayed intervention when treating chemical eye burns. *Graefe's Archive for Clinical and Experimental Ophthalmology*, 245(10), 1507-1513.

Saydjari, R., Abston, S., Desai, M. H., and Herndon, D. N. (1986). Chemical burns. *The Journal of burn care & rehabilitation*, 7(5), 404-408.

Schaefer, T. J. and Szymanski, K. D. (2020). Burn Evaluation And Management. *StatPearls* [Internet]. StatPearls Publishing; Treasure Island (FL): Aug 10, 2020.

Spoo, J., and Elsner, P. (2001). Cement burns: a review 1960-2000. *Contact Dermatitis*, 45(2), 68-71.

Vanzi, V., and Pitaro, R. (2018). Skin injuries and chlorhexidine gluconate-based antisepsis in early premature infants: A case report and review of the literature. *The Journal of perinatal & neonatal nursing*, 32(4), 341-350.

Wang, X., Zhang, Y., Ni, L., You, C., Ye, C., Jiang, R., ... and Han, C. (2014). A review of treatment strategies for hydrofluoric acid burns: current status and future prospects. *Burns*, 40(8), 1447-1457.

White, C. E., Park, M. S., Renz, E. M., Kim, S. H., Ritenour, A. E., Wolf, S. E., and Cancio, L. C. (2007). Burn center treatment of patients with severe anhydrous ammonia injury: case reports and literature review. *Journal of burn care & research*, 28(6), 922-928.

Yano, K., Hosokawa, K., Kakibuchi, M., Hikasa, H., and Hata, Y. (1995). Effects of washing acid injuries to the skin with water: an experimental study using rats. *Burns*, 21(7), 500-502.

Zhang, Y., Ni, L., Wang, X., Jiang, R., Liu, L., Ye, C., ... and Han, C. (2014). Clinical arterial infusion of calcium gluconate: the preferred method for treating hydrofluoric acid burns of distal human limbs. *International journal of occupational medicine and environmental health*, 27(1), 104-113.

Zador, P. L., and Ciccone, M. A. (1993). Automobile driver fatalities in frontal impacts: air bags compared with manual belts. *American Journal of Public Health*, 83(5), 661-666.

Zhang, Y., Wang, X., Sharma, K., Mao, X., Qiu, X., Ni, L., and Han, C. (2015). Injuries following a serious hydrofluoric acid leak: first aid and lessons. *Burns*, 41(7), 1593-1598.

Chapter 7

Electrical Injuries

Emine Emektar*, MD and Meral Yıldırım, MD

Department of Emergency Medicine, Health Science University Turkey,
Ankara, Turkey

Abstract

Electric currents are widely used as an energy source. When an electric current passes through a human body, it can cause skin lesions, organ injury, and death. The effects of electric currents depend on many factors, including the open/closed status of the electric circuit, type of current, electric voltage, current strength in amperes, tissue resistance, exposure time, and path of the current.

Electric injuries may result from the direct effect of the electric current on body tissues, deep and superficial injuries resulting from the conversion of electrical energy into thermal energy, muscle contractions due to electric shock and/or post-shock falls, and blunt trauma. Patients who are admitted for medical care after significant electric exposure should be approached as a multi-trauma patient; it should be remembered that their injuries may be quite diverse, and all organ systems should be examined in detail. There is no specific treatment for electric injury, necessitating a symptomatic approach depending on the affected organ.

Keywords: electrical injury, emergency

Introduction

Electric injuries usually occur as a result of accidents. Electric injuries occur due to the direct effect of electric current or the conversion of electrical energy into thermal energy, resulting in tissue injury and organ dysfunction. Furthermore, possible concurrent blunt trauma may cause additional injuries. The emergency management of patients should aim at both direct injuries and trauma.

---

* Corresponding Author's Email: emineakinci@yahoo.com.

In: Environmental Emergencies and Injuries in Nature
Editors: Murat Yücel, Murat Güzel and İbrahim İkizceli
ISBN: 978-1-68507-833-1
© 2022 Nova Science Publishers, Inc.

In such patients, multiple surgical interventions such as fasciotomy, as well as long-term supportive treatments, may sometimes be necessary. Approximately 35-40% of serious electric shocks can be fatal (Wick, 2006).

The majority of injuries due to electric shocks in adults occur as occupational accidents whereas in children they mostly occur at a house or places where electric cables pass, or due to climbing electric poles (Taylor, 2002).

General Information and Terms

An electric current is defined as a stream of electrons carrying electrical charge from a cross-sectional unit of high concentration to a unit of low concentration. The ampere is the unit of intensity of the electric current. Electrical charge passing per unit time is termed as the intensity of the electric current. Alternating current (AC) is an electrical current with periodically changing amplitude and direction. Currently, it is mostly used as industrial electricity. Direct current (DC) is the constant flow of electrical charges from a high potential to a low potential. Electric charges being in the same direction separates direct current from alternating current. Although AC is a much more effective means of production and distribution of electricity, it is more dangerous (nearly three times) than DC, and causes tetanic contractions, prolonging the contact of the victim with the source (Gomez, 2007). Voltage is the potential difference in the electron concentration between the two tips, and this provides the driving force for the flow of electrons.

The unit of voltage is the volt (V). Irrespective of AC or DC, the greater the voltage, the greater is the electrical damage. High-voltage current typically causes deep burns whereas low-voltage current is more likely to cause tetany.

A low-voltage electric injury occurs via direct contact of the victim with the source, whereas in the case of a high-voltage injury, an electric arc can carry the current from the source to the person, resulting in injury (Jain, 1999; Wright, 1980).

The most important determinant of the injury is the amount of current passing through the body. The potential clinical effects of electric shock by the amount of current are given in Table 1 (Geddes, 1967).

Table 1. Potential clinical effects by the amount of current

Amount of current	Potential effects
1 mA	Unnoticed by most people
3 mA	Tingling sensation
16 mA	Maximum dropout current that a human can grasp
16-20 mA	Skeletal muscle contraction and spasm
20-50 mA	Respiratory muscle paralysis and respiratory arrest
50-100 mA	VF threshold
>2 ampere	Asystole
mA: milliampere	

Despite being dependent on multiple variables, electric injuries occur by three mechanisms:

1. The direct effect of electric current on body tissues;
2. Deep and superficial burns that occur as a result of the conversion of electrical energy into thermal energy; and
3. Blunt trauma resulting from muscle contractions due to electric or lightning shock and/or post-shock falls.

Classification of Electric Injuries

Electric injuries are generally divided into two, namely high-voltage (>1000V) injuries and low-voltage (<1000V) injuries. Energy in high-voltage lines is 10.000V or greater, while household energy typically ranges between 110V and 220V. On the other hand, lightning strikes can generate voltages greater than 10 million V. High-voltage injuries are more commonly associated with serious musculoskeletal, visceral, and nervous system injuries than low-voltage injuries (Jain, 1999).

The Effects of Electric Injuries on Different Systems

The clinical signs of electric injuries can vary widely, ranging from mild superficial skin burns to severe multiorgan failure and death. Classical injuries have entry and exit wounds, and the body virtually becomes an electric circuit.

Cardiovascular System

In addition to arrhythmias and other electrical abnormalities, electric injuries can also cause direct myocardial injury. Cardiac arrest and ventricular fibrillation are the most serious cardiac complications of electric injuries and are always fatal unless cardiac resuscitation is provided. However, various dysthymias with a better prognosis can also be observed. Although the most common ones are sinus tachycardia and nonspecific ST and T wave changes, conduction disorders such as various heart blocks, bundle branch blocks, and a prolonged QT interval are also common (Spies, 2006). Their pathogenesis is likely multifactorial. Plausible mechanisms include the emergence of arrhythmogenic foci after myocardial necrosis, Na-K-ATPase changes, and altered myocyte membrane permeability. Patients suffering respiratory arrest can also develop cardiac arrest and rhythm disorders due to anoxic injury (Lichtenberg, 1993; Bailey, 2007; Akkaş, 2012).

Electric injury can cause direct and indirect effects on the vascular bed, which is an excellent conductor due to its high content of water. These effects depend on vessel size. Acute effects on great arteries are not expected because the high blood flow rate dissipates heat generated by the electric current; however, medial necrosis can still develop, which may subsequently lead to aneurysm formation and rupture. Smaller vessels, on the other hand, can be acutely affected due to coagulation necrosis that usually occurs as a result of a high-voltage injury (Hunt, 1974).

Skin Injuries and Burns

In electric injuries, various skin injuries and burns can occur as a result of the conversion of electrical energy into thermal energy. Severity of injury may vary from superficial redness to full-thickness burns, depending on the density of current, surface area, and time of exposure. Since skin resistance can be dramatically altered by moisture, electric current can be conducted to deeper structures before it causes significant injury. Thus, unlike thermal injuries, the severity of skin burns cannot be used to judge the severity of any internal injury. Severe burns occur by exposure to arcs that usually develop in accidents involving high voltage electricity (ten Duis, 1995). In such circumstances, the severity of a burn not only depends on temperature, but also the energy within the arc. Exposure to such an electric arc causes rapid disintegration of the epidermis in as short as 1 msec, causing internal organ injury due to a fall in body resistance (Wright, 1980).

Burns are also common in lightning injuries. However, despite enormous energy and heat generated by lightning, deep burns are rare because it is of very short duration and its flashing effect predominates. In a study, deep burns were detected in only 5% of victims (Wright, 1980).

In small children, electric injury most commonly occurs from chewing or biting electric cables. In orofacial injuries, a burn can be of full thickness, involving the mucosa, submucosa, muscles, nerves, and blood vessels (Donly, 1988; Banks, 1988). Marked edema and scar formation may be observed in the wound area within hours after injury. Wounds are usually replaced by granulation tissue and scar by 2-3 weeks. In this type of injury, labial artery injury below the scar tissue may cause serious bleeding. In orofacial injuries, care should be taken in terms of bleeding that may develop in the next days.

Respiratory System

Although respiratory arrest is one of the most common causes of sudden death in serious electric injuries, electric current has no direct destructive effect on lungs or respiratory tract. Respiratory arrest usually occurs as a result of direct injury to the respiratory center or electric injury causing tetanic contractions of respiratory muscles while it passes through the thorax. Pulmonary contusion and associated respiratory dysfunction may occur as a result of blunt trauma (fall, victim thrown away by electric shock, etc.) during electric injury. Like almost any critical disease, electric injury may also be complicated by respiratory complications due to the injury itself or the treatment (e.g., ARDS secondary to ischemia or aggressive fluid resuscitation, ventilator-associated pneumonia) (Karamanlı, 2016; Kasana, 2016; Chawla, 2016).

Nervous System

Although nervous system injury is common in electric injuries, there is no sign that it is considered pathognomonic. Nervous system injury is mostly caused by trauma or dysfunction of other organ systems (usually cardiorespiratory) rather than the direct effect of electrical current.

Household electricity can cause continuous tetanic contractions in muscles by creating an indefinite refractory state in the neuromuscular junction even with relatively low-density currents (30 mA). These tetanic contractions are responsible for the "locking-on" phenomenon that prevents the victim's hand from being detached from the electric source.

Among the direct effects of electric current on the CNS, the most serious one is respiratory center injury resulting in respiratory arrest (Ramati, 2019; Cherington, 2005). Apart from this, cranial nerve deficits and seizures may also occur. If a horizontal electric current is formed from hand to hand, the direct effect of electric current can cause spinal injury by spinal transection at the level of C4-C8. The most common nervous system injuries caused by the direct effect of electric current are anoxia secondary to cardiac/respiratory arrest and cerebral or ischemia coupled with trauma-induced spinal injury.

Loss of consciousness, confusion, and amnesia are common after electric shock. When there is no associated injury, they usually recover without sequela (Cherington, 2005; Davis, 2012).

Seizures, vision problems, and deafness may also occur (Patten, 1992; Liew, 2006). Peripheral nerve injuries may cause various motor and sensory deficits.

Renal System

Among other organ systems that can suffer significant damage from electric injury, the kidneys are particularly important. Although direct kidney injury from electric current is usually not expected, the kidneys are very sensitive to anoxic/ischemic injury. Additionally, rhabdomyolysis, myoglobin and creatine phosphokinase release cause renal tubular injury that results in renal failure.

Although myoglobinuria is common among patients with serious electric injuries, the incidence of renal failure is low (Browne, 1992; Jain, 1999).

Other Systems

A fall from height or severe muscle contractions may cause skeletal system injuries. Fractures of the long bones of the upper extremity and vertebrae are more common. Vertebral injuries may cause spinal injury and further complicate the situation.

In muscles, deep tissue necrosis and edema may cause rhabdomyolysis and compartment syndrome (Jain, 1999).

Physical Examination

Patients who are admitted to medical care after significant electrical exposure should be approached in the same way as multi-trauma patients; it should be remembered that they may have diverse types of injuries, and a detailed physical examination involving all systems should be performed.

After serious electrical exposures, some injuries may not be initially apparent, and frequent reviews of a patient's status are essential. There is no specific treatment for electric injury, and a symptomatic approach tailored to the affected organ is essential.

Key areas to consider include:

- *Airway, respiration, and circulation*: After the scene of accident is secured, it is essential to evaluate airway, breathing, and circulation and to establish a secure airway as early as possible to prevent the possible effects of anoxia, one of the major causes of death. In the circulation step, spinal immobilization should be considered in the case of a possible blunt trauma, as with the evaluation of trauma victims.
- *Cardiovascular system*: Heart rhythm and arterial pulses should be evaluated, and an ECG should be rapidly obtained.
- *Skin*: A burn check should be performed; blisters, charred skin and other lesions should be sought; and extra attention should be paid to skin folds and regions around the joints, and in small children, to the mouth.
- *Neurological system*: Level of consciousness and pupil reflexes should be evaluated, and a motor and sensory examination should be performed.
- *Eyes*: Visual acuity should be evaluated, and a detailed eye examination including fundoscopic examination should be performed.
- *Ears*: Tympanic membrane and hearing should be evaluated.
- *Musculoskeletal system*: Signs of injury (e.g., fracture, acute compartment syndrome) should be sought, and the four extremities, the pelvis, and the spine should be manually examined.

Diagnostic Studies

There are no clear guidelines as to which studies should be performed after electric injury; therefore, every case should be individually managed based on clinical findings (Zemaitis, 2021).

The following diagnostic studies are usually performed for patients who require hospital admission:

- Electrocardiogram
- Full blood count
- Renal function tests (creatinine and BUN)
- Basic serum electrolytes (including potassium and calcium)
- Creatine phosphokinase (for rhabdomyolysis)

- Troponin
- Imaging studies for regions with suspected or overt trauma.

Evaluation and Approach

There is no specific treatment for an electric injury, and a symptomatic approach is needed, depending on the affected organ. Since the true severity of an electric injury is dependent on the path of the electric current, it is important to determine how the injury took place (Fish, 1999; Fish, 2000).

Before intervening in the person exposed to electrical injury, it is imperative to make sure that the victim is separated from the source. No medical intervention should be commenced before the electric source is shut off or the victim is taken away from it. If the electric source cannot be shut off rapidly, necessary measures should be taken to prevent injury to the rescuer. The rescuer should wear gloves and shoes suitable for the power line voltage. Resuscitative efforts should be started at once, and the victim's spine should be stabilized if possible.

Following the primary evaluation, rapid fluid resuscitation should be started in patients with significant burns or suspected rhabdomyolysis (myoglobinuria). Since internal injury may also be present irrespective of external skin lesions in electric injuries, the Parkland formula does not correctly guide fluid resuscitation. While a urine output target of 0.5-1mL/kg is the aim in thermal burns, a urine output target of twice this rate (initially 100mL/hour) is the aim in electric injuries, due to the expected myoglobin burden. After myoglobinuria resolves, fluid therapy should be adjusted to a urine output target of 30-50mL/hr. Ringer lactate is usually preferred for fluid resuscitation.

If sufficient urine output cannot be achieved, then osmotic diuretics, such as mannitol, or sodium bicarbonate, which cause urine alkalization, can be used. The presence of overt myoglobinuria is a sign of severe muscle injury, and such patients may require fasciotomy. The prognostic factors associated with the need for fasciotomy within 24 hours after injury include: (1) myoglobinuria, (2) a burn area larger than 20% of body surface area, and (3) a full thickness burn area larger than 12% of body surface area.

The presence of any of these three factors predicts the need for fasciotomy. Tetanus toxoid administration and appropriate wound care should also not be forgotten in the emergency department (Cancio, 2005).

Every patient presenting with electric injury should undergo ECG testing for a rhythm analysis. Cardiac monitorization and close follow-up are recommended for patients with cardiac arrest, chest pain, ECG abnormalities, or an exposure to high voltage. Many studies to date have shown that cardiac involvement mostly occurs at an early stage, and life-threatening cardiac dysthymias do not develop in the subsequent hours to days.

Patients who are injured by a low voltage and have a normal admission ECG can be discharged without performing additional tests when a detailed physical examination shows no additional abnormality. Similarly, children without any cardiac disease history, who are exposed to a low voltage electric current, can be discharged after a detailed physical examination (Bailey, 2007).

In addition, computerized tomographic (CT) imaging may be needed to evaluate falls or potential ischemic or anoxic brain injury. If signs of trauma to other systems exist, additional imaging may be necessary. Tissue injury should be evaluated, and possible associated complications should be determined. A detailed vascular and neurological examination of the affected extremities should be performed. A normal initial evaluation does not necessarily exclude the possibility of serious injury or delayed spinal cord injury following high-voltage contact. Children are more likely to suffer household electric injuries rather than high-voltage electric injuries. Children need amputation and fasciotomy less than adults. Serious oral injury may ensue in a child who has inserted an electric cable in his/her mouth. The electric field and electric current that are formed between the two wires near the end of the cord can cause high temperatures and significant tissue injury. Oral burns have few systemic complications.

Although the true risks of electric injuries in pregnant women are not entirely clear owing to a small number of case reports published in the literature, fetal mortality varies between 15% and 73%. In addition to previously recommended measures, fetal heart rate and uterine activity should be monitored for at least 4 hours in patients with 20 to 24 weeks of gestation, owing to potential mechanical trauma and electrical discharge to the fetus (Fish, 2000; Fatovich, 1993; Awwad, 2013).

Follow-up in the Emergency Department

Low-Voltage İnjuries

Although there is no universally accepted protocol for the treatment of patients with low-voltage injuries, asymptomatic patients who have been exposed to 240 V AC shock can generally be discharged home if they have a normal ECG and physical examination on admission (Blackwell, 2002, Bailey, 2007). Patients who do not feel well or who have a new ECG abnormality should be monitored and re-assessed.

High-Voltage İnjuries

All patients exposed to ≥600V AC should be monitored even in the absence of an apparent injury. If the patients are asymptomatic and the initial ECG is normal, routine cardiac monitoring is not mandatory. Patients exposed to low-voltage injury, who have superficial skin injury and symptoms, irrespective of abnormal laboratory or ECG signs, may have systemic injury and need hospital admission. Patients with large cutaneous burns should be transferred to a burn center after the first trauma stabilization.

Conclusion

Although electric shocks are not very common nowadays, they are an important problem in terms of the high mortality and morbidity they cause. While electrical injuries mostly occur at work in adults, electrical injuries in children mostly occur at home. Electrical injuries may occur due to the direct effect of electrical current on body tissues, deep and superficial burns resulting from the conversion of electrical energy to thermal energy, muscle contractions due to electrical shocks and/or blunt traumas due to falls after impact. Clinical signs of electrical injuries; These range from mild superficial skin burns to severe multiorgan failure and death. The best treatment for electric shocks is still prevention. There is no specific treatment for electrical injury and a symptomatic approach is required according to the affected organ.

References

Akkaş M et al. (2012). Cardiac monitoring in patients with electrocution injury. *Turkish Journal of Trauma & Emergency Surgery: TJTES*, 18(4), 301-305.

Awwad J et al. (2013). Accidental Electric Shock during Pregnancy: Reflection on a Case. *AJP Reports*, 3(2), 103-104.

Bailey B, Gaudreault P & Thivierge RL. (2007). Cardiac monitoring of high-risk patients after an electrical injury: A prospective multicentre study. *Emergency Medicine Journal: EMJ*, 24(5), 348-352.

Banks K & Merlino PG. (1998). Minor oral injuries in children. *The Mount Sinai Journal of Medicine*, New York, 65(5-6), 333-342.

Blackwell N & Hayllar J. (2002). A three-year prospective audit of 212 presentations to the emergency department after electrical injury with a management protocol. *Postgraduate Medical Journal*, 78(919), 283-285.

Browne BJ & Gaasch WR. (1992). Electrical injuries and lightning. *Emergency Medicine Clinics of North America*, 10(2), 211-229.

Cancio LC et al. (2005). One hundred ninety-five cases of high-voltage electric injury. *The Journal of Burn Care & Rehabilitation*, 26(4), 331-340.

Chawla G et al. (2019). A Rare Case of Neurogenic Pulmonary Edema Following High-voltage Electrical Injury. *Indian Journal of Critical Care Medicine: Peer-Reviewed, Official Publication of Indian Society of Critical Care Medicine*, 23(10), 486-488.

Cherington M. (2005). Spectrum of neurologic complications of lightning injuries. *NeuroRehabilitation*, 20(1):3-8.

Davis C et al. (2014). Wilderness Medical Society practice guidelines for the prevention and treatment of lightning injuries: 2014 update. *Wilderness & Environmental Medicine*, 25(4 Suppl), S86-S95.

Donly KJ & Nowak AJ. (1988). Oral electrical burns: etiology, manifestations, and treatment. *General Dentistry*, 36(2), 103-107.

Fatovich DM. (1993). Electric shock in pregnancy. *The Journal of Emergency Medicine*, 11(2), 175-177.

Fish RM. (1999). Electric injury, part I: treatment priorities, subtle diagnostic factors, and burns. *The Journal of Emergency Medicine*, 17(6), 977-983.

Fish RM. (2000). Electric injury, Part II: Specific injuries. *The Journal of Emergency Medicine*, 18(1), 27-34.

Fish RM. (2000). Electric injury, part III: cardiac monitoring indications, the pregnant patient, and lightning. *The Journal of Emergency Medicine*, 18(2), 181-187.

Geddes LA & Baker LE. (1967). The specific resistance of biological material--a compendium of data for the biomedical engineer and physiologist. *Medical & Biological Engineering*, 5(3), 271-293.

Jain S & Bandi V. (1999). Electrical and lightning injuries. *Critical Care Clinics*, 15(2), 319-331.

Hunt JL et al. (1974). Vascular lesions in acute electric injuries. *The Journal of Trauma*, 14(6), 461-473.

Karamanli H & Akgedik R. (2017). Lung damage due to low-voltage electrical injury. *Acta Clinica Belgica*, 72(5), 349-351.

Kasana RA, Baba PU & Wani AH. (2016). Pattern of high voltage electrical injuries in the Kashmir valley: A 10-year single centre experience. *Annals of Burns and Fire Disasters*, 29(4), 259-263.

Lichtenberg R et al. (1993). Cardiovascular effects of lightning strikes. *Journal of the American College of Cardiology*, 21(2), 531-536.

Liew L & Morrison GA. (2006). Bilateral hearing loss following electrocution. *The Journal of Laryngology and Otology*, 120(1), 65-66.

Patten BM. (1992). Lightning and electrical injuries. *Neurologic Clinics*, 10(4), 1047-1058.

Ramati A et al. (2009). Alteration in functional brain systems after electrical injury. *Journal of Neurotrauma*, 26(10), 1815-1822.

Spies C & Trohman RG. (2006). Narrative review: Electrocution and life-threatening electrical injuries. *Annals of Internal Medicine*, 145(7), 531-537.

Taylor AJ et al. (2002). Occupational electrocutions in Jefferson County, Alabama. *Occupational medicine*, (Oxford, England), 52(2), 102-106.

ten Duis HJ. (1995). Acute electrical burns. *Seminars in Neurology*, 15(4), 381-386.

Wick R et al. (2006). Fatal electrocution in adults--a 30-year study. *Medicine, Science, and the Law*, 46(2), 166-172.

Wright RK & Davis JH. (1980). The investigation of electrical deaths: A report of 220 fatalities. *Journal of Forensic Sciences*, 25(3), 514-521.

Zemaitis MR et al. (2021). *Electrical Injuries*. [Updated 2021 Aug 26]. In: *StatPearls* [Internet]. Treasure Island (FL): StatPearls Publishing; 2021 Jan-. Available from: https:// www.ncbi.nlm.nih.gov/books/ NBK448087/.

Chapter 8

Lightning Injuries

Çağdaş Yıldırım, MD, Fatih Tanrıverdi, MD and Ayhan Özhasenekler*, MD

Department of Emergency Medicine, Ankara Yıldırım Beyazıt University, Ankara, Turkey

Abstract

Lightning is a form of direct current electric energy. Fifty lightning strikes per second take place on the Earth. Worldwide, rural populations have been at greatest risk. People who work or engage in activities outside, such as campers, hikers, farmers, and hunters, are often hit by lightning strikes. The electrical current of lightning often travels over the body surface, rather than through it, in a phenomenon called "flashover." Therefore, electrical energy from lightning strikes is less likely to cause internal heart damage or muscle necrosis than electrical energy from human sources. This phenomenon is also thought to explain how victims have survived a lightning strike with little or no injury. Resuscitation efforts should be started immediately according to Advanced Cardiac Life Support (ACLS) and Advanced Trauma Life Support (ATLS) guidelines.

Keywords: environmental, emergency situation, lightning injury, ventricular fibrillation, sudden death

Introduction

Lightning is a form of direct current electric energy. The electrical potential difference between a negative electrically charged cloud and a positive electrically charged ground generates an ionization process. This process overcomes the insulating properties of the surrounding air so lightning occurs (O'Keefe, 2004).

Measurements of the lightning strike by standard photography show the diameter of the main body is about 2 to 3 cm. The core temperature of the lightning varies with the diameter of the strike and it could be approximately 8,000°C to 50,000°C. The current flow of a lightning strike rises to a peak in approximately 2 microseconds, and lasts only 1 to 2 milliseconds. The

---

* Corresponding Author's Email: drhasenek@gmail.com.

In: Environmental Emergencies and Injuries in Nature
Editors: Murat Yücel, Murat Güzel and İbrahim İkizceli
ISBN: 978-1-68507-833-1

voltage of a lightning strike may exceed 1,000,000 volts with more than 200,000 amperes of current flow. Lightning strikes have much more voltage and energy than high-voltage or low-voltage alternating current (AC) electricity (Cooper et al., 2017).

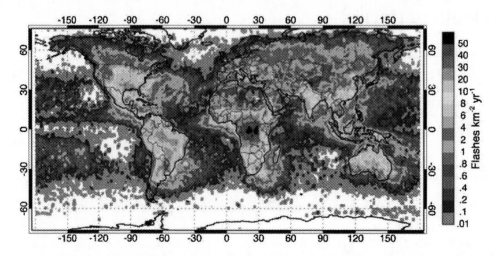

Figure 1. Worldwide density of lightning strikes http://ghrc.nsstc.nasa.gov/.

Fifty lightning strikes per second take place on the Earth. Lightning strikes are not equally distributed around the globe (Figure 1). Central Africa has a mountainous-terrain moist airflow from the Atlantic Ocean. This geographical situation makes Central Africa the region where lightning strikes are most common in the world (Christian et al., 2003). Lightning strikes occur more frequently in June, July, August and September.

Lightning can occur during dust storms, sandstorms, tornadoes, hurricanes, blizzards, nuclear explosions, and clouds over volcanic eruptions. Although rare, it is possible for lightning to occur without a single cloud in the sky (called a "bolt out of the blue"). This phenomenon occurs in sunny weather, usually after a storm. It poses a risk, especially for people who return to outdoor activity too early (Cherington, 1997). Worldwide, rural populations have been at greatest risk. People who work or engage in activities outside, such as campers, hikers, farmers, and hunters, are often hit by lightning strikes. The incidence of injury is higher because this population group does not have access to structures that can provide shelter.

Internationally, an estimated 24,000 fatalities with 10 times as many injuries occur annually as a result of lightning (Holle, 2008). It has a 10% to 30% mortality rate, with significant morbidity in most survivors (approximately 70%) (Whitcomb et al., 2002). Lightning deaths account for fewer than 3% of weather-related deaths, more commonly caused by extreme heat or cold (CDC, 2014). Most of the injured population are between the ages of 10 and 30 (Forster et al., 2012). This can be explained by the fact that most of the population engaged in outdoor activities are in this age group.

Mechanisms of Lightning Strikes

The mechanisms of lightning strikes are classified as 5 types (Davis et al., 2014):

1. *Direct hit*: Lightning strikes the victim directly.
2. *Splash strike*: Lightning first strikes an object near the victim, then the current travels through the air to the victim. A splash strike may injure multiple victims close to the object. Splash strikes account for one-third of lightning injuries.
3. *Contact strike*: Lightning first strikes an object that the victim is holding (for example, when using a phone indoors) and the current is transferred through the victim to the ground.
4. *Ground current*: In this case, the lightning's first contact point is the ground. The current is transferred from the ground to the nearby victims. The electrical voltage and current decrease as the distance between the victim and the hit point increases. Step voltage is also a variation of ground current. The current enters one of the victim's feet, is conducted through the torso, and is conducted through the other foot to the ground.
5. *Upward streamer current*: This is a newly defined lightning strike. Current passes up from the ground, without a nearby ground strike, and through the victim.

Mechanism of Injury

The electrical current of lightning often travels over the body surface, rather than through it, in a phenomenon called "flashover" (Auerbach et al., 2018). Therefore, electrical energy from lightning strikes is less likely to cause internal heart damage or muscle necrosis than electrical energy from human sources. This phenomenon is also thought to explain how victims have survived a lightning strike with little or no injury.

Lightning's shock wave can throw its victim as far as 10 m. Lightning causes internal injury mostly from blunt mechanical force. However, current can also pass through the body, although this is rare. Wet skin is a protective factor for internal injury because it helps current to pass over the skin rather than the internal organs.

The superheating of metallic objects in contact with the patient could cause thermal injury, blast-type effects and barotrauma, or shrapnel-like effects (O'Keefe and Semmons, 2018).

Injuries

Cardiovascular

The effect of a lightning strike on the cardiovascular system can range from benign electrocardiographic (ECG) changes to catastrophic conditions like sudden death. If current passes through the heart (especially from direct strikes) this could lead to simultaneous depolarization of all myocardial cells. This is thought to be the cause of asystolic arrest. Ventricular fibrillation may also be observed. Death is rare if the victim has survived the initial impact of a lightning strike (Cooper, 1980).

Table 1. Electrocardiographic changes seen with a lightning strike

ST segment elevation
QT interval prolongation
Atrial fibrillation
Inverted or flattened T waves

In the victim with spontaneous circulation, hypertension and tachycardia are common findings, presumably because of sympathetic nervous system activation. Cardiac effects reported after a lightning injury include global depression of myocardial contractility, coronary artery spasm, pericardial effusion, and atrial and ventricular arrhythmias. Changes in the ECG can be seen in Table 1 (Bailey, 2020). Transient ECG changes are seen with contact strikes or a ground current. If a victim with an automatic implantable cardioverter defibrillator is struck by a lightning strike, firing of the device could occur (O'Keefe and Semmons, 2018).

Neurologic

Most neurologic injuries related to a lightning strike can be classified as transient neurologic symptoms with immediate onset, permanent neurologic symptoms with immediate onset and delayed neurologic syndromes (Davis et al., 2014). Transient neurologic symptoms with immediate onset include loss of consciousness, seizure, headache, paresthesia, or weakness.

"Keraunoparalysis" was described by Charcot, in 1889. The victim of a strike finds himself or herself on the ground when he/she awakes and unable to move the limbs. Pulselessness, pallor or cyanosis, and motor and sensory loss are more common symptoms in the affected extremities. The lower extremities are more commonly involved. This phenomenon results from an overstimulation of the autonomic nervous system leading to vascular spasm. Symptoms may persist for up to 24 hours (O'Keefe and Semmons, 2018).

Permanent neurologic symptoms with immediate onset include heat-induced coagulation of the cerebral cortex (from direct strikes), hypoxic encephalopathy, lightning-induced intracranial hemorrhage peripheral nerve lesions, cerebral infarction, and cerebral salt-wasting syndrome.

Delayed neurologic syndromes include muscular atrophy and amyotrophic lateral sclerosis, parkinsonian syndromes, progressive cerebellar ataxia, myelopathy with paraplegia or quadriplegia, and chronic pain syndromes (Reisner, 2013). Lightning can also cause intracranial injury by secondary trauma.

Skin

A pathognomonic finding for a lightning strike is the Lichtenberg figure. It consists of a red superficial "feathering" or "ferning" pattern (Figure 2) (Dries and Marini, 2017). There are also four types of burn caused by lightning. Flash burns are mild erythema and may involve the cornea. Punctate burns are full thickness burns, usually <1 cm in diameter. These burns are thought to result from current exiting the body. Contact burns occur from the overheating of metal objects close to the skin. Superficial erythema and blistering burns have been described.

Linear burns, <5 cm wide, occur in areas of skinfolds such as the axilla or groin because of vaporization. These areas have heavy sweat concentrations (Bailey, 2020).

Eye

Ocular injuries are common in lightning strike victims. The most common ocular injury is lightning induced cataract (Norman et al., 2001). This could be attributed to damage of the lens by radiant energy. Other injuries of the eye include hyphemia, vitreous hemorrhage, corneal abrasion, uveitis, retinal detachment or hemorrhage, macular holes, and optic nerve damage.

Ear

The audio vestibular system is a low-resistance pathway for current (Jones et al., 1991). This makes this area vulnerable to injury. The tympanic membranes of patients are commonly ruptured (more than 60% of victims) due to the blast effect produced by the expansion of the air surrounding the lightning. Other effects include hearing loss, tinnitus, vertigo, and nystagmus.

Other Systems

Skeletal fractures can be seen from the blunt force injury associated with lightning strike. Rhabdomyolysis after lightning strike is unusual, and for this reason acute kidney injury is rare. Acute lung injury could develop due to lightning (Şener et al., 2019).

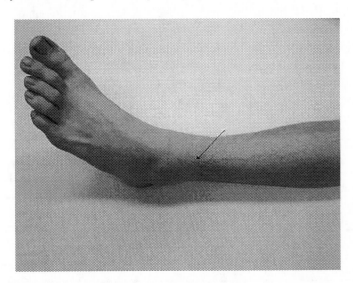

Figure 2. Lichtenberg figure of leg (Dries and Marini, 2017).

Management

Multiple victims could suffer from lightning strikes because of multiple strikes and splash strikes. It is necessary to first assess and treat those victims who are without vital signs or spontaneous respiration (Taussig, 1969) because victims become apneic and have dilated non-reactive pupils due to autonomic dysfunction. This is called "reverse triage" which is specific to lightning strike victims. Resuscitation efforts should be started immediately according to ACLS and ATLS guidelines. Responders must check for a central pulse before starting cardiopulmonary resuscitation (CPR) because keraunoparalysis may mimic a pulseless victim. Mortality is lower than in other causes of cardiac arrest. Prolonged CPR is sometimes successful (Bailey, 2020). Another important issue is the oxygenation of patients, because one of the leading causes of mortality is anoxia. The airway should be opened, and supplemental oxygen should be started immediately. The medullary respiratory center remains paralyzed after the return of spontaneous circulation (ROSC). Patients may suffer from a second cardiac arrest if ventilation is not supported (Davis et al., 2014).

Patients struck by lightning should undergo careful secondary care for occult injuries. Because of blast injuries, these patients should be approached as multi-trauma patients.

Patients with spontaneous circulation are likely to have tachycardia and hypertension. Specific treatment is not usually necessary. Pericarditis or cardiomyopathy are possible as delayed cardiac injuries. It is recommended that discharged patients reapply to the emergency department if they experience new chest pain or dyspnea (Davis et al., 2014).

If neurologic deficits of keraunoparalysis persist despite the resolution of pallor or pulselessness, the physician should rule out a spinal injury. A computed tomographic scan of the head is indicated in all lightning strike victims with loss of consciousness or a persistently abnormal neurologic examination (Cherington, 2005).

Lichtenberg figures are not true thermal burns; they disappear within 24 hours. Fewer than 5 per cent of skin burns due to lightning strikes are deep burns. Contact wounds are not commonly seen in lightning injuries. Routine burn care is recommended.

Ophthalmologic and otolaryngologic evaluations of the eye and tympanic membrane are essential for all survivors as soon as medically feasible (Davis et al., 2014).

Patients with an abnormal ECG and suffering from a direct strike should be monitored for a minimum of 24 hours (O'Keefe and Semmons, 2018).

Table 2. High-risk indicators in lightning strike victims

Suspected direct strike
Loss of consciousness
Focal neurologic complaint
Chest pain or dyspnea
Major trauma defined by a Revised Trauma Score >4
Cranial burns, leg burns or burns >10% total body surface area
Pregnancy

Prevention

Wilderness Medical Society Practice Guidelines made some recommendations for the prevention of lightning injuries (Davis et al., 2014).

- "When thunder roars, go indoors" (buildings or hard top vehicles)
- Avoid tall objects in rural areas
- Wait 30 minutes before continuing outdoor activities after hearing the last thunderclap ("bolt out of the blue")
- The lightning position (sitting or crouching with the knees and feet close together)
- Group members should be more than 20 feet away from each other (lightning can jump up to 15 feet between objects).

Conclusion

A lightning strike is an environmental injury with high rates of morbidity and mortality. Effects of lightning strike on the cardiovascular system can range from benign ECG changes to catastrophic conditions like sudden death. If current passes through the heart (especially from direct strikes) this could lead to the simultaneous depolarization of all myocardial cells. This is thought to be the cause of asystolic arrest. Ventricular fibrillation may also be observed. In addition to direct damage, the affected patients are also exposed to secondary trauma; similarly, many other mechanisms associated with lightning injury have the same risk. It will always, therefore, be a rational approach to evaluate patients as multiple-trauma patients. To avoid lightning injuries, the above-mentioned recommendations should be followed.

References

Auerbach, P. S., Donner, H. J., & Weiss, E. A. (2018). *Field guide to wilderness medicine* (pp. 440-442). Mosby.

Bailey, C (2020). Electrical and lightning injuries. Tintinalli J. E., & Ma O, & Yealy D. M., & Meckler G. D., & Stapczynski J., & Cline D. M., & Thomas S. H. (Eds.), *Tintinalli's Emergency Medicine: A Comprehensive Study Guide*, 9e. McGraw Hill.

Cherington, M. (2005). Spectrum of neurologic complications of lightning injuries. *Neuro Rehabilitation*, 20(1), 3-8.

Cherington, M., Krider, E. P., Yarnell, P. R., & Breed, D. W. (1997). A bolt from the blue: lightning strike to the head. *Neurology*, 48(3), 683-686.

Christian, H. J., Blakeslee, R. J., Boccippio, D. J., Boeck, W. L., Buechler, D. E., Driscoll, K. T., ... & Stewart, M. F. (2003). Global frequency and distribution of lightning as observed from space by the Optical Transient Detector. *Journal of Geophysical Research: Atmospheres*, 108(D1), ACL-4.

Cooper, M. A. (1980). Lightning injuries: prognostic signs for death. *Annals of emergency medicine*, 9(3), 134-138.

Cooper, M. A., Andrews, C. J., Holle, R. L., Blumenthal, R. Y. A. N., & Navarette Aldana, N. (2017). Lightning-related injuries and safety. *Auerbach's Wilderness Medicine 7th ed.* Auerbach P. Elsevier, Philadelphia, 71-117.

Davis, C., Engeln, A., Johnson, E. L., McIntosh, S. E., Zafren, K., Islas, A. A., ... & Cushing, T. (2014). Wilderness Medical Society practice guidelines for the prevention and treatment of lightning injuries: 2014 update. *Wilderness & environmental medicine*, 25(4), S86-S95.

Dries, D. J., & Marini, J. J. (2017). Management of critical burn injuries: recent developments. *Korean journal of critical care medicine*, 32(1), 9.

Forster, S. A., Silva, I. M., Ramos, M. L., Gragnani, A., & Ferreira, L. M. (2012). Lightning burn - review and case report. *Burns,* 39(2), e8-12.

Holle, R. L. (2008, April). Annual rates of lightning fatalities by country. In *20th International lightning detection conference* (Vol. 2425).

http://www.cdc.gov/nchs/data/nhsr/nhsr076.pdf. (*Centers for Disease Control and Prevention: CDC National Health Statistics Report*. July 2014.) Accessed November 27, 2021.

Jones, D. T., Ogren, F. P., Roh, L. H., & Moore, G. F. (1991). Lightning and its effects on the auditory system. *The Laryngoscope*, 101(8), 830-834.

Norman, M. E., Albertson, D., & Younge, B. R. (2001). Ophthalmic manifestations of lightning strike. *Survey of ophthalmology,* 46(1), 19-24.

O'Keefe, G. M. (2004). Lightning injuries. *Emerg Med Clin North Am*, 22, 369-403.

O'Keefe, K. P., Semmons R. (2018). Lightning and Electrical Injuries. In Walls, Ron M. (Eds.), *Rosen's Emergency Medicine: Concepts and Clinical Practice,* Ninth Edition (pp. 1765-1772.e2). Elsevier.

Reisner, A. D. (2013). Possible mechanisms for delayed neurological damage in lightning and electrical injury. *Brain injury*, 27(5), 565-569.

Şener, M. U., Demir, A., & Şener, A. (2019). Lightning-strike-induced acute lung injury: a case report. *Ulus Travma Acil Cerrahi Derg*, 25(2), 198-201.

Taussig, H. B. (1969). "Death" from lightning and the possibility of living again. *American scientist,* 57(3), 306-316.

Whitcomb, D., Martinez, J. A., & Daberkow, D. (2002). Lightning injuries. *Southern medical journal*, 95(11), 1331-1335.

Chapter 9

High Altitude Emergencies

Zülfi Engindeniz, MD and Umut Ocak*, MD

Department of Emergency Medicine, Bursa Yuksek Ihtisas Training and Research Hospital,
University of Health Sciences, Bursa, Turkey

Abstract

High altitude-related medical disturbances are generally accepted as high altitude illnesses and include both acute and chronic conditions. Our objective in this chapter is to give the readers a brief description of the most seen and life-threatening high altitude emergencies along with their pathophysiology, management, and therapeutic approaches. Rarely seen high altitude urgencies-emergencies, non-emergent and chronic conditions are beyond the scope of this chapter. High altitude emergencies typically associated with ascent to altitude include acute mountain sickness (AMS), high altitude cerebral edema (HACE), and high altitude pulmonary edema (HAPE). In this regard, principal physiologic and pathologic processes, diagnosis, and management of high altitude emergencies known to be predictable and preventable will be reviewed according to the current literature.

Keywords: high altitude, acute mountain sickness, high altitude cerebral edema, high altitude pulmonary edema

Introduction

Many people around the world travel to high altitude regions due to various reasons (occupational, recreational, sports related, etc.) at different times of the year. Especially those living around altitudes near to sea level are exposed to an increased risk of developing any form of high altitude related emergencies. High altitude is generally accepted as elevations greater than 2500 meters above sea level. Very high altitude is accepted as 3500-5500 meters and extreme altitude is 5500-8850 meters. However, the classification of altitude is arbitrary, and the clinic of the patients does not strictly follow the classification. In other words, any type of

* Corresponding Author's Email: drumutocak@gmail.com.

In: Environmental Emergencies and Injuries in Nature
Editors: Murat Yücel, Murat Güzel and İbrahim İkizceli
ISBN: 978-1-68507-833-1

acute mountain sickness may be observed at lower altitudes and being at a lower altitude does not necessarily rule out the diagnosis (Luks et al., 2019).

Physiologic and Pathologic Changes at High Altitude

Oxygen is the main metabolic fuel of the human body required for survival, both at the systemic and cellular levels. The main factor affecting oxygen availability is the partial pressure of oxygen (Po_2) and its level. Po_2 depends on several variables, but mainly on barometric pressure. Although the atmospheric oxygen level, 20.9%, remains constant up to 12000 meters, its partial pressure decreases with altitude, as atmospheric pressure decreases. While, at sea level (zero altitude) the inspired Po_2 is 159 mmHg, at the peak of mount Everest i.e., 8848 meters, Po_2 decreases exponentially to 43 mmHg (Andrew et al., 2022). This decrease in Po_2 occurs gradually as altitude increases and if the ascent is also gradual, bodies' homeostatic mechanisms have enough time to adapt themselves to hypoxia and this is called acclimatization. However, if the ascent is rapid without acclimatization, compensatory mechanisms fail to respond, and this results in pathologic processes in primarily hypoxia-sensitive central nervous and cardiopulmonary systems.

The initial reaction to hypoxia comprises a systemic acute stress response to increase oxygen delivery to tissues. The decline in arterial Po_2 triggers carotid body receptors and causes an increase in respiratory rate and heart rate. As hypoxia persists hypocapnia develops as a result of hypoventilation which in turn triggers medullary chemoreceptors to suppress hyperventilation. The excretion of bicarbonate from the kidneys goes up to compensate for respiratory acidosis. In the long term, with acclimatization, although these mechanisms are antagonistic, the result is an overall steady increase in ventilation. Cardiac output is increased because of sympathetic discharge and increased heart rate. Pulmonary vascular resistance is increased due to hypoxic pulmonary vasoconstriction. Increases in cardiac output together with pulmonary vasoconstriction result in enhanced pulmonary perfusion. On the other hand, as Po_2 is lower, the alveolar concentration of oxygen is also lower, and the alveolar-capillary diffusion gradient of oxygen is dramatically diminished at high altitudes (Andrew et al., 2022).

Erythropoietin (EPO) is highly sensitive to hypoxia and within hours of exposure, its plasma level increases, and the red blood cell quantity will increase. That increase in red blood cells is not significant in the short term; however, chronic exposure to hypoxia may result in excessive erythrocytosis. The rise of red blood cells during the first days of high altitude is mainly due to hemoconcentration secondary to diuresis. By increasing red blood cells, the human body targets an increase in oxygen delivery to tissues. However, in the long term, this effort is counteracted by increased viscosity possibly aggravating capillary perfusion. In terms of the oxygen hemoglobin dissociation curve, the initial response to hyperventilation and respiratory alkalosis is to a shift towards the left facilitating oxygen binding to hemoglobin. Within time, as alkalosis improves with renal compensation and 2,3-diphosphoglycerate levels increase, a compensatory right shift develops (Andrew et al., 2022).

Respiratory alkalosis triggers bicarbonate diuresis from the kidneys. Baroreceptors sense the volume increase due to peripheric vasoconstriction and blunt antidiuretic hormone and aldosterone secretion. As a sum, diuresis, volume, and bicarbonate losses result in hemoconcentration. Hemoconcentration, in turn, facilitates oxygen transport to a degree (Andrew et al., 2022).

The cerebral response to high altitude mainly targets the protection of highly hypoxia-sensitive brain tissue. The initial response to hypoxia is an increase in cerebral blood flow. Hyperventilation resulting in hypocapnia then triggers cerebral vasoconstriction and intracranial pressure increases. With acclimatization, cerebral blood flow will decrease but it remains higher than that of sea level (Andrew et al., 2022; Sanborn et al., 2015; Wilson et al., 2009).

As a result, the human body creates a cascade of events, to protect itself from hypoxia which escalates with altitude and the speed of altitude gain. This stress response, to a degree, varies not only among individuals but also the organ systems of a single person. These individual differences together with environmental conditions (altitude, latitude, temperature, humidity, atmospheric pressure, etc.) affect the probability of an individual developing a condition related to high altitude.

Acute Mountain Sickness

Acute mountain sickness (AMS) is a collection of symptoms after a recent ascent or altitude gain, including at least a mild headache as a prerequisite and a total of three or more points in the four rated symptoms of the Lake Louise AMS score (Table 1) (Roach et al., 2018).

Table 1. 2018 Lake Louise Acute Mountain Sickness Score[*]

Headache
0—None at all
1—A mild headache
2—Moderate headache
3—Severe headache, incapacitating
Gastrointestinal symptoms
0—Good appetite
1—Poor appetite or nausea
2—Moderate nausea or vomiting
3—Severe nausea and vomiting, incapacitating
Fatigue and/or weakness
0—Not tired or weak
1—Mild fatigue/weakness
2—Moderate fatigue/weakness
3—Severe fatigue/weakness, incapacitating
Dizziness/light-headedness
0—No dizziness/light-headedness
1—Mild dizziness/light-headedness
2—Moderate dizziness/light-headedness
3—Severe dizziness/light-headedness, incapacitating
AMS Clinical Functional Score
Overall, if you had AMS symptoms, how did they affect your activities?
0—Not at all
1—Symptoms present, but did not force any change in activity or itinerary
2—My symptoms forced me to stop the ascent or to go down on my own power
3—Had to be evacuated to a lower altitude

[*] Adapted from Roach et al. (2018).

Earlier versions of the Lake Louise score included sleep disturbance as another scoring category, however, the use of it has been abandoned as sleep disturbance has shown poor correlation with other symptoms of AMS. The Lake Louise score is designed mainly for standardizing scientific research rather than as a diagnostic tool. 3-5 points of the score is accepted as mild, 6-9 points as moderate, and 10-12 points as severe AMS (Roach et al., 2018).

AMS has been reported in 10-70% of people traveling to high altitudes in different regions of the world (Andrew et al., 2022; Bärtsch & Swenson, 2013). The prevalence and severity of AMS increase as altitude increases. Major risk factors for developing AMS were reported as a previous history of AMS, rapid ascent, exertion, young age, genetic predisposition, and a lack of previous acclimatization. Symptoms generally develop within hours to days of the ascent. The main symptom, headache, is characterized as a throbbing bitemporal headache which worsens with movement and the Valsalva maneuver. With headache, varying degrees of nausea and/or vomiting, dizziness, and general weakness may accompany the symptoms. Symptoms generally resolve within 1 to 4 days with acclimatization; however, severe cases may need a descent to resolve. After acclimatization and resolution of symptoms, further altitude gains may trigger another attack or even progress to HAPE or HACE (Andrew et al., 2022; Bärtsch & Swenson, 2013; Davis & Hackett, 2017).

Several mechanisms were proposed about how AMS develops and progresses to HACE; however, a clear causal relationship was not established on hypoxia triggered pathophysiological mechanisms that evolve to AMS. Proposed mechanisms include trigeminovascular activation, increased intracranial pressure, disruption of the blood-brain barrier, abnormal fluid balance, cerebral venous outflow obstruction, and inflammation (Andrew et al., 2022; Bärtsch & Swenson, 2013; Davis & Hackett, 2017; Wilson et al., 2009).

Physical examination is generally non-specific. Blood pressure and pulse rate are variable among patients and are usually normal. A mild increase in body temperature may be observed. Oxygen saturation (SP_{O2}) is generally normal or slightly lower than expected for the current altitude. There may be rales on lung auscultation. Peripheral or fascial edema may also be observed in some patients (Andrew et al., 2022; Bärtsch & Swenson, 2013; Davis & Hackett, 2017; Dünnwald et al., 2021).

Differential diagnosis of AMS includes carbon monoxide poisoning, alcohol hangover, acute migraine attack, dehydration, hypothermia, infection, caffeine withdrawal, intracranial hemorrhage, mass or aneurysm, venous sinus thrombosis, and hyponatremia. Although AMS should be the initial suspect with high altitude settings, all these conditions may cause similar symptoms to AMS and should not be overlooked.

High Altitude Pulmonary Edema

High altitude pulmonary edema (HAPE) is the most common cause of death from high altitude illness and is a form of non-cardiogenic pulmonary edema. HAPE is characterized by decreased exercise capacity, exertion, fatigue, weakness, and dry cough early in the progress of two to four days of ascent. As the condition deteriorates, exercise capacity declines, and resting dyspnea and pulmonary edema may develop. AMS symptoms are usually present simultaneously with HAPE. Resting dyspnea is a major warning sign and hypoxia may lead to neurological findings like ataxia and mental status change with or without HACE. Without intervention the condition rapidly progresses to coma and death within hours (Andrew et al., 2022; Bärtsch & Swenson, 2013; Davis & Hackett, 2017; Luks et al., 2019).

The underlying mechanism of HAPE is pulmonary hypertension due to hypoxic vasoconstriction at the pulmonary vascular bed. Left ventricle functions are generally preserved but the right ventricular load is increased. High pulmonary pressure causes shear stress on capillary walls resulting in endothelial leakage of plasma and red blood cells first at the interstitial and then the alveolar space (Andrew et al., 2022; Bärtsch & Swenson, 2013; Davis & Hackett, 2017).

Physical examination findings are that of respiratory distress. Tachypnea, tachycardia, fever up to 38.5°C and decreased SPo_2 with cyanosis may be observed. Rales are heard most commonly in the right middle lung, and may become widespread along with the progress of the disease. If available, chest x-ray or computed tomography shows patchy alveolar opacities (Andrew et al., 2022; Bärtsch & Swenson, 2013; Davis & Hackett, 2017). Extravascular lung water also increases and can be assessed by lung ultrasonography as B-lines (Lichtblau et al., 2021).

Pneumothorax, pneumonia, pleural effusion, pulmonary embolism, acute coronary syndrome, cardiogenic pulmonary edema, chronic obstructive pulmonary disease, or asthma exacerbation should be considered as the differential diagnosis of HAPE. Given the setting of high altitude, as medical intervention chances are scarce, and the life-threatening potential of all differential diagnoses is considered, descent should be strongly considered for severe cases of HAPE whenever feasible.

High Altitude Cerebral Edema

HACE is the most severe form of high altitude illness characterized by progressive neurologic deterioration of AMS or HAPE. Mental status change, confusion, psychiatric changes, ataxia, and stupor progressing to coma and death from brain herniation may be observed during the course. Third and six cranial nerve involvements due to adjacent brain edema were reported (Andrew et al., 2022; Bärtsch & Swenson, 2013; Davis & Hackett, 2017; Wilson et al., 2009).

HACE usually develops after 2 days at altitudes higher than 3000 to 4000 meters. It may be seen together with HAPE, and most cases are preceded by AMS. The postulated mechanism of edema is vasogenic rather than cytotoxic. In severe cases of vasogenic edema, hemorrhagic transformation may be observed (Andrew et al., 2022; Bärtsch & Swenson, 2013; Davis & Hackett, 2017; Wilson et al., 2009).

Differential diagnoses of HACE include hypoglycemia, hyponatremia, hypothermia, central nervous system infection, postictal state, complex migraine, psychosis, stroke, space-occupying lesion of the central nervous system, intracranial hemorrhage, carbon monoxide poisoning, drugs, alcohol, and toxin exposure.

Prevention and Management of High Altitude Illness

As medical capabilities at high altitudes are generally scarce, preventive measures are highly important especially for planned travels for high altitudes. Along with medications and interventions that are used either to prevent or treat high altitude illness planning a schedule allowing acclimatization is also recommended (Luks et al., 2019). Table 2 summarizes the medications used for the prevention and treatment of high altitude illnesses.

Allowing acclimatization by controlling the rate of ascent especially controlling sleeping altitude is recommended by the Wilderness Medical Society to prevent high altitude illness (Luks et al., 2019). Pulse oximetry may be used as an adjunct not only for the evaluation of acclimatization but also for the follow-up of patients with high altitude illnesses (Dünnwald et al., 2021).

In terms of medical therapy, acetazolamide is recommended to prevent and treat AMS and HACE especially for those who have a moderate to high risk of AMS. Risk categories for AMS are shown in Table 3. Preventive and treatment doses are shown in Table 2. The AMS treatment dose may also be used together with dexamethasone for the treatment of HACE keeping in mind that dexamethasone is the first-line therapy for HACE (Luks et al., 2019).

The acetazolamide therapy can be used for 2 days in people who record a recommended daily altitude. However, people who ascend more than the recommended one should continue the acetazolamide for 2 to 4 days and discontinue after the optimum loss of altitude following a rapid descent. Prophylactic use of dexamethasone is also shown to be effective, but dexamethasone does not have an acclimatization effect like acetazolamide. Ibuprofen may also be used as an alternative for the prophylaxis of AMS (Luks et al., 2019).

Table 2. Recommended dosages for medications used in the prevention and treatment of altitude illness[*]

Medication	Indication	Route	Dosage
Acetazolamide	AMS, HACE prevention	Oral	62.5[a]-125 mg every 12 h Pediatrics: 2.5 mg/kg every 12 h
	AMS treatment	Oral	250 mg every 12 h Pediatrics: 2.5 mg/kg every 12 h (maximum: 125 mg per dose)
Dexamethasone	AMS, HACE prevention	Oral	2 mg every 6 h or 4 mg every 12 h Pediatrics: Should not be used for prophylaxis
	AMS, HACE treatment	Oral, IV, IM	AMS: 4 mg every 6 h HACE: 8 mg once, then 4 mg every 6 h Pediatrics: 0.15 mg/kg-/dose every 6 h (maximum: 4 mg per dose)
Ibuprofen	AMS prevention	Oral	600 mg every 8 hour
Nifedipine	HAPE prevention	Oral	30 mg ER version, every 12 h or 20 mg ER version every 8 h
	HAPE treatment	Oral	30 mg ER version, every 12 h or 20 mg ER version every 8 h
Tadalafil	HAPE prevention	Oral	10 mg every 12 h
Sildenafil	HAPE prevention	Oral	50 mg every 8 h

[*] Adapted from (Luks et al., 2019). [a] 62.5 mg dose of acetazolamide shown to be as effective as 125 mg (McIntosh et al., 2019).

Inhaled budesonide, Ginkgo biloba, and acetaminophen have already been studied for AMS prevention (Kotwal et al., 2015; Sridharan & Sivaramakrishnan, 2018; Yang et al., 2021; Zhu et al., 2020). As studies have contradictory results, they are not recommended for AMS prophylaxis. Hypoxic tents, coca derivatives, antioxidants, iron, dietary nitrates, leukotriene receptor blockers, phosphodiesterase inhibitors, salicylic acid, spironolactone, and sumatriptan do not have enough evidence to be recommended for AMS prevention for the time being (Luks et al., 2019).

In terms of HAPE prevention, acclimatization, and staged ascent, nifedipine, tadalafil, and sildenafil are recommended. Dexamethasone (8mg every 12 hours) can be used as an alternative to the above medications, in persons who cannot use nifedipine or tadalafil. Acetazolamide is not recommended for HAPE prophylaxis, but it can be used for the prevention of reentry of HAPE in people with a previous history of HAPE (Luks et al., 2019).

Table 3. Risk categories for AMS[*]

Risk category	Description
Low	• Individuals with no history of altitude illness and ascending to ≤ 2800 m • Individuals taking ≥ 2 days to arrive at 2500-3000 m with subsequent increases in sleeping elevation < 500 m/day and an extra day for acclimatization every 1000 m
Moderate	• Individuals with a history of AMS and ascending to 2500-2800 m in 1 day • No history of AMS and ascending to > 2800 m in 1 day • All individuals ascending > 500 m/day (increase in sleeping elevation) at altitudes above 3000 m but with an extra day for acclimatization every 1000 m
High	• Individuals with a history of AMS and ascending to >2800 m in 1 day • All individuals with a history of HACE or • HAPE • All individuals ascending to > 3500 m in 1 day • All individuals ascending > 500 m/day (increase in sleeping elevation) above > 3000 m without extra days for acclimatization • Very rapid ascents (e.g., < 7 d ascents of Mt. Kilimanjaro)

[*]Adopted from (Luks et al., 2019).

Descent is the single best treatment for AMS, HACE, and HAPE. Descent should be considered in all cases of HACE and HAPE, for severe cases of AMS, and AMS cases that do not respond to other measures. When available, supplemental oxygen with a target SPo_2 of more than 90% is recommended when descent is not possible. Portable hyperbaric chambers (Gamow bag) may be useful for the treatment of severe AMS, HACE, and HAPE where supplemental oxygen is unavailable, or descent is not possible. Acetazolamide and dexamethasone are recommended for the treatment of AMS and HACE but not recommended for the treatment of HAPE. Acetaminophen and ibuprofen can be used to relieve headaches at high altitude. For the treatment of HAPE, nifedipine or phosphodiesterase inhibitors can be used when descent is not possible or delayed and supplemental oxygen or portable hyperbaric chamber is not available. Continuous positive airway pressure (CPAP) or expiratory positive airway pressure systems (EPAP) may be used as adjunctive therapy of HAPE in patients who are not responding to supplemental oxygen alone. CPAP and EPAP are not recommended for the treatment of AMS or HACE, due to lack of evidence (Luks et al., 2019).

Physicians' initial incentive, along with the supportive therapy, should be the descent of the patients with high altitude illnesses. In patients who do not respond to treatment and even descent, hospitalization and possible differential diagnoses should be considered. It should always be kept in mind that other than high altitude illnesses; standard emergencies may also occur at high altitudes.

Conclusion

High altitude illnesses are preventable and somehow predictable conditions. Given the nature of the settings where they are observed, emphasis should be on the prevention part. The healthcare providers should have detailed knowledge in terms of the diagnosis, prognosis, management, and treatment of those high altitude related life-threatening conditions. Descent is the definitive therapy for all those high altitude emergencies in AMS, HAPE, and HACE.

References

Andrew M. L., Schoene, R.B, & Swenson, E. (2022). High Altitude. In *Murray & Nadel's Textbook of Respiratory Medicine, 7 ed* (pp. 1460-1474). Elsevier Inc.

Bärtsch, P., & Swenson, E. R. (2013). Clinical practice: Acute high-altitude illnesses. *N. Engl. J. Med.*, *368*(24), 2294-2302. https://doi.org/10.1056/NEJMcp1214870.

Davis, C., & Hackett, P. (2017). Advances in the Prevention and Treatment of High Altitude Illness. *Emerg. Med. Clin. North Am.*, *35*(2), 241-260. https://doi.org/10.1016/j.emc.2017.01.002.

Dünnwald, T., Kienast, R., Niederseer, D., & Burtscher, M. (2021). The Use of Pulse Oximetry in the Assessment of Acclimatization to High Altitude. *Sensors (Basel)*, *21*(4). https://doi.org/10.3390/s21041263.

Kotwal, J., Kotwal, A., Bhalla, S., Singh, P. K., & Nair, V. (2015). Effectiveness of homocysteine lowering vitamins in prevention of thrombotic tendency at high altitude area: A randomized field trial. *Thromb. Res.*, *136*(4), 758-762. https://doi.org/10.1016/j.thromres.2015.08.001.

Lichtblau, M., Bader, P. R., Carta, A. F., Furian, M., Muralt, L., Saxer, S., . . . Ulrich, S. (2021). Extravascular lung water and cardiac function assessed by echocardiography in healthy lowlanders during repeated very high-altitude exposure. *Int. J. Cardiol.*, *332*, 166-174. https://doi.org/10.1016/j.ijcard.2021.03.057.

Luks, A. M., Auerbach, P. S., Freer, L., Grissom, C. K., Keyes, L. E., McIntosh, S. E., . . . Hackett, P. H. (2019). Wilderness Medical Society Clinical Practice Guidelines for the Prevention and Treatment of Acute Altitude Illness: 2019 Update. *Wilderness Environ. Med.*, *30*(4s), S3-s18. https://doi.org/10.1016/j.wem.2019.04.006.

McIntosh, S. E., Hemphill, M., McDevitt, M. C., Gurung, T. Y., Ghale, M., Knott, J. R., . . . C, K. G. (2019). Reduced Acetazolamide Dosing in Countering Altitude Illness: A Comparison of 62.5 vs 125 mg (the RADICAL Trial). *Wilderness Environ. Med.*, *30*(1), 12-21. https://doi.org/10.1016/j.wem.2018.09.002.

Roach, R. C., Hackett, P. H., Oelz, O., Bärtsch, P., Luks, A. M., MacInnis, M. J., & Baillie, J. K. (2018). The 2018 Lake Louise Acute Mountain Sickness Score. *High Alt. Med. Biol.*, *19*(1), 4-6. https://doi.org/10.1089/ham.2017.0164

Sanborn, M. R., Edsell, M. E., Kim, M. N., Mesquita, R., Putt, M. E., Imray, C., . . . Martin, D. S. (2015). Cerebral hemodynamics at altitude: effects of hyperventilation and acclimatization on cerebral blood flow and oxygenation. *Wilderness Environ Med.*, *26*(2), 133-141. https://doi.org/10.1016/j.wem.2014.10.001

Sridharan, K., & Sivaramakrishnan, G. (2018). Pharmacological interventions for preventing acute mountain sickness: a network meta-analysis and trial sequential analysis of randomized clinical trials. *Ann Med*, *50*(2), 147-155. https://doi.org/10.1080/07853890.2017.1407034.

Wilson, M. H., Newman, S., & Imray, C. H. (2009). The cerebral effects of ascent to high altitudes. *Lancet Neurol*, *8*(2), 175-191. https://doi.org/10.1016/s1474-4422(09)70014-6.

Yang, H. L., Deng, M. J., Zhang, W., & Huang, S. (2021). [The preventive effect of four drugs on acute mountain sickness: a Bayesian network meta-analysis]. *Zhonghua Jie He He Hu Xi Za Zhi*, *44*(11), 953-960. https://doi.org/10.3760/cma.j.cn112147-20210330-00211.

Zhu, X., Liu, Y., Li, N., & He, Q. (2020). Inhaled budesonide for the prevention of acute mountain sickness: A meta-analysis of randomized controlled trials. *Am. J. Emerg. Med.*, *38*(8), 1627-1634. https://doi.org/10.1016/j.ajem.2019.158461.

Chapter 10

Dysbarism and Diving Emergencies

Suleyman Turedi and Mustafa Cicek[*]

Turkish Ministry of Health, University of Health Sciences Kanuni Education and Research Hospital, Trabzon, Turkey

Abstract

By nature, the human body did not evolve to live in water or to spend a long time in water. But for thousands of years, humans have been benefiting from the possibilities of the sea for feeding, hunting, and sheltering. Diving activities involve some risks in terms of health. Underwater has a structure that does not contain air that the human body can breathe, and the pressure increases as the depth increases. This causes the volume of gases to decrease. As you go deeper, the volume of gases decreases due to pressure, and this means that inhalation is more and more compressed, which is why diving is a challenging activity in itself.

The underwater environment contains various difficulties due to its natural structure. We cannot speak underwater, we cannot see because the light decreases as we go deeper, we cannot breathe, and we may experience many medical problems due to high pressure. Injuries can be minimized when underwater sports are performed by the rules of physics and with appropriate training. Dysbarism is any adverse medical condition resulting from changes in ambient pressure. If these changes in pressure occur at a rate or time that exceeds the body's capacity to adapt safely, certain medical problems can occur. In an underwater environment, the pressure increases linearly with depth. Barotrauma, on the other hand, is a clinical problem that occurs during volume changes in gas-filled organs, which we usually see after moving quickly or descending too deep during underwater descents and ascents without complying with the adaptation mechanisms. Arterial gas embolism happens when a diver is advancing to the surface underwater, after the panicked, uncontrolled use of the BC, etc. If the lungs make a sudden rise when they are full of air after a situation like this, the air in the lungs expands with decreasing pressure. Damage occurs if a tensile force occurs above the elastance level that the lung alveoli can withstand. In the injured alveoli, air enters the pulmonary venous circulation. Circulating air moves into the left atrium. If the air that enters the systemic circulation by following the left ventricle and aorta paths disrupts the circulation in the microvascular bed, clinical findings occur in the affected divers. Usually, air bubbles travel through the carotid and vertebral arteries to the brain.

---

[*] Corresponding Author's Email: mustafacicek1989@gmail.com.

In: Environmental Emergencies and Injuries in Nature
Editors: Murat Yücel, Murat Güzel and İbrahim İkizceli
ISBN: 978-1-68507-833-1
© 2022 Nova Science Publishers, Inc.

When the diver starts to rise after the bottom time, the pressure will decrease and the amount of nitrogen dissolved in the blood and tissues will decrease in the same parallel. This cleaning process is not immediate but takes place at a certain speed through the lungs. This process, which we call the decompression stage, may differ from person to person. Therefore, waiting should be allowed for certain periods during the rise to clear the dissolved nitrogen in the blood and tissues after this pressure-nitrogen relationship. If the diver does not comply with these times and makes a rapid rise, the dissolved nitrogen turns into gas form with the effect of decreasing pressure and causes functional and circulatory problems due to mechanical effects in whichever organ or system.

Keywords: barotrauma, gas embolism, decompression

Introduction

Although there are many types, underwater diving activities are carried out for recreational, sportive, scientific, and military purposes today. Diving can also be done by simply holding the breath or by using closed-circuit systems with tubes containing an oxygen-nitrogen mixture. Recreational dives are usually made to a depth of 40 meters. People with technical experience and equipment knowledge and experience go deeper. These people are underwater commandos, coast guard teams, licensed athletes, underwater construction divers and search and rescue teams.

The number of recreational divers in the USA is around 2.7-3.5 million (Buzzacott, 2018). Despite such a serious number, the accident and death rate is at an acceptably low level. While the average mortality rate in recreational dives is 16.4 per 100,000 divers, the death rate per dive is 0.48 (Denoble, 2008, Richardson, 2010). As the access to diving equipment has increased, the attractiveness of the underwater environment has attracted even less experienced people to dive.

By nature, the human body did not evolve to live in water or to spend a long time in water. But for thousands of years, humans have been benefiting from the possibilities of the sea for feeding, hunting, and sheltering. There is evidence that Neanderthals dived for shells 40,000 years ago (Bachrach, 1975). Herodotus records a mention of the diving of Scyllis and his daughter Cyana for the Persian king Xerxes during the 50-year war between the Greek and Persian states in 500 BC. In addition, it is seen in many cultures that soldiers conduct military operations such as cutting the anchor chains of enemy ships and drilling holes in their hulls by diving. It is recorded in Ariston's records that Alexander the Great used a glass barrel called a "Colimpha" to watch the divers who did not clean the underwater military remains. Spanish explorers enslaved native divers in the caravans who were reportedly forced to dive and collect pearls. Diving throughout history, up to the past 300 years, has always been done by holding the breath. The only method that has been used for many years is that of the bell, called the diving bell, which is filled with air and immersed with the diver and a few more breaths can be taken with the air inside. Aristotle referred to this device when talking about problems with the ears in his work called "Problemse" in the 300s BC.

The first diving suit was produced by Augustus Siebe in 1837 (Davis, 1955). In this model, normal room air was supplied to the diver by a manual pump operated out of the water. With this outfit, the underwater construction part of bridges built over streams, namely the caissons, could be made more easily. The workers working in these caissons experienced some problems such as joint pain and paralysis after getting out of the water, and this was called Caisson disease at that time. This clinical condition is now known as decompression sickness (Jarcho, 1968; Butler, 2004). As time and technology progressed, the needs changed and the question of how to be more comfortable underwater led to discoveries. In 1865, French engineers developed a regulator that could supply air according to the increasing pressure change in the underwater environment. This regulator required a connecting hose providing air delivery from the outside environment (Bachrach, 1975). This regulator was later integrated to pilots operating at high altitudes. In 1943, Jacques-Yves Cousteau and Emile Gagnan invented a demand regulator and a valve system that provides the interconnection, besides the compressed air cylinders, called the Aqua-Lung. This system is the forerunner of the system we still use today, namely SCUBA (self-contained underwater breathing apparatus).

Diving activities involve some risks in terms of health. Underwater has a structure that does not contain air that the human body can breathe, and the pressure increases as the depth increases. This causes the volume of gases to decrease. As you go deeper, the volume of gases decreases due to pressure, and this means that inhalation is more and more compressed, which is why diving is a challenging activity in itself. All primary care and emergency physicians should know about diving injuries. In addition to simple medical conditions, it should be possible to provide access to hyperbaric oxygen therapy in serious conditions such as decompression sickness or arterial gas embolism.

Dive Types

Breath-Holding Freediving

Freediving ranges from the times when people made a living by underwater hunting to today's entertainment and sportive competition environment. To be precise, it means diving without the use of an air supply. Using flippers, goggles or a snorkel makes no difference. A snorkel is equipment used with a connecting hose that provides a free field of view and breathes atmospheric air from a short distance without coming to the surface. It is mostly used for viewing the underwater world, photographing, and performing short-distance dives. Freediving is a sport that includes different disciplines for open water and pool diving, determined by the World Confederation of Underwater Activities (CMAS). It is an exciting yet extreme sport in which the limits of the human body are tested and adaptation to high pressure is at the highest level. Today, world record-holding free divers can cover a depth of more than 200 meters vertically and a distance of more than 300 meters horizontally in a single breath. Herbert Nitsch holds the world record in the men's No limits category with 253.2 meters. The athlete broke this record on the island of Santorini on 6 June 2012. During this dive, he suffered from decompression sickness and suffered a stroke. This record for women belongs to Tanya Streeter, who reached a depth of 160 meters on August 17, 2002.

In freediving, athletes may encounter clinical conditions such as hypothermia, hypoxia, barotrauma (ear, sinus, lung), and decompression sickness. Sometimes it can occur in injuries caused by vehicles and marine animals.

Scuba Diving

Scuba diving is a system that allows open-circuit breathing, which includes a regulator system that delivers air at a pressure equal to the water pressure in the diver's environment. In other words, the person breathes the air coming from the tube and the breath goes out to the environment he is in. Air bubbles may be seen. In addition, a swimming mask is worn that covers the nose and eyes. In addition, a swimming suit (wetsuit) is worn, which makes it less affected by the season and the water temperature. Weight plates are attached to the waist area of this suit with a belt that can provide a suitable diving maneuver according to the weight of the person. The buoyancy compensator (BC, buoyancy compensator) is worn in the form of a vest, which can fill with air while in the water and rise to the surface when this amount of air is increased, and sinking is enabled by decreasing the amount of air. When the amount of equipment is large, it is recommended and preferred to install pallets to facilitate movement. Dive computers that display data such as time spent underwater, pressure exposed, compass, and direction information can be used.

Closed Circuit (Rebreather) Diving

Its working principle and difference from Scuba are that the air exhaled remains in the system and the bubbles do not come out. When scuba diving first started in the late 1800s, those first systems that pumped air from the outside with a connecting hose were closed-circuit systems. Over time, the development of technology has made these systems more electronic and useful. Having a structure that does not send bubbles to the external environment, it is mostly used in military operations, scientific observation studies, and special areas such as animal photography. In closed-circuit systems, the most problematic parts are hypoxia and hypercarbia. The system works as follows; With inhalation, a mixture of oxygen and nitrogen enters the lungs. After the gas exchange, air containing a small amount of oxygen and carbon dioxide is sent to the outside. The exhaled air moves through the circuit and passes through the carbon dioxide absorber (soda lime). At this stage, there is no carbon dioxide in the air and the oxygen concentration in the mixture is controlled. An automatic solenoid valve introduces the deficient amount of oxygen from the oxygen tank into the system according to the measured oxygen concentration, and the diver re-breathes the oxygen-optimized air. Today, there are different models of different brands that calculate the basal oxygen consumption of divers with the developing technology, adjust the gas mixtures more optimally according to the depth, bring the gas mixture to the appropriate temperature, and switch to the open scuba system in the case of failures such as carbon dioxide removal from the circuit.

The advantages of closed-circuit systems are; Due to lower and efficient oxygen consumption, you can stay underwater longer, the risk of decompression sickness is less due to less nitrogen exposure, it does not form bubbles, it is quieter, and has a structure that does not frighten living animals.

In closed-circuit systems, there are different types of equipment under the name of manual, semi-closed, and electronic closed-circuit systems. They have several advantages over each other. There is an approach and belief that the more manual ones have less potential to cause electronic malfunctions. However, it should not be forgotten that the safest closed-circuit system is the one that is well maintained and the user knows best.

Users of closed-loop systems must be well-trained. They should pay attention to steps such as the maintenance of the system, the control of the carbon dioxide trap, and the consideration of the sensor warnings. Frequent calibrations are required. Otherwise, serious clinical problems may be encountered. In the studies, the causes of death in divers using closed-circuit systems are hypoxia, carbon dioxide necrosis, and hyperoxia-induced seizures. Between 2005 and 2010, 20 divers died while using a closed-circuit system (Fock, 2014). Here you can see the important of the maintenance of the equipment.

Surface Assisted Diving

These are systems that allow the diver to breathe and stay underwater for a very long time with a system that pumps air on the water (on the shore or a ship) and a connection hose. It is generally used in scientific research and the construction industry. This equipment is quite heavy and is very difficult to move out of the water. Medical problems that may occur in scuba diving can also occur in this type of diving.

Mixed Gas Dive

As we explored the underwater world, divers and researchers researched the question of how we could stay longer, and it was discovered that the use of mixed gases could be a solution. Oxygen, nitrogen, and helium are the gases used in mixed gas diving. While such applications were initially used in military and scientific diving due to costs, they have been preferred in recreational diving in recent years and can be authorized with a separate certification.

The purpose of mixed gases is to reduce the narcotic effect of nitrogen, to reduce the toxic effect of high oxygen, and to dive with less risk of decompression sickness. Therefore, it is aimed to increase the underwater stay time with less nitrogen and oxygen at a level that will not reach toxic effects. A third alternative is helium gas. Helium gas can be used here instead of nitrogen or in a combination where all 3 gases are together.

Enriched Nitrox (Enhanced Air Nitrox)
Reduction of nitrogen ratio; This is applied to reduce the narcotic effect caused by the use of excess nitrogen and to reduce the risk of decompression sickness that occurs when rising to the surface after more nitrogen dissolves in the blood. The air we breathe in the atmosphere contains 21% oxygen and 78% nitrogen. Two different nitrox mixtures are commonly used today. These are nitrox 1 (EAN32-32% oxygen, 68% nitrogen) and nitrox 2 (EAN36-36% oxygen, 64% nitrogen). Bottom time refers to the time the diver will spend at the deepest point during a dive. In a routine dive, the gas mixture used by the person, the amount of gas, and the basal oxygen consumption affect the diver's bottom time, as there is a need to spend time at certain intervals until the surface in order not to be exposed to decompression sickness after the bottom time is over. The use of nitrogen provides an advantage in dives not deeper than 40 meters. In deeper dives, it does not have much advantage over normal air. While it takes 60 minutes to stay in normal air in a dive at 18 meters, when nitrox is used, this time increases to 105 minutes and gains 45 minutes. This difference decreases as you go deeper and decreases to 8 minutes at 30 meters (Lang, 2006). Another problem is oxygen toxicity. In the use of nitrox,

more oxygen is used than atmospheric air. In particular, the increase in external pressure with deeper penetration further increases oxygen toxicity. Therefore, EAN32 should be used for dives shallower than 40 meters, and EAN36 for dives shallower than 34 meters. In the case of oxygen toxicity, the central nervous system is affected and it is a clinical condition that can go up to the loss of peripheral vision, vision as if we are in a tunnel, ringing in the ears, nausea, vomiting, muscle twitching, confusion, agitation, anxiety, coordination disorders, weakness, and seizures. The use of enriched nitrox reduces the risk of nitrogen narcosis and decompression sickness but carries a risk of oxygen toxicity (Souday, 2016). It should not be forgotten that it should be used at the appropriate depth and at the appropriate times.

Heliox
This is a mixture created by using helium instead of nitrogen in atmospheric air. It is especially preferred for dives deeper than 40 meters. The most important problems encountered by divers when inhaling helium gas are chills and speech problems. In addition, a clinical condition called high-pressure neurological syndrome (HPNS) can be seen when heliox is inhaled and a rapid descent is deeper than 150 meters.

Trimix
The gas produced by mixing oxygen, nitrogen, and helium is called trimix. The main aim here is to reach deeper points in addition to reducing the risk of nitrogen narcosis and decompression sickness. Today, it is especially preferred for diving deeper than 60 meters. Adding nitrogen to the mix reduces the risk of HPNS. In scuba diving, which has entered the Guinness Book of Records today, athletes prefer trimix during the deepest dive. It has started to be used in recreational diving, but it seems that it will take time to become widespread.

Saturation Diver

As diving accidents occur, their causes have been understood and serious studies have been carried out on how to adapt to the high pressure environment of the underwater and how to return from this adaptation to the normal atmosphere without any problems. Such studies are pioneered by commercial, scientific, and military activities. The logic of saturation diving, which is a technique used especially by divers working in deep seas, is simple. The dive is initiated in a pressure chamber located on the ships. At however many meters depth the diver will work, the ambient pressure is provided on the ship. Divers sometimes have to work for days at a depth of 200 meters, and this pressure equality is maintained throughout this period, aiming to pass the time without decompression. This type of business is high risk and requires serious investment. Divers need to take care of their daily life and health because they cannot leave such a high-pressure environment immediately unless there is an emergency.

Polar Diving

After the requirements of scientific research, there was a need for underwater research in the polar regions and divers had to work in much colder waters. In such environments, the coldness of the water is not the only problem, as another important issue is that the aquatic creatures are dangerous for divers due to wildness and untouched nature. The cold environment creates the risk of hypothermia underwater and may cause this risk of hypothermia to continue after divers get out of the water. Sometimes divers can become confused and trapped under the thick ice sheet. In this case, divers may need to break through this layer of ice, and if this is not achieved, death may result. In addition, due to the extremely dry environment in the camping areas on the surface, attention should be paid to the risk of fire.

Atmospheric Diving

This system, which allows for a longer and safer stay in deep waters, is used in deep-sea research and search and rescue operations. The equipment has the durability to protect the body against the water pressure of hundreds of meters and to keep the pressure of 1 atm at the seaside constant in the clothes.

Diving Physiology

The underwater environment contains various difficulties due to its natural structure. We cannot speak underwater, we cannot see because the light decreases as we go deeper, we cannot breathe, and we may experience many medical problems due to high pressure. Injuries can be minimized when underwater sports are performed by the rules of physics and with appropriate training.

No matter how durable the human body, some medical problems may occur when entering the aquatic environment. Situations such as motion sickness, drowning, hypothermia, heatstroke, allergic reactions, irritant dermatitis, and infections can be seen due to environmental exposure while swimming. Medical problems such as barotrauma, arterial gas embolism, decompression sickness, dysbaric retinopathy, dysbaric osteopathy, and immersion pulmonary edema may be experienced in diving individuals. Due to the gas types used by divers, problems such as hypoxia, hypercapnia, carbon monoxide poisoning, and gas narcosis may occur. Divers can be attacked by creatures living in the marine environment and be injured or there may be accidents resulting in death.

Pascal's law was defined in the 1700s and states that liquids transmit the same pressure they are exposed to. When a diver dives into the water, the pressure of the water in contact with his body is the same in all parts of the body that contain fluid. In organs containing gas, on the other hand, there is a volumetric reduction with the effect of pressure (Boyle's law). And the change is reversed in a diver who comes to the surface. Pressure-related clinical problems occur by these laws.

Dysbarism and Barotrauma

Dysbarism is any adverse medical condition resulting from changes in ambient pressure. If these changes in pressure occur at a rate or time that exceeds the body's capacity to adapt safely, certain medical problems can occur. In an underwater environment, the pressure increases linearly with depth. That is, for every 33 feet (10.06 meters) of depth, the pressure increases by 1 atm, and the volume of the gases decreases in the same proportion. In other words, there is a pressure of 3 atm at 99 feet (30.17 meters), and the volume of a gas that is 100 cm3 at sea level decreases to 33 cm3 (Auerbach 2016).

Barotrauma, on the other hand, is a clinical problem that occurs during volume changes in gas-filled organs, which we usually see after moving quickly or descending too deep during underwater descents and ascents without complying with the adaptation mechanisms.

Mask Barotrauma

The mechanism described in Boyle's law is valid. To see underwater, divers use goggles with a layer of clear glass at eye level that covers their eyes and nose. For the image to be clear, there should be a layer of air in front of the eyes. In other words, the mask contains some air in front of the eyes. As divers go deeper, the volume of this air will gradually decrease with the effect of pressure. This will create a vacuum effect in the areas that the mask touches and covers. As experienced divers go deeper, they breathe a certain volume of air through their nose into this cavity of the mask, thus preventing barotrauma of the mask.

These patients are generally inexperienced divers and may present with facial pain, redness, bruising periorbital swelling, and subconjunctival hemorrhage at the point of contact with the mask. In more serious clinical situations, there may be a pain in the eye, proptosis, limitation of eye movements, diplopia, and visual changes. If patients describe diplopia, abnormal vision, proptosis, or limitation of eye movements, they should be evaluated with CT or MRI (Latham, 2011). Systemic complaints should not be ignored by focusing on the facial complaints of the patient and decompression sickness should not be overlooked.

Most of the cases are mild and no additional treatment is required in cases such as skin swelling, redness, bruising, or subconjunctival hemorrhage. These usually heal spontaneously within 1-2 weeks. In cases that compress the optic nerve and increase intraocular pressure, such as subperiosteal orbital hematoma, which are more serious conditions, an emergency ophthalmology opinion should be sought and drainage with needle aspiration or orbitotomy should be planned (Ergözen, 2017).

Sinus Barotrauma

As divers descend in the water, the air volume in the gas-filled sinuses (ethmoid, maxillary, frontal) will decrease with the effect of increasing pressure. If there is no air supply in the respiratory tract, this reduced air creates a vacuum effect in the sinus cavity. This vacuum effect can cause problems such as edema, bleeding, and hematoma in the sinus mucosa. In addition, the pressure gradually decreases as divers approach the surface. The volume of air in the sinuses increases, putting pressure on the sinus mucosa and causing pain. The incidence of paranasal barotrauma in divers is around 27% (Uzun 2009). During diving, pain occurs in the affected sinus. If such a situation occurs, the dive should be canceled and the diver returned to the surface. Some different clinical conditions can be seen according to the affected paranasal sinus. If the sphenoid sinus is affected, vision loss due to optic neuropathy may occur, and if the maxillary sinus is affected, toothache, cheek, and upper lip numbness may occur (Schipke, 2018; Neuman, 1975).

In sinus barotraumas, divers' allergic structures, active sinusitis, and anatomical obstructions such as nasal polyps, etc. function as a unilateral valve which is a predisposing cause and should be checked before diving. In general, the picture of sinusitis is seen. It should not be skipped, especially in patients who present with pain in the sinuses after diving. Systemic pain relievers, antihistamines, corticosteroids, and topical antihistamines can be used for treatment. Antibiotics may be preferred if there is an infected condition.

Ear Barotrauma

The ear is anatomically divided into three as the outer ear, middle ear, and inner ear. Each has a different pathophysiology of barotrauma. Inner ear barotrauma affects 40% of all divers (Green, 1993). There are various maneuvers for equalizing inner ear pressure through the eustachian tube. The Valsalva maneuver is to increase the pressure in the nasopharynx when the nose is closed and the glottis is left open and to increase the pressure by injecting air into the inner ear through the eustachian tube. The Toynbee maneuver is performed by trying to swallow while the nose and glottis are closed. The Frenzel maneuver, when the nose is closed and the glottis is open, pushes the chin forward and downward to open the eustachian canal and pressure equalization is achieved.

The natural structure of the external ear canal contains some air. If this air is disconnected from the underwater environment (plug, diving suit covering the ear, earplugs), the volume of the diver will decrease during descent. In this case, pain, swelling, and erythema may occur in the external ear canal. Very rarely, rupture of the tympanic membrane may occur. Here the tympanic membrane has curved outward. Since the first symptom is pain, the diver feels the need to equalize his ear, and when he performs the Valsalva maneuver, the pressure in the inner ear increases, and rupture of the tympanic membrane may occur. In the treatment, it is sufficient to wash the external ear canal with warm water. If there is a rupture of the tympanic membrane, antibiotic drops containing fluoroquinolones and hydrocortisone drops should be used.

Middle ear barotrauma occurs more frequently. During the descent, the tympanic membrane curves inward due to the effect of increasing water pressure and the decrease in volume in the inner ear. This causes pain, ear fullness, and decreased hearing. If the diver cannot add air to the inner ear with the ear equalization maneuver, the risk will increase. If the ear continues to descend without equalization, the difference between the inner ear pressure and the external ambient pressure will gradually increase and the contraction power of the eustachian tube will increase. This makes basic ear equalization maneuvers increasingly useless. If the pain does not go away and there is no relief after the ear equalization maneuver, it is necessary to rise again, perform the equalization and then descend. Due to the pressure difference between them, edema in the inner ear, rupture, and bleeding in the vascular structures can be seen. A further increase in the pressure difference causes a rupture of the tympanic membrane (Fismen, 2012). The rupture eliminates the pressure difference and reduces pain, but the seawater contacts the middle ear. In this case, clinics such as vertigo, vomiting, and disorientation can be seen. The first thing to do is to get to the surface. Patients should be seen by an otolaryngologist. Findings that may be encountered in the examination are graded according to the TEED classification. Bleeding in the inner ear causes conductive hearing loss.

Middle ear barotrauma, if there is no complication, can heal within 3-7 days of taking painkillers and decongestants. Antihistamines can be used in cases with an allergic picture and thought to have eustachian dysfunction. Intermittent application of the Frenzel maneuver during treatment can help to clear accumulated collections. If tympanic membrane rupture is accompanied, drops containing a combination of fluoroquinolones and hydrocortisone should be used. Tympanic membrane ruptures heal in an average of 1-3 months. Defects that do not close spontaneously within 1 month should be surgically repaired.

Inner ear barotrauma occurs much less frequently. Due to the structures it contains, it can cause much more serious and permanent problems. Complications such as labyrinth window rupture, or perilymphatic fistula may damage the cochleovestibular system and may be accompanied by permanent deafness. As divers begin to descend underwater, the tympanic membrane curves inward. In this case, the stapes novel is pushed into the window. If the middle ear pressure equalization maneuver is performed forcefully, middle ear pressure will increase. This pressure increase will cause a rupture of the oval pen, followed by a rupture of the Reissner membrane, and mixing of the endolymph and perilymph (Parell, 1985). Divers may experience ear pain, ear fullness, hearing loss, nausea, vomiting, nystagmus, diaphoresis, disorientation, and ataxia during descent. A sensorineural hearing loss occurs. Bed rest with the head elevated at 30 degrees is recommended for treatment. Activities that will increase intracranial pressure should be avoided. Perilymphatic fistulas and hearing problems usually heal spontaneously within 3-12 weeks (Parell, 1985). Surgery may be an option for non-closure fistulas. The most basic way to prevent inner ear barotrauma is to do the ear equalization maneuver softly and calmly. In addition, it must be differentiated from inner ear decompression disease, as in the presence of decompression sickness, hyperbaric therapy is applied. In the distinction of these two entities, it will be sufficient to detail whether their complaints started during the descent or the ascent.

Clothing Barotrauma

This is damage to the skin by the vacuum effect due to the principle of decreasing gas volume as the pressure increases during the dives made after air is trapped between the diving suit and a part of the body. Ecchymosis and erythema may occur on the skin. No additional treatment is needed, as it heals spontaneously in a few days.

Dental Barotrauma

Dental caries can result from several dental conditions, including defective restorations, oral tissue tears, new extractions, periodontal abscesses, pulpal or apical lesions or cysts, and endodontic (root canal) treatment (Peker 2009). In these disorders, air may be present in the tooth. This presence of air can cause pain or even eruption in the tooth after increasing pressure underwater, after a decrease in volume, or after an increase in air volume during the ascent.

Lung Barotrauma

This can occur by two different mechanisms. The first is pulmonary barotrauma during descent. The freediver style occurs when diving with breath-holding. When the diver dives into the water and goes deeper, the volume of air remaining in the lungs gradually decreases due to the increasing water pressure. Transpulmonic pressure exceeds interalveolar pressure when the total lung volume decreases to the residual volume and exceeds this threshold. In this case, the reduced volume of the alveolar space draws fluid and blood from the pulmonary bed like a vacuum. Affected individuals may have dyspnea and cough up blood. It usually goes away on its own when it comes to the surface.

The second and most dangerous of all barotraumas is pulmonary barotrauma, which occurs during ascent. The alveoli enlarge inversely with the pressure they are exposed to. When divers think they are suffocating, in the moment of panic, when they experience a rapid rise after reasons such as uncontrolled positive BC (buoyancy controller), falling weight plates, etc. the air in the alveoli suddenly expands and damage occurs if it exceeds the alveolar wall tension. The extent of this damage may be a local alveolar injury, pneumomediastinum, pneumothorax, or tension pneumothorax. The worst-case scenario is that these gas bubbles enter the circulation and form an arterial gas embolism. Local alveolar damage occurs as a result of a rupture of the alevoles and can usually cause chest pain, cough, and hemoptysis. In this case, if there is no arterial gas embolism clinic and the neurological examination is normal, it is sufficient to follow up with supportive treatment. Air escaping from the ruptured alveoli can sometimes travel to the mediastinum and from there to the neck region and cause pneumomediastinum. In this case, chest pain, subcutaneous crepitation, dyspnea, and dysphagia may develop. The treatment of pneumomediastinum is mostly resting in a head-up position. Oxygen may be required. Entering low-pressure environments (air travel, high altitude) is not recommended. Pneumothorax is a rare clinical practice. Pneumothorax is detected in 4%-10% of cases with arterial gas embolism (Pearson, 1984). Generally, diving-associated pneumothorax has symptoms such as shortness of breath and pleuritic chest pain, and is of small volume. It is followed conservatively and supportive treatment is applied. If the patient is to undergo recompression therapy, tube thoracostomy is required.

Facial Baroparesis

The seventh cranial nerve passes through the temporal bone. As a result of the mechanisms in inner ear barotrauma, if eustachian dysfunction accompanies the event, inner ear pressure increases, and nerve compression may occur (Iaovlev, 2014). As a result of this pressure, a feeling of fullness and ipsilateral peripheral facial paralysis is seen in the affected ear. Ear equalization maneuvers, oral or topical decongestants, or sometimes recompression can be used for treatment.

Gastrointestinal Barotrauma

The gastrointestinal structures have an elastic and expandable structure. A gastrointestinal clinic is rarely seen, as the volume of gases decreases during dive descents. When the rise begins, the gases expand and cause an increase in the volume where they are. Those who do excessive Valsalva maneuvers, consume carbonated beverages before diving, eat legumes, and chew gum during diving have excessive gas accumulation. In this case, the expanding gas may cause colic-like abdominal pain, cramps, belching, abdominal distention, and sometimes even perforations (Molenat, 1995).

Arterial Gas Embolism

This is the worst prognostic form of pulmonary barotrauma. It is an important cause of death and disability, especially in recreational diving (Kizer, 1987). A diver advances to the surface underwater, after the panicked, uncontrolled use of the BC, etc. If the lungs make a sudden rise when they are full of air after a situation like this, the air in the lungs expands with decreasing pressure. Damage occurs if a tensile force occurs above the elastance level that the lung alveoli can withstand. In the injured alveoli, air enters the pulmonary venous circulation. Circulating air moves into the left atrium. If the air that enters the systemic circulation by following the left ventricle and aorta paths disrupts the circulation in the microvascular bed, clinical findings occur in the affected divers. Usually, air bubbles travel through the carotid and vertebral arteries to the brain. Here, a mechanical obstruction occurs in small- and medium-sized arteries, and the brain's blood supply is impaired. Ischemia begins in the brain parenchyma fed by the occluded vessels. The vascular endothelium is disrupted and this picture is followed by cerebral edema. Systemic hypertension occurs as a response.

Loss of consciousness, apnea, and sudden death occur in 4% of divers with arterial gas embolism. In these cases, there is no response to resuscitative interventions or compressive approaches. The reason for this may be serious arrhythmias, coronary artery occlusions, and brain stem infarcts (Evans, 1981). In addition, the main problem is that a significant amount of excess air enters the circulation. As a result of autopsy studies, it is thought that the mechanism in cases with fatal outcomes is obstruction caused by a significant amount of air in the central vascular bed (Neuman, 2003, Neuman, 1998). Approximately 10% of cases with AGE are lost. 50% recover without sequelae and sequelae are seen in the remaining group. Clinical findings occur in direct proportion to the amount of air that enters the circulation. Loss of consciousness, focal paralysis, plegia, convulsion, aphasia, visual disturbance, vertigo, and headache are the most common symptoms. The general approach should be considered as AGE, especially in the presence of neurological signs (loss of consciousness) that occur during a dive or within 10 minutes of surfacing. In this case, transfer to the nearest health institution and the next stage, the hyperbaric oxygen therapy clinic, should be arranged.

Anamnesis is the most important criterion when these patients apply. It is necessary to think about AGE and act quickly in a patient describing a diving history and a consciousness problem. This consciousness problem can sometimes occur while the diver is still in the water and the risk of aspiration can be added to the table. The first step is primarily ABC assessment and airway safety. Afterward, transfer to the nearest health institution should be planned. The transplant should be in the supine position. Trendelenburg is not recommended. It is necessary to start 100% oxygen therapy during the transplant. Oxygen therapy will benefit from reducing ischemia caused by circulating bubbles. Land or air vehicles can be used to transport patients. Helicopters should be preferred in aircraft and the transfer should be low flying, the altitude of which does not exceed 305 meters. Otherwise, the volume of the circulating bubbles will increase further and the occlusive effect will become evident. Circulating bubbles cause endothelial damage after ischemia, and this causes plasma extravasation, resulting in hemoconcentration. In addition, a predisposition to hypovolemia occurs due to plasma loss. For this reason, intravenous fluid therapy should be given to avoid hypotension and to achieve adequate volume. Fluid therapy should be given so that the hourly urine output is 1-2 cc/kg/hour. When the hospital application is made, the first evaluation is made and initial laboratory tests are requested. Routines such as hemoglobin, creatine phosphokinase, chest X-ray, and ECG should be seen.

It is very important to enter hyperbaric therapy early, even in cases with neurological findings or spontaneous recovery. In addition, the delay does not eliminate the indication for hyperbaric therapy. In the literature, some cases received hyperbaric treatment more than 6-24 hours later and showed improvement (Mader, 1979, Kizer, 1983). Hyperbaric therapy increases the ambient pressure and raises the oxygen concentration. After this effect, the volume of circulating air bubbles decreases, and their occlusive effect decreases. This helps to improve ischemia. Shrinking air bubbles are more likely to be cleared from the circulation. It also reduces ischemia-reperfusion injury and modifies inflammation. Hyperbaric therapy should initially be performed in the presence of 100% oxygen below 2.8 atm. It is also important to know how late the diver enters the hyperbaric treatment. If the time is prolonged, sessions can be adjusted by starting with low pressure and increasing it to a pressure of 6 atm with clinical status monitoring in certain periods.

As drug therapy, many experts use heparin, low-molecular-weight heparin, aspirin, and corticosteroids. But there is no proven effect of these drugs. It has been shown that the use of lidocaine alone has cerebroprotective and anti-inflammatory effects and also reduces brain edema (Mitchell, 1999).

Decompression Sickness

The air we breathe in the atmosphere contains 21% oxygen and 78% nitrogen. Due to the atmospheric pressure in the environment we live in, the nitrogen in the air we breathe is dissolved in the blood, albeit in a small amount. There are 3 stages in diving: descent, bottom time, and ascent. When a diver dives, the external pressure increases, and, according to Henry's law, the solubility of gases in liquids increases in direct proportion to the pressure and surface area, and the amount of nitrogen in the blood and tissues increases as the solubility increases. Since this nitrogen is in a dissolved form, it has no mechanical effect. It can only cause the previously mentioned nitrogen narcosis. When the diver starts to rise after the bottom time, the pressure will decrease and the amount of nitrogen dissolved in the blood and tissues will decrease in the same parallel. This cleaning process is not immediate but takes place at a certain speed through the lungs. This process, which we call the decompression stage, may differ from person to person. Therefore, there should be an allowance for certain waiting periods during the rise to clear the dissolved nitrogen in the blood and tissues after this pressure-nitrogen relationship. If the diver does not comply with these times and makes a rapid rise, the dissolved nitrogen turns into a gas form with the effect of decreasing pressure and causes functional and circulatory problems due to the mechanical effect in whichever organ or system. It is necessary to comply with the tables called "dive tables", which are determined according to each depth and include the maximum dive time and appropriate decompression times according to the diving depth.

Due to this problem caused by the use of nitrogen, divers use gas mixtures such as less nitrogen or more oxygen (EAN 32, EAN 36), helium instead of nitrogen, or a mixture of oxygen, nitrogen, and helium in different ratios (trimix) in deep dives. The aim here is to reduce the decompression sickness effect of inhaled inert gas. When we go from high pressure to low pressure, air bubbles form in the venous system. This can be observed in asymptomatic divers after diving. It filters these bubbles that come from the pulmonary venous route and prevents them from joining the arterial circulation. If the number of air bubbles is high or there is a right-to-left shunt, there is a transition to the arterial system, and AGE may occur. Decompression sickness is a disease with multisystemic effects. It can cause pathology in the musculoskeletal system, central nervous system, and lungs, inner ear, etc. systems.

The incidence of decompression sickness is rare. In sports diving, the rate is 3/10000 and in recreational diving 1.5-10/10000 (Pollock, 2017). The greater the depth of the dive, the greater is the risk of DCS. The risk in men is 2.5 times higher than in women.

Musculoskeletal Decompression Disease

This is the most common type of decompression sickness, accounting for 70% of cases. Generally, the shoulders and elbows are the most commonly affected areas. The hip and knee are the most commonly affected areas in saturation divers. While this pain is mild, throbbing, and squeezing in nature, it can sometimes increase with tearing and joint movement. Sometimes it spreads around the joint and hypoesthesia can be seen. Sometimes there may be erythema and edema on the joint. Traumatic events should be excluded from the differential diagnosis. If DCS is suspected, when a manometer is placed around the joint and inflated to 150-220 mmHg, the bubbles spread to the surrounding tissues and the diagnosis becomes clear if the joint pain is relieved after this procedure (Rudge, 1991). Divers with these complaints should be treated with hyperbaric oxygen at an early stage. Otherwise, these bubbles may enter the venous circulation and cause more serious problems. In addition, hyperbaric oxygen therapy is recommended even if there are isolated joint diseases or even pain that goes away on its own. Untreated patients are at risk of developing osteonecrosis of large joints in the future. In addition, signs of severe fatigue should be carefully examined. If fatigue is thought to be unrelated to underwater activity, early symptoms of DCS should be considered.

Cutaneous Decompression Disease (Skin Bend)

This condition, which is rarely seen in diving, usually creates a mottled redness on the skin, a cutis marmorata-like picture. The mechanism of its formation is not clear. The complaint is in the form of a tingling sensation throughout the body. Other clinics related to marine exposure (wetsuit barotrauma, skin rash, plankton dermatitis) should be distinguished.

Pulmonary Decompression Disease

This is a rare but serious form that is seen after inadvertent increases in decompression times. Air bubbles accumulate in the pulmonary bed. This causes dyspnea, cyanosis, chest pain, and cough. In this picture, hemodynamics may be impaired and neurological findings may be added to the picture with the passage of bubbles into the arterial system.

Neurological Decompression Disease

In this form, which has a wide range of symptoms, it is vital not to miss the patients and to evaluate the symptoms after diving well. Neurological findings are seen in the majority of cases with diving injuries. The spinal cord, especially the thoracic and lumbar regions, is most commonly affected. As a result, clinics such as weakness, paresis, plegia, loss of sphincter tone, widespread pain and fatigue, and loss of reflexes can be seen in the feet. The mechanism is that air bubbles formed in the spinal cord impair circulation and cause infarction. Of course, the brain can also be affected. In this case, it is not possible to distinguish it from AGE.

Vestibular Decompression Disease

This is the form of DCS seen in the inner ear. Typically, the vestibular apparatus is affected. Nausea, dizziness, vomiting, tinnitus, and nystagmus are seen. It can be distinguished from inner ear barotrauma by pain and the absence of the hemorrhagic image seen in inner ear evaluation. It is mostly seen in saturation dives or very deep dives.

Vasomotor Decompression Sickness

This is the most serious form of DCS. A severe shock picture is observed and the cause is not fully elucidated. Mechanisms such as a fluid shift due to endothelial damage and the occlusive effect of air bubbles in the pulmonary bed are predicted. If hyperbaric treatment is not taken in a very early period, the probability of a mortal course is high.

There are limited biochemical markers that can be used in the diagnosis of decompression sickness. Urine density, hematocrit, and albumin can be used. An increase in urine density after plasma volume loss after vascular endothelial injury, an increase in hematocrit in the range of 50-60 and a decrease in albumin value may be signs. It is not appropriate to wait for laboratory analysis to diagnose DCS. Diagnosis is made by clinical findings and necessary transplantation procedures should be arranged for early hyperbaric treatment. Divers should be ventilated with 100% oxygen from the time that symptoms are noticed to the initiation of hyperbaric therapy. The aim here is to reduce the rate of inert gas in the circulation and to reduce possible tissue hypoxia. In addition, due to plasma volume loss after endothelial damage, intravenous isotonic fluid therapy should be initiated to preserve hemodynamics. The target urine output is 1-2 ml/kg/hr. A urinary catheter should be inserted if spinal DCS is suspected. Air vehicles may be preferred for transport. If there is no vehicle that can adjust the interior cabin pressure, or if there is no such vehicle, low-flying transportation should be provided that will not exceed 305 meters. Hyperbaric therapy should not be delayed in DCS. In the literature, even in cases delayed up to 48 hours, recovery was observed after hyperbaric therapy (Hadanny, 2015). In affected divers, symptom monitoring should be performed during hyperbaric therapy, and repeated sessions should be applied when necessary.

The most important thing that can be done for protection is to comply with the decompression times and not to make a fast ascent. In addition, there are opinions that regular exercise, aerobic exercise performed 2-24 hours before diving, applications such as antioxidants, and sauna reduce the possibility of decompression sickness.

Conclusion

All primary care and emergency physicians should know about diving injuries. In addition to simple medical conditions, it should be possible to provide access to hyperbaric oxygen therapy in serious conditions such as decompression sickness or arterial gas embolism.

References

Auerbach, P. S., Cushing, T. A., & Harris, N. S. (2016). Auerbach's Wilderness Medicine E-book. Elsevier Health Sciences.

Bachrach, A. J. (1975). A short history of man in the sea. The physiology and medicine of diving and compressed air work. Bailliere and Tindall. London.

Butler, W. P. (2004). Caisson disease during the construction of the Eads and Brooklyn Bridges: A review. *Undersea Hyperb Med*, 31(4), 445-59.

Buzzacott, P., Schiller, D., Crain, J., & Denoble, P. J. (2018). Epidemiology of morbidity and mortality in US and Canadian recreational scuba diving. *Public health*, 155, 62-68.

Davis, S. R. H. (1955). Deep Diving and Submarine Operations, Etc.. Siebe Gorman & Company.

Denoble, PJ., Pollock, NW., Vaithiyanathan, P. (2008). Scuba injury death rate among insured DAN members. *Diving Hyperbaric Medicine.*, 38, 182.

Ergözen, S. (2017). Preventable diving-related ocular barotrauma: a case report. *Turkish journal of ophthalmology*, 47(5), 296.

Evans, D. E., Kobrine, A. I., Weathersby, P. K., & Bradley, M. E. (1981). Cardiovascular effects of cerebral air embolism. *Stroke*, 12(3), 338-44A.

Fismen, L., Hjelde, A., Svardal, A. M., & Djurhuus, R. (2012). Differential effects on nitric oxide synthase, heat shock proteins and glutathione in human endothelial cells exposed to heat stress and simulated diving. *European journal of applied physiology*, 112(7), 2717-2725.

Fock, A. W. (2013). Analysis of recreational closed-circuit rebreather deaths 1998–2010. *Diving Hyperb Med*, 43(2), 78-85.

Green, S. M., Rothrock, S. G., Hummel, C. B., & Green, E. A. (1993). Incidence and severity of middle ear barotrauma in recreational scuba diving. *Journal of Wilderness Medicine*, 4(3), 270-280.

Hadanny, A., Fishlev, G., Bechor, Y., Bergan, J., Friedman, M., Maliar, A., & Efrati, S. (2015). Delayed recompression for decompression sickness: retrospective analysis. *PloS one*, 10(4), e0124919.

Iakovlev, E. V., & Iakovlev, V. V. (2014). Facial baroparesis: a critical differential diagnosis for scuba diving accidents--case report. *Undersea and hyperbaric medicine*, 41(5), 407-409.

Jarcho, S. (1968). Alphonse Jaminet on caisson disease (1871). *The American journal of cardiology*, 21(2), 258-260.

Kizer, K. W. (1982). Delayed treatment of dysbarism: a retrospective review of 50 cases. *Jama*, 247(18), 2555-2558.

Kizer, K. W. (1987). Dysbaric cerebral air embolism in Hawaii. *Annals of emergency medicine*, 16(5), 535-541.

Lang, M. A. (2006). The state of oxygen-enriched air (nitrox). *DIVING AND HYPERBARIC MEDICINE-SOUTH PACIFIC UNDERWATER MEDICINE SOCIETY*, 36(2), 87.

Latham, E., van Hoesen, K., & Grover, I. (2011). Diplopia due to mask barotrauma. *The Journal of emergency medicine*, 41(5), 486-488.

Mader, J. T., & Hulet, W. H. (1979). Delayed hyperbaric treatment of cerebral air embolism: report of a case. *Archives of neurology*, 36(8), 504-505.

Mitchell, S. J., Pellett, O., & Gorman, D. F. (1999). Cerebral protection by lidocaine during cardiac operations. *The Annals of thoracic surgery*, 67(4), 1117-1124.

Molenat, F. A., & Boussuges, A. H. (1995). Rupture of the stomach complicating diving accidents. *Undersea & hyperbaric medicine: journal of the Undersea and Hyperbaric Medical Society*, Inc, 22(1), 87-96.

Neuman, T. (1975). Maxillary sinus barotrauma with cranial nerve involvement: Case report.

Neuman, T. S. (2003). Arterial gas embolism and pulmonary barotrauma. Bennett and Elliott's physiology and medicine of diving. 5th ed. London: Saunders, 557-77.

Neuman, T. S., Jacoby, I., & Bove, A. A. (1998). Fatal pulmonary barotrauma due to obstruction of the central circulation with air. *The Journal of emergency medicine*, 16(3), 413-417.

Parell, G. J., & Becker, G. D. (1985). Conservative management of inner ear barotrauma resulting from scuba diving. *Otolaryngology—Head and Neck Surgery*, 93(3), 393-397.

Pearson, R. R. (1984). Diagnosis and treatment of gas embolism. In *The physician's guide to diving medicine*, (pp. 333-367). Springer, Boston, MA.

Peker, I., Erten, H., & Kayaoglu, G. (2009). Dental restoration dislodgment and fracture during scuba diving: a case of barotrauma. *The Journal of the American Dental Association*, 140(9), 1118-1121.

Pollock, N. W., & Buteau, D. (2017). Updates in decompression illness. *Emergency medicine clinics*, 35(2), 301-319.

Richardson, D. (2010, April). *Training scuba divers: a fatality and risk analysis. In RecReational Diving Fatalities WoRkshop pRoceeDings*, (p. 119).

Rudge, F. W., & Stone, J. A. (1991). The use of the pressure cuff test in the diagnosis of decompression sickness. SCHOOL OF AEROSPACE MEDICINE BROOKS AFB TX.

Schipke, J. D., Cleveland, S., & Drees, M. (2018). Sphenoid sinus barotrauma in diving: case series and review of the literature. *Research in sports medicine*, 26(1), 124-137.

Souday, V., Koning, N. J., Perez, B., Grelon, F., Mercat, A., Boer, C., ... & Asfar, P. (2016). Enriched air nitrox breathing reduces venous gas bubbles after simulated SCUBA diving: A double-blind cross-over randomized trial. *PloS one*, 11(5), e0154761.

Uzun, C. (2009). Paranasal sinus barotrauma in sports self-contained underwater breathing apparatus divers. *The Journal of Laryngology & Otology*, 123(1), 80-84.

Chapter 11

Injuries with Sea Creatures

Okan Bardakçı*, MD, Gökhan Akdur, MD and Okhan Akdur, MD

Department of Emergency Medicine, Çanakkale Onsekiz Mart University, Çanakkale, Turkey

Abstract

Venomous marine animals can be dangerous to swimmers, divers, and fishers. Most marine envenomations are not severe, and victims may delay seeking emergency care. These mild envenomations include weever fish, lionfish, starfish, and coral abrasions. Also, severe envenomation from stonefish, stingray, blue-ringed octopus, cone snail, and box jellyfish (Irukandji) can be life-threatening. Rapid treatment in these cases can increase survival rates and minimize systemic (anaphylaxis) and local complications (allergic response, infections, pain) by venoms.

Keywords: marine toxins, fish venoms, emergency treatment

Introduction

Marine injuries increase with the summer season. These are one of the reasons for applying to the emergency service in the coastal settlements and especially in the winter season for fishers. Injuries occur in the form of trauma and poisoning. Toxins of sea creatures exert their effects through neurotoxic, cytotoxic, myotoxic, and hematotoxic mechanisms. Toxins from marine animals are thermolabile due to their high protein content. They are generally produced in cold environments (Haddad et al., 2009), but the potential for toxicity should not be ignored as they do not denature until 48 hours after the death of the source (Rensch and Murphy, 2021). This chapter outlines the management and treatment recommendations for marine envenomations in emergency medicine settings. Common sea creatures and injuries are discussed.

---

* Corresponding Author's Email: drokanbardakci@gmail.com.

In: Environmental Emergencies and Injuries in Nature
Editors: Murat Yücel, Murat Güzel and İbrahim İkizceli
ISBN: 978-1-68507-833-1

Coral

Corals are the most common cause of marine injury, and they are living organisms with a calcium carbonate exoskeleton that cling to the seafloor and reproduce by structures called nematocysts. By skin contact, nematocysts can be injected into the subcutaneous tissue. The soles of the feet, hands, knees, and forearms are the most frequently injured areas. Itching, pain, and erythema may occur, and cellulitis and ulceration may develop (Taylor et al., 2006).

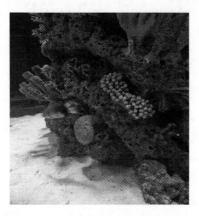

Figure 1. Coral (https://pxhere.com).

The injured area should be immobilized, and elevation should be applied. In order to prevent nematocyst activation, the wound site should be washed with 5% acetic acid for 15-30 minutes after washing with normal saline. In the case of clinical suspicion, a foreign body evaluation should be performed with direct radiography (Farrar et al., 2013).

Stingray

There are 150 different stingrays, which live in shallow waters on the seafloor and have a flat body structure. The stingray with its venomous stings has evolved for defense, and it can extend to 30 cm, extending parallel from the body-tail junction to the upper part of the tail (Pedroso et al., 2007). In its poisonous structure, orpotrin causes vasoconstriction, while porflan causes inflammation and tissue necrosis. Injury often occurs due to feet stepping on them and fishing with nets or grazing.

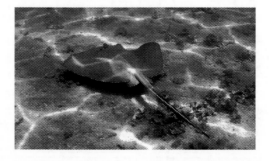

Figure 2. Stingray (https://pxhere.com).

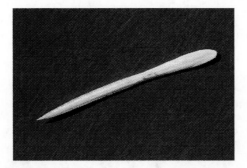

Figure 3. Stingray Spine (https://www.greelane.com).

Injury is toxin-mediated caused by direct damage of the needle. The clinical course varies according to the size of the needle and the location of the injury. Within minutes after injury, very severe pain progresses through the extremity to the trunk, reaches its peak in 30-90 minutes, and lasts for 48 hours (Auerbach, 2001). Rhabdomyolysis has been reported with the myotoxic effect of the toxin (Masson et al., 2012). It has been reported to cause great vessel, thorax, and intra abdominal injuries.

Injuries to the trunk require an approach like stab wounds. Mortality has been reported after heart and abdominal cavity penetration and significant artery injury and this is rare (Cooper, 1991). Extremity injuries carry a risk of late infection. The needle may remain in the soft tissue, so the wound site should be evaluated for a foreign body after cleaning the wound site (Cappa et al., 2020).

After the injury, the toxin should be removed by first washing the wound with sterile saline. For pain and toxin denaturation, hot water (>45°C) should be applied for 30-60 minutes. If pain control cannot be achieved, non-steroidal anti-inflammatory drugs or opiates can be used. After pain control, foreign body evaluation in the soft tissue should be performed with radiography, and antibiotic therapy (tetracycline, ciprofloxacin) should be started.

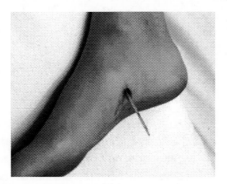

Figure 4. Stingray Spine (https://www.bayareaorthofl.com).

Stonefish

In recent years, the stonefish has been reported in the Pacific coasts, Indonesia, India, the Red Sea, and the Mediterranean (Bilecenoğlu, 2012). It is the most venomous fish known. Its appearance is very similar to the seafloor and coral rocks, and it is reported that contact is usually made by feet stepping on them. Stonefish can stay alive for 24 hours outside the sea (on the coast, on the rocks). Poisoning occurs after contact with 11-17 dorsal fins containing neurotoxin (verrucotoxin) (Smith and Wheeler, 2006).

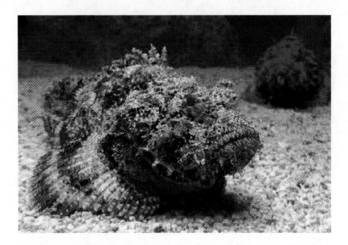

Figure 5. Stonefish (https://www.flickr.com).

Post-exposure symptoms begin with severe pain and warmth. Increasing the amount of injected venom may result in cardiovascular system damage, convulsions, muscle paralysis, respiratory arrest, and death (Khoo, 2002).

The mechanism of action of the venom varies according to the amount taken. It has an effect with an increase in β-receptor activity at 3 μg/ml, and it has been shown that a β-blocker can suppress this effect (propranolol), and negative inotropic and negative chronotropic effects were observed at 5 μg/ml (Sauviat et al., 1995). However, β-blockers are of no use in muscle paralysis and convulsions. It has been reported that the application of hot water (>45°C) at the time of contact provides toxin denaturation and reduces tissue necrosis and systemic toxicity (Barnett et al., 2017).

Anti-venom developed by Commonwealth Serum Laboratories (CLS) in Australia neutralizes the venom effect in severe poisonings.

Lionfish

The Pacific Ocean coasts, the Red Sea, and the Mediterranean are the main habitats (Church and Hodgson, 2000). Their flashy and colorful appearance and being hunted for aquariums increase injury frequency. Injuries have often been reported in divers. The dorsal and lateral fin spines are poisonous.

Symptoms are seen with severe pain and tissue edema at the time of contact. Systemic effects are seen with nausea-vomiting and sweating. The toxin's negative chronotropic and inotropic effects were observed in animal experiments (Cohen and Olek, 1989).

After cleaning the wound site after contact, it should be ensured that there is no foreign body belonging to the fish in the tissue. The toxin is heat-sensitive, and hot water (>45°C) should be applied quickly to the contact area for 30-90 minutes.

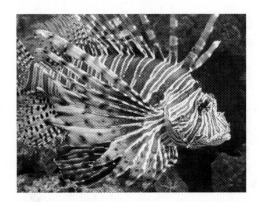

Figure 6. Lionfish (https://pxhere.com).

Weever Fish

Two poisonous species (T. draco, T. vipera) of Weever fish belonging to the Trachinidae family, were seen in the Mediterranean Black Sea and Scandinavia. These two species were described by their injuries (Dehaan et al., 1991).

The dorsal fin needles contain toxins. Although injuries have been reported due to stepping on these fish living at the bottom of the sea, fishers frequently encounter them. T. vipera usually causes superficial injuries and severe pain. Pain starts 2-3 minutes after exposure and intensifies, and it can last up to 24 hours (Bonnet, 2000, Borondo et al., 2001). The complete resolution of edema may take up to a month. T. draco has reported swelling, redness, pruritus, nausea, vomiting, hypotension, hallucinations, abdominal cramps, and rarely local tissue necrosis (Gorman et al., 2020). The only reported case of mortality was a fisherman in the USA.

In the treatment, the application of hot water (>45°C) for 30-90 minutes until the area can withstand the exposure, limits the denaturation of the protein-based venom and the toxin effect. After pain control following hot water application, it should be checked that there is no needle in the tissue of the injury area. Tetanus prophylaxis is recommended. At discharge, non-steroidal anti-inflammatory drugs are sufficient for pain and edema (Ziegman and Alevood, 2015).

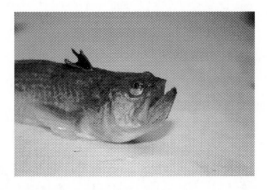

Figure 7. Weever fish (https://commons.wikimedia.org).

Patients who apply to the emergency department with severe pain suspected of toxin exposure at sea should first have their vital signs evaluated. Patients with deterioration in their vital signs should be followed closely with cardiac monitoring, and attention should be paid to the possibility of respiratory depression. Complete blood count and biochemical tests should be studied. Patients with extremity injuries should be followed up with extremity elevation, peripheral circulation control, and a neurological examination, and care should be taken for rhabdomyolysis. Since toxins originating from sea creatures are heat sensitive, the first approach in studies is the application of hot water heated to at least >45°C, which is accepted as the first intervention to prevent the denaturation of the toxin and the continuation of toxicity. If the pain persists after a hot application, it can be repeated. Non-steroidal anti-inflammatory and, if necessary, opiate group drugs can also be used for pain control. Patients without serious injuries can be discharged from the emergency room after 4-6 hours of follow-up after bleeding, and pain control is achieved. The wound site is evaluated for foreign bodies (Noonburg and Greer, 2005).

The dominant bacteria in the marine flora are gram (-) rods (vibrio, clostridium). Infective injuries are conditions that require careful attention due to late admission and inappropriate use of antibiotics. Wound culture should be taken in late infections. 2nd generation cephalosporins or fluoroquinolones are the antibiotics that should be preferred in treatment (Noonburg and Greer, 2005).

Cephalopoda (Octopuses)

Cases of poisoning can be seen in the Indo-Pacific region. Blue octopus bites cause poisoning in people swimming or walking on the coast or in tide pools in Australia (Cavazzoni, 2008, Hirshon, 2018).

Octopus bites are rarely life-threatening, except for three blue-ringed octopus species from the genus Hapalochlaena (Walker, 1983; Flachsenberger, 1986-87).

Hapalochlaena fasciata grows up to 20 cm in length. Typically, there are dark brown bands and blue rings. They can be distinguished by the blue and black rings on their yellowish skin that change color when the animal is threatened. Its venom is effective by injection into the skin after biting people (Kizer, 1983-84; Auerbach, 1991; McGoldrick, Marx, 1992; Nimorakiotakis, Winkel, 2003).

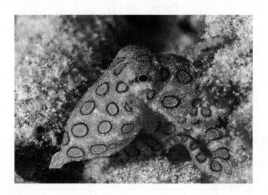

Figure 8. Blue-ringed octopus (https://www.flickr.com).

Tetrodotoxin and other chemicals (such as acetylcholine, dopamine) are found in the saliva of the blue-ringed octopus.

10-20 minutes after the bite, there are neurological symptoms such as paresthesia, muscle weakness, and respiratory arrest rather than pain. This is thought to be insignificant, as pain is not usually prominent at the time of the first bite (Lorentz et al., 2016). This tetrodotoxin, can cause death from paralysis and respiratory failure by blocking voltage-dependent fast sodium channels in peripheral nerves and preventing conduction. The effects of tetrodotoxin on the central nervous system are nausea and vomiting, miosis, diabetes insipidus, and suppression of cortical activities (Hirshon, 2018).

The prognosis is good as long as severe hypoxia does not occur in octopus poisoning. Mortality is rare. If appropriate precautions are taken, full recovery is expected. Patients should be informed that symptoms such as joint pain and effusions may continue for up to a few weeks after poisoning (Hirshon, 2018).

Although the bite of a blue-ringed octopus is usually painless, a bee sting-like reaction may occur. The bite of a blue-ringed octopus is not usually painful. Symptoms are likely to begin about 10 minutes after the bite. If severe poisoning occurs, nausea, vomiting, blurred vision, ataxia, muscle paralysis, cardiac arrest, and death may occur. Anaphylaxis and similar reactions have not been reported. Generally, a person who is bitten on one extremity has one or two lesions on the skin of the bite. It may remain as a local reaction, but there may also be a progression of edema and erythema involving the entire extremity. Paralysis may develop in patients. If respiratory arrest is not treated in a timely manner, death is possible.

Bite area irrigation should be performed and there is no evidence that local aspiration without incision is beneficial (Hirshon, 2018).

It has no anti-venom. Supportive treatment is given until the effect of the poison wears off (including endotracheal intubation and respiratory support). It is generally recommended to follow up in the intensive care unit for 4-10 hours. Recovery is usually rapid if significant hypoxia has not occurred. Although it has been shown in animal experiments that 4-Aminopyridine (non-depolarizing neuromuscular blocking agent antagonist) reverses the effects of tetrodotoxin in pharmacological treatment, there is no established therapeutic dose for use in octopus poisoning in humans (Flachsenberger, 1986-87; Hirshon, 2018; Chang et al., 1997).

Cone Snail

Most of these cone snails live in temperate and tropical oceans, especially in the Indo-Pacific regions. However, a few species are also found in cooler waters. Their poisoning has been most commonly described in divers and shell collectors (Isbister, 2004; Andresen, 1997; Norton, 2006). Poisoning may occur while walking in shallow tropical waters, swimming, or collecting for aquariums, and poisoning may develop when diver collectors come into contact with the cone snails in their collection bag (Vearrier, 2019).

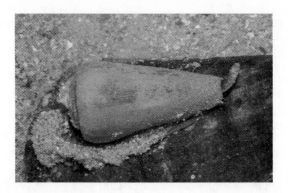

Figure 9. Cone Snail (https://www.flickr.com).

The C. geographus species is responsible for 50% of human poisonings and all reported deaths (Vearrier, 2019). Their venom is a complex protein mixture that has an overall effect on several different types of ion channels (Andresen, 1997). Numerous conotoxin peptides have been identified (Layer et al., 2004). Cone bark toxins inhibit the transmission of neuromuscular signals. C. geographus can produce the most potent toxins known, thus rapidly causing cerebral edema, coma, respiratory arrest, and heart failure. Due to this rapid effect, it is called the "smoking snail" because it gives the people it bites only as much time as it takes to smoke a cigarette. In non-fatal poisonings, symptoms may take a few weeks for recovery (Veraldi et al. 2011).

A total of 139 cases of cone snail poisoning have been documented worldwide (Kohn, 2016). Usually, stings by cone snails occur on people's fingers when held in their hands or on swimmers' feet when swimming in shallow water. Poisoning can also occur when people who collect the shells come in contact with their collection bags. The proboscis of the cone can quickly extend more than a shell length to poison its victim. The cone radula can pass through a 5 mm neoprene wet suit. Paresthesia and ischemia can be seen in the poisoned area within minutes. In severe poisonings, nausea, cephalgia, speech disorder, increased salivation, ptosis, double vision, cloudy vision, general paralysis and respiratory insufficiency may occur and develop within hours. Death occurs due to diaphragmatic paralysis or cardiac insufficiency (Kapil, 2018).

A high mortality risk is associated with C. geographus, C. textile, and C. marmoreus. After exposure, morbidity symptoms such as nausea, weakness, and double vision may occur for a few hours. It was reported that death occurred within an hour after poisoning in 33% of the 15 cases with a known post-poisoning death time. More wound care may be required to heal ulcerations developing in the poisoning area (Kohn, 2016).

The time of exposure and, if possible, the type of cone should be determined. After exposure, symptoms such as paresthesias (local, peroral or general), burning, a stinging sensation at the time of the poisoning, nausea, headache, diplopia, dysphagia, aphonia, paralysis, and respiratory arrest can be seen. In the physical examination, vital signs, and cardiopulmonary and neurological examination should be performed in detail and repeated sequentially.

Before arriving at the hospital, the necessary treatment should be done by focusing on protecting the patient's vital functions and preventing the transport of the toxin from the injection site. First, the person should be removed from the water to avoid drowning. The patient should remain still, and the limb should be held in an adequately restrained position.

Correct and careful application of the lymphatic occlusion pressure immobilization bandage may benefit. Systemic symptoms may develop within half an hour and death within an hour. Paralysis may develop in the oropharyngeal muscles. An appropriate position and support should be given to prevent aspiration. These precautions should be continued during patient transport. Applying a tourniquet to the patient's wound area or removing the toxin from the inserted area does not provide any benefit (Vearrier, 2019).

Cardiovascular and respiratory support are essential elements in the initial management of suspected cone bark poisoning for which there is no antidote in emergency care. The wound site should be adequately cleaned, and tetanus prophylaxis should be evaluated appropriately. Excision of the inserted area has no role in the treatment. The patient's wound site is contaminated, so prophylaxis with doxycycline and ceftriaxone is recommended. The extremity can be immersed in warm water for pain relief of the affected extremity. Local anesthesia without epinephrine (lidocaine) and/or oral or intravenous analgesia can be applied if the pain is not relieved. Suppose a lymphatic occlusive pressure immobilization bandage has been placed on the wound area on the extremity before arrival at the hospital. In this case, it should be removed for more than 4-6 hours to disturb the circulation in the distal bandage. Do not remove this tourniquet until you prepare for situations that may occur with the dispersion of conotoxins (Vearrier, 2019).

Priority should be given to the airway, and it should be considered that a mechanical ventilator may be required longer than 24 hours. There are case reports that edrophonium 10 mg IV can be used as an empirical treatment for stroke. If a 2 mg test dose of edrophonium is of benefit, an additional 8 mg dose should be administered. In an adverse reaction to edrophonium, naloxone may help treat severe hypotension. Central venous access should be considered for fluid resuscitation in severe poisoning cases. Seizures secondary to hypoxia may occur. In mild cases of poisoning, the patient can be discharged if they have recovered within 6-8 hours (Vearrier, 2019).

Jellyfish

Jellyfish are members of the phylum Cnidaria. An invertebrate swims in brackish and brackish water, with a central bowl and long, easily detachable tentacles. Jellyfish prey by injecting venomous nematocysts. Nematocytes found in jellyfish tentacles are rapidly discharged upon touch.

Jellyfish do not actively move and attack people. Because it is not often seen in the water, after skin contact, jellyfish nematocysts inject a mixture of proteinaceous toxins into the skin of victims, leaving a hollow barbed tube (Jouiaei et al., 2015; Wilcox et al., 2017). The poison passes into the systemic circulation. Jellyfish can cause local and systemic symptoms, depending on the type (Piontek et al. 2020). Jellyfish venom includes cytolytic toxins, neurotoxins that affect various ion channels, and non-protein bioactive components (Cegolon et al., 2013; Wilcox et al., 2017).

Although local effects of pain, redness, and swelling of the skin are generally seen in jellyfish poisonings, serious and life-threatening systemic effects may occur when the tentacles touch a large surface area of the skin (for example, the whole trunk or extremity) or stings of certain jellyfish species (Vimpani et al., 1988).

Dangerous Jellyfish Species

- *Chironex fleckeri*: Found in tropical Australia and the Indo-Pacific regions (O'Reilly et al. 2001; Ramasamy et al. 2004). The tentacles of this jellyfish are covered with venom-containing nematocysts. It can cause cardiac arrest, cardiogenic shock, and dermonecrotic damage in humans (Ramasamy et al., 2003; Huynh TT et al., 2003).
- *Carukia barnesi*: It is a box jellyfish found in the northern regions of Australia. It is one of the species that cause the Irukandji syndrome. Other jellyfish species that can cause this syndrome are Carybdea, Malo, Alatina, Gerongia, and Morbakka. This syndrome is characterized by a delayed onset of generalized back and abdominal pain that can last up to one hour after the complaint of pain. This is often accompanied by nausea, vomiting, sweating, tachycardia, and severe hypertension similar to sympathomimetic toxicity, most likely due to the release of endogenous catecholamines. In severe cases, cardiomyopathy with pulmonary edema and cardiogenic shock has been reported (Macrokanis et al., 2004; Little et al., 2006; Grady, Burnett, 2003).
- *Physalia physalis*: Earth is a common Hydrozoa (not a true jellyfish). Also known as Portuguese man of war, the man of war of the Pacific, or bluebottle; and has a blue or purplish, boat-like pneumatophore (bell-equivalent) up to 25 cm long and has multiple tentacles up to 30 m long on the back (Vimpani et al., 1988). Physalia forms colonies. They are large (Portuguese man of war) in the Atlantic and smaller (bluebottle jellyfish) in the Pacific. Poisoning by *P. fizalis* usually has local effects consisting of moderate to severe pain and skin lesions with erythema or necrosis. However, systemic symptoms such as vomiting, abdominal pain, muscle spasms, headache, syncope, confusion, dyspnea, and chest pain rarely develop (Vimpani et al., 1988). However, death due to respiratory arrest has been defined (Boulware, 2006).

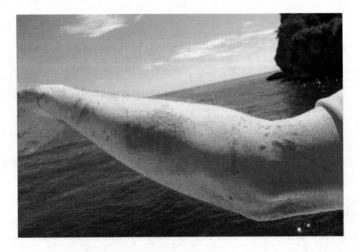

Figure 10. Jellyfish skin lesion (https://www.flickr.com).

The clinical presentation of a patient with a jellyfish sting depends on the type of jellyfish, the patient's characteristics, the exposure time, the skin area exposed, and the type of treatment administered at the time of exposure. Most jellyfish cause local symptoms. (Vimpani et al., 1988). However, jellyfish stings of certain species can rarely cause severe pain, systemic symptoms, and even death.

People usually don't see the jellyfish or tentacles, but feel the pain right away. Urticarial lesions usually appear within a few minutes. The lesions are usually burning and itching. Pain may radiate from the extremity to the whole body. Skin manifestations include tentacle scars, ecchymosis and vesicles (Kain, 1999). Skin necrosis can be seen with severe stings, including stings by *C. Fleckeri* and *P. physalis*. The papular urticaria rash may recur after 7-14 days and be intensely itchy. Lesions usually heal within ten days, but sometimes it can take weeks (Lippmann et al. 2011).

Irukandji Syndrome

It typically begins with a mild to moderately painful local stinging sensation, followed within minutes to an hour by severe generalized back, chest, and abdominal pain, vomiting, sweating, agitation, severe hypertension, and tachycardia (Macrokanis et al., 2004; Little et al., 2006; Little et al., 2003).

Patients may develop myocardial damage and pulmonary edema a few hours after stings. Fatal intracranial hemorrhage due to severe hypertension has also been reported (Currie et al., 2005).

Cases of box jellyfish (e.g., *C. fleckeri*) stings have been reported in Australia and the Indo-Pacific region (Bailey et al., 2003). *C. fleckeri* (Australian box jellyfish) tentacles can cause immediate cardiac arrest or severe shock if they contact a large area of skin (Bengtson et al., 1991).

Although rare, death has also been reported following stings by *P. physalis* (Portuguese man of war) due to respiratory arrest (Boulware, 2006; Kain, 1999; Bengtson et al., 1991). Anaphylaxis rarely occurs after a jellyfish sting (Pereira et al., 2018).

When the eyes are affected, it causes burning pain, photophobia, keratitis, corneal edema, endothelial cell swelling, and anterior chamber inflammation. These usually disappear within two days.

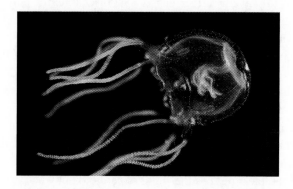

Figure 11. Box jellyfish (https://www.flickr.com).

In most cases, the diagnosis of a jellyfish sting is clinical. For many patients, the specific species of stinging jellyfish is unclear, and management is based on known common species in the area. Clues such as knowing the common jellyfish species found in that geographical area and knowing the characteristics of the tentacle pattern on the skin can be used to identify the jellyfish species. In particular, the *C. fleckeri* tentacles give the insertion site a characteristic "icy ladder" appearance. When a definitive diagnosis is needed, nematocysts can be examined under the microscope and compared to known nematocysts from various jellyfish. The nematocysts can be obtained from skin scrapings or by applying adhesive tape to the sting site (Vimpani et al., 1988; Yu Yao et al., 2016). Skin scraping is the preferred method for removing nematocysts but it is somewhat painful. The skin is scraped over the sting site to collect any remaining nematocysts and then placed in 1-4% formalin. Applying adhesive tape to the sting is suitable for tentacle stings and causes less pain. Adhesive tape is placed over the area and then pulled to remove nematocysts. The tape is then applied to a microscope slide (Ramasamy et al., 2004; Australian Resuscitation Council, 2018).

Pre-hospital health personnel should take the necessary precautions to protect themselves and ensure the patient's decontamination. Wet clothing and protective clothing with gloves are ideal for this. It is not recommended to catch jellyfish in order to recognize the species (Greene, 2017).

Steps to be taken for patient decontamination (Greene, 2017):

- Inactivation of nematocytes: Applying vinegar or 4-6% acetic acid solution is first recommended. Pour vinegar over the sticking tentacles for at least 30 seconds. Especially in *C. barnesi* and physalia poisonings, applying hot water (42-45°C) for twenty minutes effectively reduces pain. Ethyl alcohol, methyl alcohol, or urine should not be used for this.
- After applying vinegar, the tentacles can be safely removed using a glove or with a tool such as forceps.

The severity of the injury determines the treatment. Emergency care should focus on treating life-threatening poisonings (occurring primarily in Australia and the Indo-Pacific region), ensuring that appropriate first aid is given, and pain control. Respiratory and cardiovascular support may be required if severe systemic symptoms are present. Neutralize and remove tentacles as directed in pre-hospital care. If not yet done, the patient should also take first aid measures to prevent further nematocyst discharge, including irrigating the sting site with vinegar, removing the tentacles, and applying cold packs or ice in a dry plastic bag for pain. Management of anaphylaxis includes reducing airway mucosal edema, additional oxygen, volume resuscitation, and adrenaline. Wound care is critical because both freshwater and saltwater contain many microorganisms. Cultures for both aerobes and anaerobes should be obtained from infected wounds. Prophylactic antibiotics usage is not recommended. Tetanus immunization should be administered if needed. Local anesthetics and corticosteroids can be useful choices for pain management. Ice application can be effective for pain relief after applying 5% acetic acid (vinegar). Recurrent and delayed urticarial reactions may occur after 30 days at the wound area, which can be managed with steroids (Greene, 2017).

For patients with cardiac arrest or other signs of cardiotoxicity occurring several times after being stung by *C. fleckeri* (Australian box jellyfish), a specific sheep serum anti-venom is recommended (Bengtson et al., 1991). For anti-venom to be effective, it must be administered quickly (ideally within one hour of the sting). The physician should administer one vial (20,000 units) intravenously over 5-10 minutes as an initial dose. For adults and children in cardiogenic shock or cardiac arrest, dosing may be repeated up to a maximum of three vials in 5 to 20 minutes after the contact (Li et al., 2013).

Treatment of Irukandji Syndrome

There is no available antidote. Emphasizing airway, breathing, and circulation is the main goal of treatment. Nitroglycerin and phentolamine may be used for anti-hypertensive treatment. Benzodiazepines can alleviate adrenergic toxicity and anxiety. Magnesium is recommended for pain relief (Greene, 2017).

Delayed hypersensitivity reactions are common after *C. fleckeri* stings. In case reports, patients who did not resolve spontaneously benefited from oral antihistamines and topical corticosteroids (Ramasamy et al., 2004).

Prevention of jellyfish stings is best accomplished by wearing a wetsuit or other protective clothing. Sunscreen lotions containing jellyfish sting inhibitors have been shown to reduce the risk of sting injuries by 82% (Bailey et al., 2003).

Poisoning with Echinodermata

Echinoderms do not cause a significant public health problem. Toxic ones are found mostly in the Indo-Pacific reefs. Starfish poisoning is rare and the most common course is contact with the crown of thorns starfish (Acanthaster planci). Sea urchins, which are poisonous, are concentrated in tropical and subtropical marine regions (Gallagher, 2017).

Phylum Echinodermata. This includes brittle stars (class Ophiuroidea), starfish (class Asteroidea), sea urchins (class Echinoidea), and sea cucumbers (class Holothuroidea). They were named Echinodermata, which means prickly skin, because of the spines that cover the outside of the skeleton. Swimmers, divers, and fishers are at risk (Kapil, 2018).

Most echinoids have spines and venom that can cause injury, but few cause toxic injuries to humans (Williamson et al., 1996; Marsh et al., 1986).

Brittle stars (class *Ophiroidea*) do not usually cause injury, but the crown of thorns starfish (*Acanthaster planci*) is responsible for most human injuries. They have spiny protrusions that are extremely sharp and long. These protrusions are covered with three layers containing the glandular structures that produce the toxins. When broken during their penetration, toxins are released with local and systemic effects in humans.

Sea urchins (*Echinoidea*) use their unique spines and pedicellaria (a sensitive catching structure equipped with pincer-like jaws) to inject the venom. In poisoning, the active pedicellaria leaves the body and continues venom secretion, so it must be removed from the skin quickly.

Sea cucumbers (*Holothuroidea*) are generally non-toxic. Some species may cause intense skin and ocular irritation on contact (Williamson et al., 1996; Marsh et al., 1986).

Significant local and systemic effects may occur following the poisoning of echinoderms from any of the three poisonous classes. However, no deaths directly related to them have been reported.

The crown of thorns starfish, and sea urchin species cause sudden pain after puncture wounds. In addition, chestnuts containing pedicellaria can cause severe pain at the slightest touch without any puncture. Topical exposure of venomous sea cucumbers to holothurin toxins may result in significant ocular inflammation, dermatitis, and pain (Marsh et al., 1986; Freyvogel, 1972; Edmonds, 1986).

Crown of Thorn Starfish (Acanthaster Planci)

Intoxication occurs with the penetration of the epidermis. A sudden unbearable and burning pain may occur in this area. A single injury may cause pain for hours, while multiple or intra-articular punctures may cause pain, and limitation of joint movement for weeks. No anaphylaxis or death was reported. Common complications are secondary infection due to foreign material and granuloma formation (Gallagher, 2017).

Sea Urchins

The mechanism of poisoning varies between 3 groups.

Long-spined sea urchins (*Diadema spp., Echinothrix spp.*) can cause deep penetrating injuries. Intoxication may initially be in the form of severe burning pain, localized edema, and erythema, localized at the puncture site. Systemic symptoms (such as nausea, vomiting, paresthesia) occur in the most severe cases (Gallagher, 2017).

Some short-spined sea urchins (*Asthenosoma spp., Araeosoma spp.*) have spines covered with balloon-like venom sacs that can cause a severe sting which can be effective without causing a piercing wound (Gallagher, 2017).

Poisoning may occur if there is sufficient contact with pedicellar sea urchins. The flower sea urchin (*Toxopneustes pileolus*) is the most venomous species. In contact, severe pain, paresthesias, hypotension, respiratory distress, and muscle paralysis may occur for 6-8 hours (Gallagher, 2017).

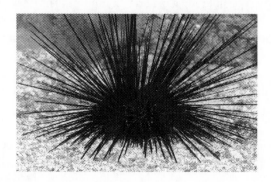

Figure 12. Sea Urchin (https://www.flickr.com).

Sea Cucumber

Poisoning occurs after contact with the body wall or by contact with the tubular organ of Cuvier located in the anus. It can cause contact dermatitis on the skin, severe ocular inflammation in the eye, and blindness (Gallagher, 2017). The severity of poisoning varies depending on the type of creature, the number of stings, and the age and underlying diseases of the victim.

After penetrating injuries, pain, erythema, edema, bleeding, ecchymosis, pruritus, chronic pain, granuloma, and secondary infections can be seen. Pain and systemic effects may occur without these local manifestations. Poisoning by the sea cucumber and some sea urchin species occurs without puncture wounds. Contact with Cuvier's venomous tentacle structures or scattered parts can cause severe dermatitis, conjunctivitis, and keratitis (Gallagher, 2017).

Systemic effects can be seen in echinoderm poisonings including vomiting, paresthesia, general weakness, respiratory distress, and delirium. The most severe echinoderm poisoning is seen due to the sting of the sea urchin flower (Toxopneustes pileolus). No mortality has been reported for the crown of thorns starfish (Acanthaster planci). Neurological disorders have been reported in two cases (Guillain-Barre syndrome and encephalitis) with long-spined black sea urchins. Anaphylaxis has not been reported in the literature. Delayed sequelae, chronic pain, and secondary infections are reported. Tetanus may develop in poisonings accompanied by penetrating wounds (Gallagher, 2017).

Recognition of severe systemic symptoms and prompt administration of vital treatments such as CPR and treatment are crucial in pre-hospital care. Pressure immobilization is recommended as an early first-aid measure in suspected severe allergic reactions such as anaphylaxis. The limb should be splinted and immobilized (Gallagher, 2017).

There is no antidote for any of the venomous echinoderms. Emergency room care includes rapid analgesia, wound management and monitoring of major systemic symptoms, and supportive treatment. After removing visible spines and sheaths, it is recommended to first immerse in hot, non-boiling water. Hot water immersion is recommended to neutralize heat-resistant toxins as an effective treatment for venomous marine spine injuries. Local anesthesia is an auxiliary analgesia method that is recommended if immersion therapy is insufficient. Additional local or regional anesthesia also allows simultaneous debridement of the wound. Parenteral analgesics can be used in cases where these are not sufficient (Gallagher, 2017).

Wound management includes the immediate removal of foreign bodies, debridement if necessary, appropriate antibiotics, and treatment for tetanus. Loose spines, spicules, and pedicels should be carefully debrided immediately to avoid further exposure to the venom.

Ultrasound or radiography can help to identify the remaining parts that may require surgical treatment. Buried spines near joints, nerves, or vessels must be surgically removed with the appropriate anesthesia. Most embedded spines are absorbed or extruded from the skin within 5-10 days. After adequate anesthesia, abundant irrigation should always be done to remove the foreign body. As in all traumatic sea injuries, the patient should be evaluated for tetanus immunization. Ocular exposure to sea cucumber (holothurin) toxins necessitates careful ophthalmological examination. Copious irrigation should be provided following topical anesthesia and prompt referral for ophthalmologic evaluation. Appropriate surgical consultation is recommended for anything close to the articular and neurovascular tissues (Gallagher, 2017).

Conclusion

All marine envenomations should be assessed in the worst scenario (anaphylaxis). We presume that patients must have a close follow-up (circulation, airway, breathing) if the source of the toxin is not clear. After bleeding control, 45°C hot water immersion (30-90 minutes) must be the first treatment for pain control and venom denaturation. Local anesthetics and nerve blocking can be the choice in pain control. Acetic acid 5% (vinegar) can be applied topically for sting decontamination. If needed, the wound must be assessed for foreign bodies (spines, teeth, coral particles) with radiography. Antibiotic prophylaxis recommended for puncture wounds should cover vibrio, staphylococcus and streptococcus (ciprofloxacin 500 mg BID or doxycycline 100 mg BID). Tetanus prophylaxis is recommended for all wounds.

References

Auerbach, P. S. (1991) Marine envenomations. *New England Journal of Medicine*, 325, 486-93.

Auerbach, P. S. (2001). *Wilderness medicine* (No. Ed. 4). Mosby Inc.

Australian Resuscitation Council. Guideline 9.4.5. (2010). *Envenomation: Jellyfish stings.* file:///C:/Users/Pc/Downloads/guideline-9-4-5-july-10.pdf.

Bailey, P. M., Little, M., Jelinek, G. A. and Wilce, JA. (2003) Jellyfish envenoming syndromes: unknown toxic mechanisms and unproven therapies. *Medical Journal of Australia*, 178, 34.

Barnett, S., Saggiomo, S., Smout, M., & Seymour, J. (2017). Heat deactivation of the stonefish Synanceia horrida venom - implications for first-aid management. *Diving and hyperbaric medicine*, 47(3), 155–158.

Bengtson, K, Nichols, M. M, Schnadig, V. And Ellis, M. D. (1991) Sudden death in a child following jellyfish envenomation by Chiropsalmus quadrumanus. Case report and autopsy findings. *The Journal of the American Medical Association*, 266, 1404.

Bilecenoğlu, M. (2012). First sighting of the Red Sea originated stonefish (Synanceia verrucosa) from Turkey. *Coral reefs*, 18(1).

Bonnet, M. S. (2000). The toxicology of Trachinus vipera: the lesser weeverfish. *British Homeopathic Journal*, 89(02), 84-88.

Borondo, J. C., Sanz, P., Nogué, S., Poncela, J. L., Garrido, P., & Valverde, J. L. (2001). Fatal weeverfish sting. *Human & experimental toxicology*, 20(2), 118-119.

Boulware, D. R. (2006) A randomized, controlled field trial for the prevention of jellyfish stings with a topical sting inhibitor. *Journal of travel medicine*, 2006, 13, 166.

Cappa G, Barcella B, Pettenazza P. Extraction procedure of a stingray spine. *Journal of Travel and Medicine* 2020 Sep 26;27(6).

Cavazzoni, E., Lister, B., Sargent, P. and Schibler. (2008) A. Blue-ringed octopus (Hapalochlaena sp.) envenomation of a 4-year-old boy: a case report. *Clinical toxicology* (Phila), 46, 760-761.

Cecil, R. L., Goldman, L. And Bennet, J. C. (Ed.). (2000). *Cecil Textbook of Medicine*, (21st ed.). WB Saunders, Philadelphia.

Cegolon, L., Heymann, W. C, Lange, J. H and Mastrangelo, G. (2013) Jellyfish stings and their management: a review. *Marine drugs*, 11, 523.

Chang, F. C. T., Spriggs, D. L., Benton,. B. J., Keller, S. A. and Capacio, B., R. (1997) 4-Aminopyridine reverses saxitoxin (STX)- and tetrodotoxin (TTX)-induced cardiorespiratory depression in chronically instrumented guinea pigs. *Fundamental and applied toxicology: official journal of the Society of Toxicology*, 38, 75-88.

Church J. E., Hodgson W. C. Dose-dependent cardiovascular and neuromuscular effects of stone fish venom. *Toxicon* 2000a; 38: 391.

Cohen, A. S., & Olek, A. J. (1989). An extract of lionfish (Pterois volitans) spine tissue contains acetylcholine and a toxin that affects neuromuscular transmission. *Toxicon*, 27(12), 1367-1376.

Cooper, N. K. Stonefish and stingrays: Some notes on the in- 28 juries they cause man. *Journal of the Royal Army Medical Corps* 1991; 137, 136- 140.

Currie, B. J. and Jacups, S. P. (2005) Prospective study of Chironex fleckeri and other box jellyfish stings in the "Top End" of Australia's Northern Territory. *Medical Journal of Australia*, 183, 631.

De Donno, A., Idolo, A. and Bagordo, F. (2009) Epidemiology of jellyfish stings reported to summer health centres in the Salento peninsula (Italy). *Contact Dermatitis*, 60,330.

Dehaan, A., Ben-Meir, P., & Sagi, A. (1991). A "scorpion fish" (Trachinus vipera) sting: fishermen's hazard. *Occupational and Environmental Medicine*, 48(10), 718-720.

Edmonds, C. (Ed.). (1989). *Dangerous Marine Creatures*. (1st ed) Reed Books Pty Ltd, Frenchs Forest, Australia.

Farrar, J., Hotez, P. J., Junghanss, T., Kang, G., Lalloo, D., & White, N. J. (2013). *Manson's Tropical Diseases E-Book*. Elsevier health sciences.

Fegan, D. and Andresen, D. (1997) Conus geographus envenomation. *Lancet*, 349, 1672.

Fenner, P. J. and Hadok, J. C. (2002) Fatal envenomation by jellyfish causing Irukandji syndrome. *Med Medical Journal of Australia*, 177,362.

Flachsenberger, W. A. (1986) Respiratory failure and lethal hypotension due to blue-ringed octopus and tetrodotoxin envenomation observed and counteracted in animal models. *J Toxicol Clin Toxicol*, 24, 485-502.

Freyvogel, T. A. (1972) Poisonous and venomous animals in East Africa. *Acta tropica*, 29, 401-451

Gallagher, S. A. and VanDeVoort, J. T. (2017, July). Echinoderm Envenomation. *Medscape* https:// emedicine.medscape.com/article/770053-overview.

Gorman, L. M., Judge, S. J., Fezai, M., Jemaà, M., Harris, J. B., & Caldwell, G. S. (2020). The venoms of the lesser (Echiichthys vipera) and greater (Trachinus draco) weever fish–A review. *Toxicon: X*, 6, 100025.

Grady, J. D. and Burnett, J. W. (2003) Irukandji-like syndrome in South Florida divers. *Annals of emergency medicine*, 42, 763.

Greene, S. (2017, April). Cnidaria envenomation differential diagnoses. *Medscape* https://emedicine. medscape.com/article/769538-overview.

Haddad V, Lupi O, Lonza JP, Tyring SK. Tropical dermatology: marine and aquatic dermatology. *Journal of the American Academy of Dermatology*. 2009 Nov;61(5): 733-50; quiz 751-2.)

Hirshon, JM., (2018, June). Octopus envenomation treatment & management. *Medscape* https://emedicine. medscape. com/article/771002.

Huynh, T.T, Seymour, J., Pereira, P., Mulcahy, R., Pereira P., Mulcahy R... (2003) Severity of Irukandji syndrome and nematocyst identification from skin scrapings. *Medical Journal of Australia*, 178, 38.

Isbister, G.K. (2004) Marine envenomation and poisoning. Dart RC (Ed), In: *Medical Toxicology*, (1621) 3rd ed, Lippincott Williams & Wilkins, Philadelphia.

Jouiaei, M., Yanagihara, A. A, Madio, B., Nevalainen, T. J., Alewood, P. F. and Fry, B. F. (2015) Ancient Venom Systems: A Review on Cnidaria Toxins. *Toxins* (Basel), 7, 2251.

Kain, K. C. Skin lesions in returned travelers. (1999) *The Medical clinics of North America*, 83,1077.

Kapil, S., Hendriksen, S. and Cooper, J. S. *Cone Snail Toxicity*. (2021 July). Stat Pearls Publishing. https://www.ncbi.nlm.nih.gov/books/NBK470586/.

Kaufman, M. B. (1992) Portuguese man-of-war envenomation. *Pediatric emergency care*, 8, 27.

Kizer, K. W. (1983) Marine envenomations. *Journal of toxicology. Clinical toxicology*, 21,527-55.

Kohn, A. J. (2016) Human injuries and fatalities due to venomous marine snails of the family Conidae. *International journal of clinical pharmacology and therapeutics*, 54, 524-38.

Khoo, H. E. (2002). Bioactive proteins from stonefish venom. *Clinical and experimental pharmacology and physiology*, 29(9), 802-806.

Layer, R. T., Wagstaff, J. D. and White, H. S. (2004) Conantokins: peptide antagonists of NMDA receptors. *Current medicinal chemistry*, 11, 3073-3084.

Li, L., McGee, R. G., Isbister, G. and Webster, A. C. (2013) Interventions for the symptoms and signs resulting from jellyfish stings. *Cochrane Database Syst Rev*, 12, CD009688.

Lippmann, J. M., Fenner, P. J., Winkel, K. and Gershwin, L. A. (2011) Fatal and severe box jellyfish stings, inceldin Irukandji stings, in Malaysia, 2000-2010. *Journal of travel medicine*, 18, 275.

Little, M., Pereira, P., Carrette, T. and Seymour, J. (2006) Jellyfish responsible for Irukandji syndrome. *QJM*, 99, 425.

Little, M., Pereira, P., Mulcahy, R., Cullen, P., Carrette, T. and Seymour., J. (2003) Severe cardiac failure associated with presumed jellyfish sting. Irukandji syndrome? *Anaesth Intensive Care*, 31, 642.

Lorentz, M. N., Stokes, A. N., Rößler, D. C. and Lötters, S. (2016) Tetrodotoxin. *Curr Biol*, 26, 870-872.

Loten, C., Stokes, B., Worsley, D., Seymour J. E., Jiang, S. and Isbister G. K. (2006) A randomised controlled trial of hot water (45 degrees C) immersion versus ice packs for pain relief in bluebottle stings. *Medical Journal of Australia*, 184, 329.

Macrokanis., C. J., Hall, N. L. and Mein, J. K. (2004) Irukandji syndrome in northern Western Australia: an emerging health problem. *Medical Journal of Australia*, 181, 699.

Marsh, L., Slack-Smith, S. and Gurry, D. L. (Ed.) (1986) *Sea Stingers and Other Venomous and Poisonous Marine Invertebrates of Western Australia* (1st ed.) Published by Western Australian Museum Perth, W. A.

McGoldrick, J. and Marx, J. A. (1992) Marine envenomations. Part 2: Invertebrates. *The Journal of emergency medicine*, 10, 71-77.

Masson, A.; Ormonde do Carmo, P.; Carvalho, J. Rhabdomyolysis secondary to an accident with marine stingray (Dasyatis family). *Journal of Venomous Animals and Toxins including Tropical Diseases* 2012, 18, 344–348.

Nimorakiotakis, B. and Winkel, K. D. (2003) Marine envenomations. Part 2-Other marine envenomations. *Australian family physician*, 32, 975-979.

Noonburg, Greer E. MD Management of Extremity Trauma and Related Infections Occurring in the Aquatic Environment, *Journal of the American Academy of Orthopaedic Surgeons*: July 2005 - Volume 13 - Issue 4 - p 243-253.

Norton, R. S. (2006) Olivera BM. Conotoxins down under. *Toxicon*, 2006, 48,780.

O'Reilly, G. M., Isbister, G. K., Lawrie, P. M., Treston G. T. and Currie, B. J. (2001) Prospective study of jellyfish stings from tropical Australia, including the major box jellyfish Chironex fleckeri. *Medical Journal of Australia*, 175, 652.

Pedroso C. M., Jared, C., Charvet-Almeida, P., Almeida, M. P., Neto, D. G., Lira, M. S., ... & Antoniazzi, M. M. (2007). Morphological characterization of the venom secretory epidermal cells in the stinger of marine and freshwater stingrays. *Toxicon*, 50(5), 688-697.

Pereira, J. C. C., Szpilman, D. and Haddad, J. V. (2018) Anaphylactic reaction/angioedema associated with jellyfish sting. *Revista da Sociedade Brasileira de Medicina Tropical*, 51, 115.

Piontek, M., Seymour, J. E., Wong, Y., Gilstrom, T., Potriquet, J. and Jennings, E. (2020) The pathology of Chironex fleckeri venom and known biological mechanisms. *Toxicon* X, 6, 100026.

Ramasamy, S., Isbister, G. K., Seymour, J. E. and Hodgson, W. C. (2004) The in vivo cardiovascular effects of box jellyfish Chironex fleckeri venom in rats: efficacy of pre-treatment with anti-venom, verapamil and magnesium sulphate. *Toxicon*, 43, 685.

Ramasamy, S., Isbister, G. K., Seymour, J. E. and Hodgson, W. C. (2003) The in vitro effects of two chirodropid (Chironex fleckeri and Chiropsalmus sp.) venoms: efficacy of box jellyfish anti-venom. *Toxicon*, 41, 703.

Rensch, G., & Murphy-Lavoie, H. M. (2021). Lionfish, Scorpionfish, And Stonefish Toxicity. *StatPearls* [Internet].

Sauviat, M. P., Garnier, P., Goudey-Perriere, F., & Perriere, C. (1995). Does crude venom of the stonefish (Synanceia verrucosa) activate β-adrenoceptors in the frog heart muscle?. *Toxicon*, 33(9), 1207-1213.

Smith, W. L., & Wheeler, W. C. (2006). Venom evolution widespread in fishes: a phylogenetic road map for the bioprospecting of piscine venoms. *Journal of Heredity*, 97(3), 206-217.

Taylor KS, Zoltan TB, Achar SA. Medical illnesses and injuries encountered during surfing. *Curr Sports Med Rep* 2006; 5:262.

Vearrier, D. (2019, March). Conidae. *Medscape* https://emedicine.medscape.com/ article/769638.

Veraldi, S., Violetti, S. A. and Serini, S. M. (2011) Cutaneous abscess after Conus textile sting. *Journal of travel medicine*, 18, 210-211.

Vimpani, G., Doudle, M. and Harris, R. (1988) Child accident-mortality in the Northern Territory, 1978-1985. *Medical Journal of Australia*, 148, 392.

Walker, D. G. (1983) Survival after severe envenomation by the blue-ringed octopus (Hapalochlaena maculosa). *Med J Aust*, 2, 663-665.

Williamson, J. A, Fenner, P. J and Burnett, J. W. (Ed.). (1996) *Venomous and Poisonous Marine Animals: Medical and Biological Handbook*, (4th ed.) Sydney, Australia Univ. of New South Wales Press.

Wilcox, C. L., Headlam, J. L, Doyle, T. K. and Yanagihara, A. A. (2017) Assessing the Efficacy of First-Aid Measures in Physalia sp. Envenomation, Using Solution- and Blood Agarose-Based Models. *Toxins* (Basel), 9, 149.

Ziegman, R., & Alewood, P. (2015). Bioactive components in fish venoms. *Toxins*, 7(5), 1497-1531.

Chapter 12

Hymenoptera Stings

Ahmet Baydın*, MD and Utku Türker, MD

Department of Emergency Medicine, Ondokuz Mayıs University Samsun, Samsun, Turkey

Abstract

Hymenoptera stings are an allergic reaction that is clinically simple, moderate, or life-threatening, often seen in summer and autumn. While mostly non-life-threatening local reactions are observed in the cases, large local lesions, systemic involvement, or anaphylaxis may also be seen, depending on the patient's immunoglobulin E response. Detailed history and physical examination are of great importance for diagnosis since the clinical picture is so variable in post-injection cases, and there is no specific laboratory or imaging method for diagnosis. While uncomplicated local lesions are usually treated with cold application, analgesics, steroids, and antihistamines are used to treat large local lesions. If anaphylaxis is present, adrenaline should also be used in the treatment.

Keywords: Hymenoptera stings, insect stings, sting management, environmental emergencies

Introduction

Hymenoptera stings are a medically important condition that is more common in late summer and early autumn and can cause severe body reactions (Dongol et al., 2013). When we search the literature, we see that many cases suffer from Hymenoptera stings. There are three clinically important Hymenoptera subgroups: Apidae, Vespidae, and Formicidae. In the subgroup Apidae, there are honeybees and wasps; in the subgroup Vespidae wasps and yellow jackets; and in the subgroup Formicidae (wingless Hymenoptera), there are ants (fire ants, harvester ants, bulldog ants, jack jumper ants) (Sainiet al., 2014). A small amount of poison that enters the body with the sting of the Hymenoptera causes an allergic reaction within a few seconds. This allergic reaction after a Hymenoptera sting can be attributed to a local reaction related to the sting site (redness and painful swelling at the sting site, Figure 1), and may cause systemic reaction unrelated to the sting (itching, erythema, urticaria, Figure 2) or anaphylaxis (Visscher et al., 1996). While most people experience only minor local reactions at the bite site after a

---

* Corresponding Author's Email: ahmetbaydn@yahoo.com.

In: Environmental Emergencies and Injuries in Nature
Editors: Murat Yücel, Murat Güzel and İbrahim İkizceli
ISBN: 978-1-68507-833-1

Hymenoptera sting, more serious clinical manifestations such as acute encephalomyelitis, acute ischemic stroke, rhabdomyolysis, acute renal failure, acute myocardial infarction, serum sickness, and anaphylaxis are observed in venom-allergic patients, and even death can be seen (Bilio, 2011; Boz et al., 2003; Guzel et al., 2016; Constantino et al., 2020; da SilvaJunior et al., 2016; Aminiahidashtiet al., 2016).

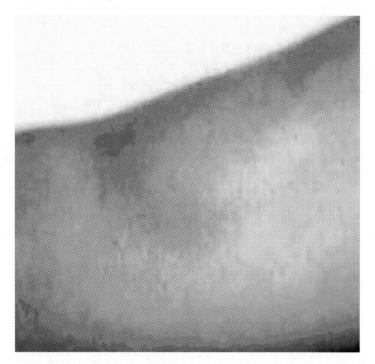

Figure 1. Local reaction associated with the sting.

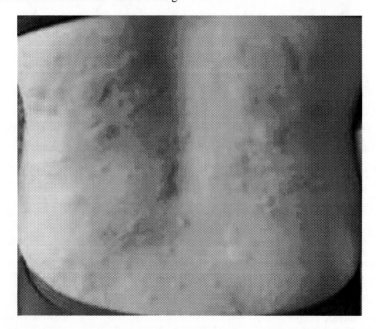

Figure 2. Systemic reaction unrelated to the insertion site.

It has been reported that cases developing a local reaction to Hymenoptera stings generally showed the same reaction in subsequent stings (Mauriello et al., 1984). In approximately 10% of cases that develop a local reaction after a Hymenoptera sting, swelling and redness may increase within 48 hours. It may take 5-10 days for this situation to return to normal (Severino et al., 2009; Golden et al., 2017). There is also a risk of developing a systemic allergic reaction after a local reaction in the inserted cases, and this risk is around 7% (Freeman, 2004). A secondary bacterial infection should be suspected if there is an increase in redness, swelling, and pain on the fifth day after the bite. This clinical picture is accompanied by fever. Cases stung by yellow jackets and fire ants have been reported to be more likely to become infected than cases stung by other species (Reisman, 2003). Since there are no reports in the literature of tetanus infection following Hymenoptera stings, we can consider these stings as "clean wounds" as long as there is no soil-contaminated injury. Therefore, tetanus vaccination is not necessary unless contamination occurs in Hymenoptera stings. Hymenoptera stinging humans is usually either for self-defense or to protect their nests. It is tough to identify the winged Hymenoptera species responsible for the sting since the local lesions on the skin after the stings of Hymenoptera are very similar in appearance.

Pathophysiology

The content of the poison in the secretion of Hymenoptera may vary depending on the development and living conditions of the insect (Przybilla and Rueff,2010). The venom of Hymenoptera generally consists of protein and peptide low molecular weight allergens and pharmacologically active compounds.

Phospholipase A2 and hyaluronidase, responsible for most systemic allergic reactions, are in a protein structure, while melittin, which causes anaphylaxis through the degranulation of basophils and mast cells, is in a peptide structure. At the same time, melittin is the most abundant substance in the poison composition. Peptides and phospholipases are responsible for the cytotoxic and neurotoxic effects, while biogenic amines and hyaluronidase are responsible for spreading the disease (Przybilla and Rueff, 2010). Allergens and active compounds found in subgroups of Hymenoptera are shown in Table 1.

Table 1. Composition of Hymenoptera Venom (Hahn 2015)

Apidae	Vespidae	Formicidae
Biogenic amines	Biogenic amines	Biogenic amines
Phospholipase A	Phospholipase A	Phospholipase A
Phospholipase B	Phospholipase B	Hyaluronidase
Hyaluronidase	Hyaluronidase	Piperidines
Acidphosphatase	Acidphosphatase	
Minimine	Kinin	
Mellitin	Mast cell degranulating peptide	
Apamin		
Mast cell degranulating peptide		

The venom found in fire ants acts differently from that of other Hymenoptera. The venom in fire ants inhibits sodium and potassium-dependent adenosine triphosphatase, reducing mitochondrial respiration and thus disrupting oxidative phosphorylation. As a result, neutrophil and platelet functions are impaired (Hahn, 2019).

Anaphylaxis, the most severe allergic reaction that may develop in 0.3-3% of cases after a Hymenoptera sting, typically occurs through immunoglobulin E and affects more than one system (Sampson et al., 2006; Graif et al., 2006). Although complaints of skin involvement are common in anaphylaxis, respiratory or circulatory system symptoms may be prominent. Hypotension, one of the complaints of the circulatory system, can be seen without any skin findings and may threaten the patient's life (Stoevesandt et al., 2012).

Clinical Findings

After the sting of the Hymenoptera, the patient knows that he has been stung because of the sudden pain and redness in the sting area. The severity of the allergic reaction in the inserted case; The type of insect that bites determines factors such as advanced age, pre-existing comorbid diseases, less severe systemic reactions to previous bites, mast cell diseases, and high basal tryptase concentration in serum (Bilio, 2011).

While local reactions are frequently observed in cases after Hymenoptera stings (uncomplicated local reaction and large local reaction), it should not be forgotten that anaphylaxis can also be seen. In uncomplicated local reactions, redness and a 1-5 centimeter in diameter painful swelling develop in the injected area, and this clinical picture regresses within a few hours.

Sometimes it may take several days for the painful swelling to resolve. Regardless of the lesion type, the location of the lesion is also essential; that is, if the insertionoccurred from the oropharynx, edema developing as a local reaction will narrow the airway, threatening the patient's life even if there is no anaphylactic reaction.

Large local reactions after the Hymenoptera sting are described as painful swelling, usually exceeding 10 centimeters in diameter, lasting longer than 24 hours, sometimes accompanied by erythema, itching, and blisters. The incidence of large local reactions after the Hymenoptera sting ranges from 2.4% to 26.4% (Bilioand Bonifazi, 2009). The swelling after the insertion gradually enlarges and reaches its peak on the second day, and returns to normal within 5-10 days. In the meantime, since compartment syndrome may develop in a patient inserted from the extremity and having a large local reaction, the physical examination of the physician evaluating the patient in terms of differential diagnosis gains importance here. Since the course of the lesions is known in large local reactions, a secondary bacterial infection should be suspected if the clinical picture worsens and fever accompanies this clinical picture in the period when we expect regression (Sampson et al., 2006). In 7% of cases that develop a significant local reaction after the insertion, there is a risk of developing a systemic allergic reaction; in other words, a widespread cutaneous reaction (Tang et al., 2009). What is meant by a systemic allergic reaction; the patient has generalized urticaria, erythema, pruritus, and/or angioedema, regardless of the insertion site, and has no symptoms other than the skin. The diagnosis of systemic allergic reaction is made when the clinic is unrelated to the lesion site, and the diagnostic criteria for anaphylaxis are not met.

Another clinical picture that can be seen after a Hymenoptera sting is anaphylaxis that develops suddenly and progresses rapidly, and threatens life. It should also be kept in mind that many different symptoms and complaints can be found in cases with anaphylaxis who apply to the emergency department after a Hymenoptera sting (see Table 2). The diagnosis of anaphylaxis in Hymenoptera stings is made based on the clinical findings in the cases (see Table 3). It has been reported that ten deaths due to anaphylaxis after a Hymenoptera sting are seen in the United States each year (Arif, 2018). For this reason, an accurate diagnosis is of great importance in patient management to prevent mortality. It should not be forgotten that the severity of anaphylaxis may increase with comorbid diseases present in the inserted cases, e.g., in patients with heart disease or respiratory tract disease, in the case of post-injection anaphylaxis development, the clinical picture of the case may worsen, or the symptoms of the existing diseases may be exacerbated. As a result of clinical studies, mast cell disease was observed in 2% of the cases that showed an anaphylaxis reaction after the Hymenoptera sting. It was stated that the risk of severe anaphylactic reaction was very high if these patients were later stung by the insect (Leendford, 2019; Akin et al., 2007). Therefore, mast cell diseaseshould be suspected in cases with severe anaphylactic reactions after the Hymenoptera sting. A clinical study reported that the onset of symptoms within 5 minutes of a Hymenoptera sting is a precursor of severe anaphylaxis. Therefore, it is necessary to be ready for advanced airway support at all times (Graft, 2006). Again, care should be taken in terms of biphasic reaction, which is a rare but typical feature of anaphylaxis.

Table 2. Symptoms and signs that can be seen in anaphylaxis (Freeman 2021)

Skin complaints and findings	Warmth, flushing (erythema), pruritus, urticaria, angioedema, and "goosebumps."
Oral complaints and findings	Itching, tingling of the lips, tongue, or palate Edema of lips, tongue, uvula, and metallic taste in mouth
Respiratory system complaints and findings	In the nose; Itching, congestion, runny nose, and sneezing In the larynx; Throat pruritus, dysphonia, hoarseness, stridor In the lower respiratory tract; Shortness of breath, chest tightness, cough, wheezing and cyanosis
Complaints and findings related to the gastrointestinal system	Difficulty swallowing (dysphagia), nausea, vomiting, abdominal pain and diarrhea
Complaints and findings related to the cardiovascular system	Feeling faint, dizziness, syncope, altered mental status, chest pain, palpitations, rhythm disturbances, hypotension and cardiac arrest
Neurological complaints and findings	Anxiety, seizure, headache, confusion, urinary or stool incontinence Sudden behavioral changes in young children, such as hugging, crying, getting angry, stopping playing
Eye complaints and findings	Itching, erythema, edema and conjunctival erythema around the orbit
Ear complaints and findings	Hearing difficulties
Other complaints and findings	Uterine cramps in women

Table 3. Anaphylaxis diagnostic criteria (Freeman 2021)

Criteria 1	Acute onset disease involving the skin, mucous membranes, or both, accompanied by at least one of the following: a) Difficulty in breathing (e.g., dyspnea, stridor, bronchospasm) b) Indicators of hypotension or end-organ perfusion disorder
Criteria 2	The rapid development of two or more of the following after exposure to the allergen a) Skin and mucosal tissue involvement b) Difficulty in breathing (e.g., dyspnea, stridor, bronchospasm) c) Indicators of hypotension or end-organ perfusion disorder d) Persistent gastrointestinal system signs and symptoms (such as cramp-like abdominal pain, vomiting)
Criteria 3	Detection of low blood pressure after the patient's exposure to the allergen a) Systolic blood pressure below 90 mmHg or a decrease of more than 30% of the person's normal blood pressure b) Low systolic blood pressure for age in children or a decrease of more than 30% from normal from 1 month to 1 year; < 70 mm Hg from 1 to 10 years old; < 70 mmHg + (age x 2) 11 to 17 years old; < 90 mmHg

*Meeting at least one of these criteria is sufficient for the diagnosis of anaphylaxis.

Cases should be kept under observation in the hospital for at least 24 hours to prevent possible mortality. Although the symptoms and signs of anaphylaxis are numerous, the skin and respiratory and cardiovascular systems are more commonly affected. Common skin, respiratory system, and cardiovascular system symptoms are generalized urticaria, flushing and angioedema, hoarseness, upper airway narrowing, dyspnea, wheezing, dizziness, syncope, and cardiovascular disease collapse (Golden, 2007). A clinical study reported that cardiopulmonary involvement was seen at a rate of 30% in anaphylaxis cases in the pediatric age group, and this involvement reached 90% in the adult age group (Bilio and Bonifazi, 2008). Therefore, we can say that anaphylaxis developing after a Hymenoptera sting may progress with a more serious clinical picture in adult patients than in children, and mortality may also be seen.

Although we do not have clinical experience on this subject, since fire ants are not found in our country, when we examine the clinical studies, we can say that exposure to these ants is frequently seen in people staying in nursing homes in the United States. There is a risk of aggravating comorbid conditions. Pustule-like and highly itchy lesions have been reported in local reactions caused by fire ants. It is reported that pustules are sterile lesions and therefore should not be drained to avoid secondary infection. However, excessive itching in the case may complicate this situation (deShazo et al., 1984).

Diagnosis

There is no laboratory test to diagnose Hymenoptera stings definitively. In the presence of local lesions after the sting, the history and physical examination are essential for diagnosis. Questions that will help the diagnosis, relating to the type of insect, are answered in the history: when the event occurred, when the lesions appeared, how long after was the hospital admission, and the applicant's profession. According to the characteristics of the lesion, the uncomplicated local or large local lesion can be differentiated. By looking at the progression of the lesion, it can be determined whether a secondary bacterial infection is also involved. If we suspect an intervening bacterial infection, a complete blood count, C-reactive protein level, and sedimentation level may be requested from the patient to support the diagnosis of infection. The complete blood count shows leukocytosis. There is an increase in C-reactive protein and sedimentation levels.

Although anaphylaxis diagnostic criteria are sufficient for the diagnosis of anaphylaxis (see Table 3), laboratory tests also help the diagnosis. High levels of mediators such as histamine and total tryptase in the blood of a patient with suspected anaphylaxis will support the diagnosis of anaphylaxis. The level of mediators such as histamine and tryptase in the blood rises within 15 minutes after the insertion and remains high for up to 3 hours. Therefore, if we look at the blood level of these mediators, we should look at the interval between 15 minutes and 3 hours after the insertion. Harmful blood levels of these mediators in laboratory tests do not exclude the diagnosis of anaphylaxis (Schwartz et al.,1989). In the laboratory examination of cases stung by Hymenoptera; anemia, thrombocytopenia, an increase in serum creatine kinase level, elevation in liver enzymes (AST, ALT), and an increase in creatinine can be observed. In a urine examination; decreased urine density, proteinuria, myoglobinuria, hemoglobinuria, hematuria, and leukocyturia may be seen (Broideset al., 2010).

Treatment

Hymenoptera stings can cause the sting patient simple injuries or life-threatening injuries requiring advanced life support. Since we do not have a specific antidote against the poison of Hymenoptera, the treatment is arranged as supportive treatment entirely according to the patient's clinical findings. There is no need to apply drugs such as antihistamines, steroids, and adrenaline to treat every allergic reaction after a Hymenoptera sting.

The first approach to treatment in local reactions developing after the sting should be a cold application to reduce swelling and itching in the lesion area. In the meantime, since keeping the wound site clean is essential in preventing secondary bacterial infections that may develop, it is necessary to pay attention to the cleanliness of the wound site. After the cold application, the needle should be removed from the skin to prevent further exposure to the poison. Suppose a cold application is insufficient to relieve pain and itching in cases withlocal reactions. In that case, a non-steroidal anti-inflammatory agent can ease pain, and an H1 receptor blocker antihistamine agent (cetirizine, diphenhydramine, and pheniramine) can be used to relieve pain-relief itching. The presence of a comorbid condition such as uncontrolled diabetes mellitus, cardiovascular diseases, respiratory diseases, peripheral venous insufficiency, chronic renal failure, liver failure, immunotherapy, and advanced age in the inserted cases predisposes to cutaneous infections, leading to the development of a secondary bacterial infection and may further complicate the lesion (Poziomkowska-Gesicka I et al., 2021). Therefore, prophylactic antibiotic treatment can be applied in cases with the comorbid disease. The drugs to be preferred for prophylactic antibiotic therapy should be ampicillin-sulbactam or amoxicillin-clavulanate. Large local reactions should be treated to improve the patient's quality of life.

For insignificant local reactions, 1 mg/kg intravenous methylprednisolone should be given with supportive therapy to reduce the inflammatory response and improve symptoms. Intravenous antihistamines can also relieve itching at or around the lesion.

Since the development of anaphylaxis in Hymenoptera stings can threaten the life of cases, the treatment approach is important. The patient suspected of anaphylaxis should be immediately monitored and evaluated regarding vital signs (blood pressure, pulse rate, respiratory rate, oxygen saturation). At the same time, at least two vascular accesses should be established to apply the treatments in these cases. In cases with anaphylaxis reactions, life-threatening airway obstruction should be prevented. Suppose the patient cannot maintain the airway patency, cannot provide oxygenation due to anaphylaxis, and the airway patency is gradually closing due to edema. In that case, permanent airway patency should be provided by endotracheal intubation. Sometimes, edema in the upper respiratory tract can make endotracheal intubation impossible. Therefore, in cases where endotracheal intubation cannot be performed, emergency cricothyrotomy may be required to ensure airway patency. Once the airway is opened, the patient should be given oxygen therapy at a rate of 8-10 liters per minute. In cases where bronchospasm has developed, administration of intramuscular adrenaline (0.5 mg of adrenaline 1:1000 from the outer thigh or deltoid muscle) and concomitant administration of the β2 agonist salbutamol by inhalation will treat bronchospasm. If the clinician sees that the bronchospasm does not improve after the administration of adrenaline and salbutamol, this treatment may be repeated. In cases with anaphylaxis, after the airway is established, the circulatory system, which is impaired due to anaphylaxis, should be supported. A bolus of fluid should be given intravenously to supportthe circulatory system. Since there is no specific fluid preferred for fluid replacement in anaphylaxis, isotonic serum physiology (0.9% NaCl) may be preferred for replacement in these cases. Antihistamines and steroids also have a place in the treatment of anaphylaxis, but by no means are antihistamines and steroids as effective as adrenaline in preventing airway hazards, hypotension, or shock caused by anaphylaxis (Sheikh et al., 2007). Antihistamines and steroids are mostly used to relieve symptoms such as itching and edema and support the effect of adrenaline. Therefore, antihistamines and steroids should not be considered as the main treatment agents in anaphylaxis. After the first application of adrenaline, the patient's clinical picture may improve within minutes or hours. However, since there is a risk of developing a biphasic reaction, the cases should be hospitalized and followed up in a monitored manner. If symptoms persist despite multiple intramuscular administrations of adrenaline, intravenous infusion of adrenaline should be considered. When administering adrenaline intravenously, extreme care should be taken with the dose given since high doses of adrenaline itself can cause death. One milligram of 1:1000 adrenaline is placed in 1 liter of isotonic saline and given as an infusion at a rate of 0.1 µg/kg/minute (Liebermanet al., 2015). Patients whose anaphylaxis is treated and whose discharge is planned should be recommended to apply to the immunology department. Suggestions should be made for obtaining an adrenaline auto-injector and learning how to use the auto-injector to receive venom immunotherapy treatment to reduce the lifetime risk in recurrent bee stings and prepare for future stings.

Conclusion

Allergic reactions are a condition that should be treated because they affect the quality of life of the cases. Although Hymenoptera stings mainly consist of non-life-threatening local lesions, it should always be kept in mind that life-threatening anaphylaxis can also develop.

References

Akin C, Scott LM, Kocabas CN, Kushnir-Sukhov N, Brittain E, Noel P and Metcalfe DD. (2007). Demonstration of an aberrant mast-cell population with clonal markers in a subset of patients with "idiopathic" anaphylaxis. *Blood*, 110, 2331-2333.

Aminiahidashti H, Laali A, Samakoosh AK and Gorji AMH. (2016). Myocardial infarction following a beesting: A case report of Kounis syndrome. *Annals of Cardiac Anaesthesia*, 19, 375-378.

Arif F and Williams M. (2018). Hymenoptera stings. *Europe PMC*.

Bilo BM and Bonifazi F. (2008). Epidemiology of insect-venom anaphylaxis. *Curr Opin Allergy Clin Immunol*, 8, 330.

Bilo MB and Bonifazi F. (2009). The natural history and epidemiology of insect venom allergy: clinical implications. *Clin Exp Allergy*, 39, 1467-1476.

Bilio MB. (2011). Anaphylaxis caused by Hymenoptera stings: from epidemiology to treatment. *Allergy*, 66, 35-37.

Boz C, Velioglu S and Ozmenoglu M. (2003). Acute disseminated encephalomyelitis after bee sting. *Neurol Sci*, 23, 313-315.

Broides A, Maimon MS, Landau D, Press J and Lifshitz M. (2010). Multiple hymenoptera stings in children: clinical and laboratory manifestations.*Eur J Pediatr*, 169, 1227-1231.

Constantino K, Pawlukiewicz AJ and Spear L. (2020). A case report on Rhabdomyolysis after multiple bee stings. *Cureus*, 12,e9501.

da Silva Junior GB, Junior AGV, Rocha AMT, de Vasconcelos VR, de Barros Neto J, Fujishima JS, Ferreira NB, Barros EJG and de Francesco Daher E. (2017). Acute kidney injury complicating bee stings – a review. *Rev Inst Med Trop Sao Paulo*, 59, e25.

deShazo RD, Griffing C, Kwan TH, Banks WA and Dvorak HF. (1984). Dermal hypersensitivity reactions to imported fire ants. *J Allergy Clin Immunol*, 74, 841-847.

Dongol Y, Shrestha RK, Aryal G, Lakkappa DB. (2013). Hymenoptera stings and the acute kidney injury. *European Medical Journal*, 1, 68-75.

Freeman T, Golden DBK and Feldweg AM. (2021). Bee, yellow jacket, wasp, and other Hymenoptera stings: Reaction types and acute management. www.uptodate.com.

Freeman TM. (2004). Hypersensitivity to hymenoptera stings. *N Engl J Med*,351,1978-1984.

Graft DF. (2006). Insect sting allergy. *Med Clin North Am*, 90, 211-232.

Golden DBK. (2007). Insectsting anaphylaxis. *Immunol Allergy Clin North Am*, 27, 261-272.

Golden DBK, Demain J, Freeman T, Randolph C, Schuller D and Wallace D. (2017). Stinging insect hypersensitivity: A practice parameter update 2016. *Annals of Allergy Asthma Immunol*, 118, 28-54.

Graif Y, Romano-Zelekha O, Livne I, Green MS and Shohat T. (2006). Allergic reactions to insect stings: Results from a national survey of 10.000 junior high school children in Israel.*J Allergy Clin Immunol*,117, 1435-1439.

Guzel M, Akar H, Erenler AK, Baydin A and Kayabas A. (2016). Acute ischemic stroke and severe multiorgan dysfunction due to multiple bee stings. *Turkish Journal of Emergency Medicine*, 16, 126-128.

Hahn I. (2015). Goldfrak's Toxicologic Emergencies. In: *Arthropods*, 10th ed, Robert S. Hoffman, Mary Ann Howland, Neal A. Lewin, Lewis S. Nelson (eds), Mc Graw Hill, New York p. 2404.

Ledford DK. (2019). Mastocytosis with Bee Sting Anaphylaxis. *J Allergy ClinImmunol Pract*, 7, 1374-1375.

Lieberman P, Nicklas RA, Randolph C, Oppenheimer J, Bernstein D, Bernstein J, Ellis A, Golden DB, Greenberger P, Kemp S, Khan D, Ledford D, Lieberman J, Metcalfe D, Nowak-Wegrzyn A, Sicherer S,

Wallace D, Blessing-Moore J, Lang D, Portnoy JM, Schuller D, Spector S and Tilles SA. Anaphylaxis-a practice parameter update 2015. (2015). *Ann Allergy Asthma Immunol*, 115, 341-384.

Mauriello PM, Barde SH, Georgitis JW and Reisman RE. (1984). Natural history of large local reactions from stinging insects. *J Allergy Clin Immunol*, 74, 494.

Poziomkowska-Gesicka I, Kostrzewska M and Kurek M. (2021). Comorbidities and Cofactors of Anaphylaxis in Patients with Moderate to Severe Anaphylaxis. Analysis of Data from the Anaphylaxis Registry for West Pomerania Province, Poland. *Int J Environ Res Public Health*, 18, 1-17.

Przybilla B, Rueff F. (2010). Hymenoptera venom allergy. *Journal der Deutschen of Dermatology*, 8, 114-129.

Reisman RE. (2003). Clinical aspects of Hymenoptera allergy. In: *Monograph on insect allergy*, 4th ed, Levine MI, Lockey RF (Eds), Dave Lambert Associates, Pittsburgh p.55.

Saini AG, Sankhyan N, Suther R and Singhi P. (2014). Acute Axonal Polyneuropathy Following Honey-Bee Sting: A Case Report. *Journal of Child Neurology*, 29, 674-676.

Sampson HA, Munoz-Furlong A, Campbell RL, Adkinson NF, Bock SA, Branum A, Brown SGA et al. (2006). Second symposium on the definition and management of anaphylaxis: Summary report-Second National Institute of Allergy and Infectious Disease/Food Allergy and Anaphylaxis Network symposium. *J Allergy Clin Immunol*, 117, 391-397.

Schwartz LB, Yunginger JW, Miller J, Bokhari R and Dull D. (1989). Time course of appearance and disappearance of human mast cell tryptase in the circulation after anaphylaxis. *J Clin Invest*, 83, 1551-1555.

Severino M, Bonadonna P and Passalacqua G. (2009). Large local reactions from stinging insects: From epidemiology to management. *Curr Opin Allergy Clin Immunol*, 9, 334-337.

Sheikh A, Ten Broek V, Brown SG and Simons FE. (2007). H1-antihistamines for the treatment of anaphylaxis: Cochrane systematic review. *Allergy*, 62, 830-837.

Stoevesandt J, Hain J, Kerstan A and Trautmann A. (2012). Over and underestimated parameters in severe Hymenoptera venom-induced anaphylaxis: Cardiovascular medication and absence of urticaria/angioedema. *J Allergy Clin Immunol*, 130, 698-704.

Tang ML, Osborne N and Allen K. (2009). Epidemiology of anaphylaxis. *Curr Opin Allergy Clin Immunol*, 9, 351.

Visscher PK, Vetter RS and Camazine S. (1996). Removing bee stings. *Lancet*, 348, 301-302.

Chapter 13

Spider and Centipede Bites

Mehmet Cihat Demir*, MD

Department of Emergency Medicine, Düzce University, Düzce, Turkey

Abstract

Spider bites usually have minor effects on humans due to their sensitive jaws, impotent venom, or inadequate toxins. Among the clinically significant ones, widow spider bites from Latrodectus species may cause muscle spasms and rigidity with pain, while recluse spider bites from Loxosceles species are initially painless and may progress to necrotic arachnidism. Bites by armed spiders in South America and funnel-web spiders in Australia are rare but cause severe poisoning and require antivenom. Most other bites have negligible and temporary effects. Centipede bites are typical in hot climates and summer months; wound care and supportive treatment are sufficient. When a spider bite is suspected, conservative treatment such as wound cleaning, the elevation of the bitten extremity, cold compress, tetanus prophylaxis, analgesics, and antihistamines should be applied. Antibiotherapy can be administered in the case of an obvious sign of infection; if systemic symptoms and dermo-necrosis have developed, hospitalization for observation and treatment is required.

Keywords: envenomation, spider bite, latrodectus, loxosceles, centipede

Introduction

Spiders in the phylum Arthropoda are found in nearly all habitats worldwide, with over 40,000 described species. Spiders, which are carnivorous hunters, undoubtedly have a crucial role in the ecological balance. Many of them also have the feature of spreading to different regions with the wind. Apart from their natural distribution, spiders can also be distributed to other areas by passenger vehicles such as cars and planes. In addition, climate change, which can have critical ecological consequences, is another factor affecting biota distribution (Walther et al., 2009).

---

* Corresponding Author's Email: mehmetcihatdemir@duzce.edu.tr.

In: Environmental Emergencies and Injuries in Nature
Editors: Murat Yücel, Murat Güzel and İbrahim İkizceli
ISBN: 978-1-68507-833-1

The probability of encountering spiders in workplaces, at home, on the street, on vacation, on a trip, and in every part of daily life is exceptionally high. No matter how many spider species, there are only a few dozen spiders of venomous species with fangs large enough to deliver venom through human skin. In spiders, like ticks, scorpions, mites, and other arachnids, the body consists of an abdomen (posterior opisthosoma) and an integrated cephalo-thorax (anterior prosoma). In the front, there is a chelicerae chin in the form of a claw which serves to take nutrients, a pedipalp with a sensory-walking-reproductive function, and four pairs of legs. While the venom is produced in a gland in the anterior prosome and transmitted by the cheliceral fang, digestion, circulation, respiration, excretion, milk, and thread production (in spinnerets) are done in the abdomen.

Spider venom to digest their prey has neurotoxic and proteolytic properties (Atkinson & Wright, 1992). On the other hand, close to 1000 different chemicals can be found in spider venom which can be helpful in drug research to treat various diseases (Escoubas & King, 2009). Arachnoserver is a good resource for high-quality information on spider venoms (Wood et al., 2009).

Most spiders either flee or pretend to be dead if threatened, known as thanatosis. They rarely bite humans and do so only for defensive purposes by nature. For this reason, spiders should be thrown gently rather than crushed (Fusto et al., 2020). The considerable majority of spider bites are harmless to humans because their teeth are too small to pass through human skin, the amount of poison is not enough for toxicity, or its effect on human cells is negligible. Although various injury mechanisms such as skin necrosis, secondary infection, allergic reactions, and host-related factors also affect Alan's outcome (Blackman, 1995). Some of the most clinically essential spider bites will be discussed in this chapter. The bites of Latrodectus and Loxosceles species, armed spiders, hobo spiders, funnel-web spiders, tarantulas, and centipedes will be covered.

Identification, General Assessment, and Management of Spider Bites

While all spiders can bite humans, only a few make any medical sense. The term araneism or arachnidism is used for systemic effects caused by spider bites. In addition, the terms latrodectism (red-back spider, widow spider) and loxoscelism (brown-recluse spider) may also be used to describe specific spider bites. Spider venom can be helpful in the identification of spider bites as it is neurotoxic (Latrodectus spp. and Atrax spp.) or cytotoxic/necrotic (Loxoxceles spp.) (Braitberg & Segal, 2009).

Spider bites are often difficult to diagnose, especially if no spider has been seen. It is crucial that the spider is caught for determining the exact species. The diagnosis is usually made clinically and by identification of the spider. The following items are required to assist in the diagnosis of a spider bite:

- Seeing the spider right next to the bitten area,
- Catching the spider quickly in an area close to the injured site,
- Systemic arachnidism.

If none of these are present, a medical record can be entered as "possible arthropod envenomation-vector unknown," assuming that the evidence is only secondary (Russell & Gertsch, 1983). Diagnosing arachnidism without direct evidence can result in inappropriate treatments and failure to recognize a more serious underlying disease (Koh, 1998; Swanson & Vetter, 2005). At the same time, the perceived threat of spider bites among healthcare professionals and the general public far exceeds the actual risk. Of course, it should not be overlooked that most spider bite notifications are overreported (Swanson & Vetter, 2005).

In spider bite diagnosis and management, airway, breathing, and circulation (ABC) safety should always be prioritized. Vital signs should be checked. Subsequently, medical history, physical examination, and laboratory evaluation are essential to rule out alternative diagnoses. In the medical history, the moment of the bite, the environment, the activity of the bitten person at the time of the incident, the examination of the patient's clothing to cause injury, whether the skin lesion is old or new, the description of the appearance of the spider, and the travel history should be questioned in the case of a spider bite. If the spider was crushed to death, it is appropriate to present its remains to the entomologist, considering the possibility of identifying the spider.

Meanwhile, the spider can be held in 70% alcohol. The lesion should be noted with all its features on physical examination. A complete systemic examination such as generalized rash, muscle fasciculations, spasms, and state of consciousness should be performed. Laboratory tests generally include complete blood count, lactate dehydrogenase, alanine aminotransferase, aspartate aminotransferase, creatine phosphokinase, and bilirubin levels as an indicator of hemolysis, urea, creatinine, sodium, potassium for acute kidney failure in cases of massive hemolysis, C-reactive protein due to cutaneous inflammatory injury, urinalysis, cardiac enzymes, electrocardiography, and coagulation tests. Usually, results are within normal limits (Malaque et al., 2011). Radiological imaging of the bitten area, and further imaging, if necessary, may be helpful.

Treatment of most spider bites is generally supportive only. The approach to spider bites is as follows:

- Removal from the dangerous environment
- Keeping the patient and doctor in a safe environment
- Ensuring airway/breathing/circulation (ABC) safety
- Ensuring wound hygiene
- Extremity elevation
- Cold application
- Tetanus prophylaxis
- Hydration
- Incision and debridement for necrotic wounds
- Analgesic and antihistamine administration
- Antibiotics in suspected wound infection
- Antivenom administration in certain spider bites.

Routine use of corticosteroids is not recommended due to unproven benefits (Mold & Thompson, 2004). In pregnant women, fetal evaluation, supportive treatment, anaphylaxis treatment, if any, and antivenom administration in the appropriate cases are seen to be safe with the available evidence (Brown et al., 2013).

Spiders Causing Dermonecrotic Arachnidism *(Loxosceles)*

Loxosceles (Araneae, Sicariidae), known as brown spiders, are common throughout the world but in temperate and tropical regions such as Africa, the Caribbean Islands, and North and South America, they pose a significant health problem, especially in Brazil (Oliveira-Mendes et al., 2020). The most distinctive feature in the appearance of many is the violin-shaped marking on the back (Figure 1) (CDC/PHIL, 1966). These spiders are not aggressive and are found among woodpiles, in attics, under rocks, or in small dark areas such as closets. They do not bite unless they perceive a threat.

The brown recluse spider is responsible for nearly all spider bites leading to significant dermonecrosis (Andersen et al., 2011; Hogan et al., 2004). While most spider bites heal on their own, some may rarely lead to a systemic disease called loxoscelism with necrotic lesions. Sphingomyelinase-D, one of the enzymes of the brown recluse spider venom, is the main culprit of dermonecrotic lesions (Kalapothakis et al., 2007; Tambourgi et al., 2004). Although the mechanism of action is not precise, its degenerative structure acting as a protease against the basal membrane and plasma can be considered as the cause of delayed wound healing, bleeding, and renal failure (Van Den Berg et al., 2002). On the other hand, the enzyme hyaluronidase is responsible for the spread of the lesion with the effect of gravity (Hogan et al., 2004). Most lesions attributed to the brown recluse spider are noted as recluse bites, although they are actually due to other causes; this exceeds the true incidence, resulting in the over-reporting of recluse bites (Vetter & Bush, 2002; Wendell, 2003). It is not easy to make a definitive diagnosis because it is painless at first. It is noticed late, and the spider is not seen; It can be confused with dermatitis, cutaneous viral infection, vasculitis, and diabetic ulcer. Although the skin ulcer usually heals spontaneously within 6-8 weeks, it may require surgery in some cases (Vetter & Isbister, 2008).

A clinically typical bite is initially painless and causes pruritus and erythema within six hours. Sporadic severe cases may progress to necrosis within 48 hours. An early sign of necrosis is the formation of painful and scarred bullae and cyanosis. While mild systemic effects are nausea, vomiting, fever, weakness, and arthralgia, the dangerous complications are pyoderma gangrenosum, intravascular hemolysis, renal failure, pulmonary edema, and systemic toxicity

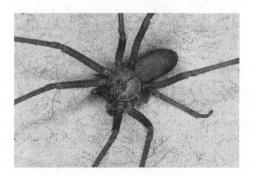

Figure 1. The characteristic violin-shaped mark of Loxosceles reclusa on the dorsal cephalothorax (CDC/PHIL, 1966).

(Andersen et al., 2011; Bey et al., 1997). Although rarely seen, necrosis can be fatal in children due to severe intravascular hemolysis (Swanson & Vetter, 2005).

It is reasonable to study the complete blood count, urea, creatinine, coagulation panel, and urinalysis in patients presenting with signs of intoxication. Most brown recluse spider bites heal without medical treatment. Mild and moderate cases are treated symptomatically, while severe cutaneous lesions and systemic complications require hospitalization, and antivenom may be considered (Oliveira-Mendes et al., 2020). There is no definitive treatment for loxoscelism yet; applications such as dapsone, colchicine, surgical excision, steroids, hyperbaric oxygen, electric shock therapy, and local nitroglycerin have no clear benefit (Andersen et al., 2011; Hogan et al., 2004). In addition to wound care, tetanus prophylaxis, hydration, antihistamines, analgesic applications, and antibiotics are applied in the presence of infection.

Widow Spiders *(Latrodectus Species)*

Latrodectus spiders are distributed worldwide, mostly in temperate and subtropical regions, and frequently seen during the summer season (Bettini, 1964). Latrodectus species are one of the most distinguishable species of all spiders, with their distinctive glossy black swollen abdomen and ventral orange-red markings. Although there are color variations between species, Latrodectus mactans (black widow) is the most well-known in the genus, with an hourglass-shaped abdomen marking (Figure 2) (CDC/PHIL, 2007). Females are responsible for the most significant bites; and males have less venom and smaller and weaker jaws. Widow spiders are not usually found inside the home but in woodpiles, garages, barns, flower pots, and garden materials.

When people accidentally injure spiders while wearing gardening gloves or gardening, they are often bitten defensively (Vetter et al., 2012). Most bites are asymptomatic or cause no symptoms other than local mild pain (Clark et al., 1992). The pain usually disappears within three days without treatment. Other symptoms include tremor, weakness, local paresthesia, headache, nausea, vomiting, tachycardia, tachypnea, hypertension, anxiety, abdominal muscle rigidity, priapism, and dyspnea (Clark et al., 1992; Müller, 1993). In a 9-year study of Latrodectus bites in the United States, it was reported that only 1.4% of 23,409 cases had serious effects but no death. It has also been reported that the antivenom is administered within the first day of the symptom period to those with moderate and severe systemic effects (Monte et al., 2011).

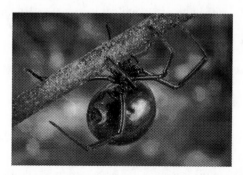

Figure 2. Latrodectus mactans with the characteristic red hourglass on its glossy black abdomen surface (CDC/PHIL, 2007).

Latrodectism, a syndrome usually caused by Latrodectus envenomation, is characterized by muscle spasms in which local tissue damage rapidly escalates and spreads (Clark et al., 1992). Severe abdominal pain may be confused with acute abdomen (Bush, 1999; White & Harbord, 1985). No laboratory test will definitively confirm the diagnosis of latrodectism, especially in mild envenomation. However, the most common abnormality observed in laboratory tests is hematuria and an elevation in white blood cell count, liver enzymes, and creatine phosphokinase (Clark et al., 1992). Further imaging and laboratory tests may be required for differential diagnosis.

The main neurotoxin responsible for the systemic clinical effects of latrodectism is α-latrotoxin. This protein binds to specific receptors on the presynaptic plasma membrane, causing the release of neurotransmitters (catecholamine and acetylcholine) through both calcium-dependent and calcium-independent mechanisms and vesicle exocytosis (Nicholson & Graudins, 2002). Latrodectus antivenom produced from horse serum can be applied mainly in children, pregnant and elderly patients with respiratory failure, seizures, uncontrolled hypertension, or severe poisoning findings unresponsive to other treatments, and its results are satisfactory (Shackleford et al., 2015; White, 1998). Slow infusion of one vial of antivenom over 30 minutes is usually sufficient.

In Latrodectus bites, tetanus prophylaxis should be routinely applied and local wound care with soap and water. In controlling pain and muscle spasms, narcotic and benzodiazepines can be administered with cardiac and respiratory monitoring. Calcium gluconate infusion is not recommended due to its limited efficacy (Clark et al., 1992; Shackleford et al., 2015). Patients should be kept under observation unless hypertension and muscle spasms resolve.

Armed Spiders *(Phoneutria)*

The genus Phoneutria, popularly known as "armed," "wandering," or "banana spiders," is limited to South America, with most bites being reported from Brazil. They are nocturnal, non-web-forming aggressive spiders. The Phoneutria nigriventer species is responsible for most human bites and does not cause significant symptoms (Lucas, 1988). The primary symptom is redness, and localized diaphoresis with an intense local pain sensation. In addition to nausea, vomiting, dizziness, and visual disturbances; systemic reactions consisting of autonomic effects may occur such as tachycardia, hypertension, general sweating, salivation, and priapism, especially in young men. Although the rate of severe envenomation is negligible, the highest risk groups are children under the age of 10 and adults over 70 (Bucaretchi et al., 2000).

In most cases, supportive treatment is sufficient. Local anesthetic can be applied near the bite area for pain control. Antivenom is available for severe envenomation (Lucas, 2015).

Hobo Spider *(Eratigena agrestis)*

This species, which is naturally found from Europe to Central Asia, is also seen on the Pacific Northwest coast (Blackman, 1995; Hänggi et al., 1995). They are fast and aggressive but rarely bite. They live in dark, moist environments such as basements. Their bites, like Loxosceles, are initially painless and continue after 15 minutes with local numbness, erythema, and stiffness at the bite site. A vesicle is seen within 36 hours, and necrosis may develop under the influence of gravity, as in Loxosceles. Scar occurs within three days, and delayed healing (Fisher et al., 1994; Swanson & Vetter, 2005). Confirmed cases experience pain, itching, and swelling (McKeown et al., 2014). The most common systemic complication is a headache with a poor response to analgesics. Visual and auditory hallucinations may accompany (Sams et al., 2001). Hobo spider bites should be considered among the differential diagnoses if the history is compatible in such neurological cases in endemic areas. Unless the spider bite is certain, attributing necrotic lesions to the hobo spider may ignore a more serious underlying condition. There is no diagnostic test or proven treatment. Wound care, tetanus prophylaxis, and symptomatic approach are applied.

Funnel-Web Spiders (Atrax/Hadronyche)

Funnel-web spiders, the most venomous spider in the world, have more than 40 species, with genera including Hadronyche, Illawarra, and Atrax. Funnel-web spiders get their name from the way they form a funnel-shaped nest that extends into a hollow to trap their prey. The Sydney funnel-web spider sits in the pocket at the entrance to the burrow, and when it senses vibrations in the web, it responds to inject venom into its prey. Funnel-web spiders have strong, sharp teeth penetrating nails and soft shoes (Binstead & Nappe, 2021). Because funnel-web spider venom is highly toxic, all species should be considered as potentially dangerous (Isbister, 2010).

Atracotoxin, the venom of one Sydney funnel-web spider, Atrax robustus, causes autonomic and neuromuscular excitation with the neurotransmitters it releases by binding to voltage-mediated sodium channels as in scorpions, and endogenous catecholaminergic discharge following early cholinergic increase (Del Brutto, 2013; Graudins et al., 2002). Findings such as nausea, vomiting, bronchorea, salivation, and lacrimation due to cholinergic increase are systemic toxicity findings; muscle fasciculations, weakness due to neuromuscular stimulation; and changes in consciousness may also occur due to the central nervous system being affected. Myocardial damage may develop with pulmonary edema due to intense catecholamine increase (Braitberg & Segal, 2009; Miller et al., 2016). Severe envenomation begins rapidly within the first two hours, but no related deaths have been reported since the start of antivenom use in 1981 (Isbister et al., 2005). Funnel-web spider antivenom; This is an effective antivenom that can be used safely as the first choice in all clinically suspected funnel-web spider bites where severe allergic reactions rarely develop (Graudins et al., 2002; Isbister et al., 2005).

In funnel-web spider envenomation, firstly, after cleaning the wound with soapy water, a pressure bandage should be quickly applied. This technique minimizes the spread of venom (Isbister, 2010). The patient should be taken to the hospital immediately. The applied pressure bandage should not be removed until the patient's vascular access is established, monitoring is provided, and the antidote is ready. Since early removal of the pressure bandage may cause the venom to enter the systemic circulation and rapidly deteriorate the patient's clinical condition, the dressing should be reapplied in this case (Braitberg & Segal, 2009). If there is evidence of systemic envenomation, antivenom should be administered immediately as the first treatment (CSL Ltd., Australian funnel-web spider antivenom; two vials, start with four if serious, 2-4 more if needed). Patients whose signs of systemic poisoning are still not developed 6 hours after bandage removal can be discharged. Follow-up is only reasonable in those with local findings (Binstead & Nappe, 2021; Braitberg & Segal, 2009). Additional treatment recommendations are as follows: tetanus prophylaxis, hydration to prevent hypotension, atropine administration in the case of salivation and bronchorea, intubation for airway safety, or continuous positive airway pressure application for pulmonary edema, benzodiazepines for tremor and agitation, and beta-blockers for tachycardia can be administered according to symptoms.

Tarantulas *(Theraphosidae)*

Tarantulas, whose body length can reach 10 cm, are known as the giants of the spider world. Although primarily found in tropical regions, they have also spread to semi-temperate areas and deserts. Tarantulas, capable of catching large and powerful prey, do not use nets to catch these prey but paralyze their prey by taking advantage of their venom's rapid and irreversible effect on the central and peripheral systems (Escoubas & Rash, 2004). Although considered to be potentially dangerous concerning their impressive size, they are generally unlikely to pose a significant human problem. Although local pain is most common, pruritus, edema, erythema, a burning sensation, and systemic effects rarely occur (Isbister et al., 2003; Lucas et al., 1994). Some species of tarantulas, which are predators like other spiders in the Americas, have hairs on their bellies that they use for defense. Although these hairs cannot penetrate human skin, they can cause ophthalmia nodosa and threaten health more than a spider bite if they get into the eyes (Belyea et al., 1998; Lasudry & Brightbill, 1997). Although these hairs are absent in older tarantula species in Asia and Africa, they can cause more severe and resistant pain through their venom (Ahmed et al., 2009).

The treatment of tarantula bites is symptomatic, but in ocular exposure, an immediate ophthalmology consultation is required after copious intraocular irrigation. Ophthalmic antibiotics and steroids can be given with ophthalmology follow-up and recommendations. Elevation of the bitten extremity, local cold application, wound cleansing, tetanus prophylaxis, oral antihistamines, and analgesics are helpful. There is no antivenom for tarantula bites. There is insufficient evidence for the efficacy of benzodiazepines and intravenous calcium gluconate administration to control muscle spasms (Key, 1981). Dantrolene reduces intracellular calcium concentration by inhibiting the ryanodine receptor, the main calcium release channel of the skeletal muscle sarcoplasmic reticulum; It is used to treat malignant hyperthermia, neuroleptic malign syndrome, spasticity, and ecstasy intoxication (Krause et al., 2004). The use of dantrolene can also be considered in benzodiazepine-resistant spasms caused by tarantula spider envenomation (Ahmed et al., 2009).

Other Spiders

Daddy long-leg spiders (Araneae, Pholcidae) are found on every continent except Antarctica. There are no cases of their bites poisoning people, and their effects are minimal. *Yellow sac spiders (Cheiracanthium)* are distributed worldwide and found in sheds, garages, window sills, and skirting boards (Vetter et al., 2006). They are very aggressive and can bite suddenly. Since the bites are very painful, like a bee sting, the spider is usually immediately noticed and caught (McKeown et al., 2014). The effect of their bites is limited to local pain, swelling, and erythema. Skin necrosis is extremely rare (Vetter et al., 2006). *Wolf spiders (Lycosidae)* have spread around the world and have minor effects. They do not cause necrotic ulcers or systemic symptoms (Isbister & Framenau, 2004). The result of the bites of *Jumping spiders (Salticidae)* consists of minor traumas that pass within two days, and they do not cause dermonecrosis (Isbister et al., 2001).

Centipede Bites

Centipedes are a group of arthropods that includes many-legged creatures of the Myriapoda family belonging to the Chilopoda class. Different centipedes have between 30 and 354 legs and vary from a few millimeters to 30 cm. The vast majority are carnivorous animals. Cases related to the bites of centipede species living in temperate climates worldwide, especially those living in Asia, Indonesia, India, Hawaii, South America, and Australia, have been reported (Ross et al., 2021).

Centipede bites occur predominantly at night, usually as extremity bites. Pain, localized erythema, and edema may develop. Two small punctures are recognized at the bite site. Although cases with local infection, allergic reactions, anaphylaxis, lymphangitis, rhabdomyolysis, necrosis, renal failure, and myocardial infarction have been reported, they mostly heal without complications (Essler et al., 2017; Fenderson, 2014; Ross et al., 2021; Yildiz et al., 2006). In a 10-year retrospective study conducted in Bangkok, 99.5% of 245 cases had no clinical features other than local effects, the most common being localized pain and swelling, and no deaths were reported (Niruntarai et al., 2021).

There is no diagnostic laboratory test and no specific antivenom. Supportive treatments such as cleaning the bite area, cold application, tetanus prophylaxis, analgesic, and antihistamine administration are performed. The local anesthetic injection can be applied in very painful bites. In endemic areas, the patient should be followed up for complications. Cases with specific symptoms such as chest pain require cardiac evaluation (Ross et al., 2021).

Conclusion

Spider and centipede bites are rare, and most of them have no medical significance. Diagnosis is highly dependent on whether the spider was caught at that time. Conservative treatment, such as wound care, tetanus prophylaxis, analgesic, and antihistamine applications, is sufficient for suspected spider bites. Patients with signs of systemic envenomation require hospitalization and the use of antivenom for bites of some specially defined species.

References

Ahmed, N., Pinkham, M., & Warrell, D. A. (2009, Dec). Symptom in search of a toxin: muscle spasms following bites by Old World tarantula spiders (Lampropelma nigerrimum, Pterinochilus murinus, Poecilotheria regalis) with review. *Qjm, 102*(12), 851-857. https://doi.org/10.1093/qjmed/hcp128.

Andersen, R. J., Campoli, J., Johar, S. K., Schumacher, K. A., & Allison, E. J., Jr. (2011, Aug). Suspected brown recluse envenomation: a case report and review of different treatment modalities. *J Emerg Med, 41*(2), e31-37. https://doi.org/10.1016/j.jemermed.2009.08.055.

Atkinson, R. K., & Wright, L. G. (1992, Jul). The modes of action of spider toxins on insects and mammals. *Comp Biochem Physiol C Comp Pharmacol Toxicol, 102*(3), 339-342. https://doi.org/10.1016/0742-8413(92)90124-p.

Belyea, D. A., Tuman, D. C., Ward, T. P., & Babonis, T. R. (1998, Jun). The red eye revisited: ophthalmia nodosa due to tarantula hairs. *South Med J, 91*(6), 565-567. https://doi.org/10.1097/00007611-199806000-00011,

Bettini, S. (1964, Oct). Epidemiology Of Latrodectism. *Toxicon, 2*, 93-102. https://doi.org/10.1016/0041-0101(64)90009-1,

Bey, T. A., Walter, F. G., Lober, W., Schmidt, J., Spark, R., & Schlievert, P. M. (1997, Nov). Loxosceles arizonica bite associated with shock. *Ann Emerg Med, 30*(5), 701-703. https://doi.org/10.1016/s0196-0644(97)70092-1,

Binstead, J. T., & Nappe, T. M. (2021). Funnel Web Spider Toxicity. In *StatPearls*. StatPearls Publishing Copyright © 2021, StatPearls Publishing LLC.

Blackman, J. R. (1995, Jul-Aug). Spider bites. *J Am Board Fam Pract, 8*(4), 288-294.

Braitberg, G., & Segal, L. (2009, Nov). Spider bites - Assessment and management. *Aust Fam Physician, 38*(11), 862-867.

Brown, S. A., Seifert, S. A., & Rayburn, W. F. (2013, Jan). Management of envenomations during pregnancy. *Clin Toxicol (Phila), 51*(1), 3-15. https://doi.org/10.3109/15563650.2012.760127.

Bucaretchi, F., Deus Reinaldo, C. R., Hyslop, S., Madureira, P. R., De Capitani, E. M., & Vieira, R. J. (2000, Jan-Feb). A clinico-epidemiological study of bites by spiders of the genus Phoneutria. *Rev Inst Med Trop Sao Paulo, 42*(1), 17-21. https://doi.org/10.1590/s0036-46652000000100003.

Bush, S. P. (1999, May). Black widow spider envenomation mimicking cholecystitis. *Am J Emerg Med, 17*(3), 315. https://doi.org/10.1016/s0735-6757(99)90137-7.

CDC/PHIL. (1966). Centers for Disease Control and Prevention. Public Health Image Library of the US. Loxosceles reclusa. https://phil.cdc.gov/Details.aspx?pid=1125 accessed December 2021.

CDC/PHIL. (2007). Centers for Disease Control and Prevention. Public Health Image Library of the US. Latrodectus mactans. https://phil.cdc.gov/Details.aspx?pid=9854 accessed December 2021.

Clark, R. F., Wethern-Kestner, S., Vance, M. V., & Gerkin, R. (1992, Jul). Clinical presentation and treatment of black widow spider envenomation: a review of 163 cases. *Ann Emerg Med, 21*(7), 782-787. https://doi.org/10.1016/s0196-0644(05)81021-2.

Del Brutto, O. H. (2013). Neurological effects of venomous bites and stings: snakes, spiders, and scorpions. *Handb Clin Neurol, 114*, 349-368. https://doi.org/10.1016/b978-0-444-53490-3.00028-5.

Escoubas, P., & King, G. F. (2009, Jun). Venomics as a drug discovery platform. *Expert Rev Proteomics, 6*(3), 221-224. https://doi.org/10.1586/epr.09.45.

Escoubas, P., & Rash, L. (2004, Apr). Tarantulas: eight-legged pharmacists and combinatorial chemists. *Toxicon, 43*(5), 555-574. https://doi.org/10.1016/j.toxicon.2004.02.007.

Essler, S. E., Julakanti, M., & Juergens, A. L. (2017, Mar). Lymphangitis From Scolopendra heros Envenomation: The Texas Redheaded Centipede. *Wilderness Environ Med, 28*(1), 51-53. https://doi.org/10.1016/j.wem.2016.11.003.

Fenderson, J. L. (2014, Nov). Centipede envenomation: bringing the pain to Hawai'i and Pacific Islands. *Hawaii J Med Public Health, 73*(11 Suppl 2), 41-43.

Fisher, R. G., Kelly, P., Krober, M. S., Weir, M. R., & Jones, R. (1994, Jun). Necrotic arachnidism. *West J Med, 160*(6), 570-572.

Fusto, G., Bennardo, L., Duca, E. D., Mazzuca, D., Tamburi, F., Patruno, C., & Nisticò, S. P. (2020, Oct 2). Spider bites of medical significance in the Mediterranean area: misdiagnosis, clinical features and management. *J Venom Anim Toxins Incl Trop Dis, 26*, e20190100. https://doi.org/10.1590/1678-9199-jvatitd-2019-0100.

Graudins, A., Wilson, D., Alewood, P. F., Broady, K. W., & Nicholson, G. M. (2002, Mar). Cross-reactivity of Sydney funnel-web spider antivenom: neutralization of the in vitro toxicity of other Australian funnel-web (Atrax and Hadronyche) spider venoms. *Toxicon, 40*(3), 259-266. https://doi.org/10.1016/s0041-0101(01)00210-0.

Hänggi, A., Stöckli, E., & Nentwig, W. (1995). Habitats of Central European Spiders. Characterisation of the habitats of the most abundant spider species of Central Europe and associated species. *Miscellanea Faunistica Helvetiae, 4*, 1-459.

Hogan, C. J., Barbaro, K. C., & Winkel, K. (2004, Dec). Loxoscelism: old obstacles, new directions. *Ann Emerg Med, 44*(6), 608-624. https://doi.org/10.1016/j.annemergmed.2004.08.028.

Isbister, G. K. (2010, Feb 9). Antivenom efficacy or effectiveness: the Australian experience. *Toxicology, 268*(3), 148-154. https://doi.org/10.1016/j.tox.2009.09.013.

Isbister, G. K., Churchill, T. B., Hirst, D. B., Gray, M. R., & Currie, B. J. (2001, Jan 15). Clinical effects of bites from formally identified spiders in tropical Northern Territory. *Med J Aust, 174*(2), 79-82. https://doi.org/10.5694/j.1326-5377.2001.tb143159.x.

Isbister, G. K., & Framenau, V. W. (2004). Australian wolf spider bites (Lycosidae): clinical effects and influence of species on bite circumstances. *J Toxicol Clin Toxicol, 42*(2), 153-161. https://doi.org/10.1081/clt-120030941.

Isbister, G. K., Gray, M. R., Balit, C. R., Raven, R. J., Stokes, B. J., Porges, K., Tankel, A. S., Turner, E., White, J., & Fisher, M. M. (2005, Apr 18). Funnel-web spider bite: a systematic review of recorded clinical cases. *Med J Aust, 182*(8), 407-411. https://doi.org/10.5694/j.1326-5377.2005.tb06760.x.

Isbister, G. K., Seymour, J. E., Gray, M. R., & Raven, R. J. (2003, Mar). Bites by spiders of the family Theraphosidae in humans and canines. *Toxicon, 41*(4), 519-524. https://doi.org/10.1016/s0041-0101(02)00395-1

Kalapothakis, E., Chatzaki, M., Gonçalves-Dornelas, H., de Castro, C. S., Silvestre, F. G., Laborne, F. V., de Moura, J. F., Veiga, S. S., Chávez-Olórtegui, C., Granier, C., & Barbaro, K. C. (2007, Dec 1). The Loxtox protein family in Loxosceles intermedia (Mello-Leitão) venom. *Toxicon, 50*(7), 938-946. https://doi.org/10.1016/j.toxicon.2007.07.001.

Key, G. F. (1981, Jan). A comparison of calcium gluconate and methocarbamol (Robaxin) in the treatment of Latrodectism (black widow spider envenomation). *Am J Trop Med Hyg, 30*(1), 273-277. https://doi.org/10.4269/ajtmh.1981.30.273.

Koh, W. L. (1998, Apr). When to worry about spider bites. Inaccurate diagnosis can have serious, even fatal, consequences. *Postgrad Med, 103*(4), 235-236, 243-234, 249-250. https://doi.org/10.3810/pgm.1998.04.459.

Krause, T., Gerbershagen, M. U., Fiege, M., Weisshorn, R., & Wappler, F. (2004, Apr). Dantrolene--a review of its pharmacology, therapeutic use and new developments. *Anaesthesia, 59*(4), 364-373. https://doi.org/10.1111/j.1365-2044.2004.03658.x.

Lasudry, J. G., & Brightbill, F. S. (1997, May-Jun). Ophthalmia nodosa caused by tarantula hairs. *J Pediatr Ophthalmol Strabismus, 34*(3), 197-198.

Lucas, S. (1988). Spiders in Brazil. *Toxicon, 26*(9), 759-772. https://doi.org/10.1016/0041-0101(88)90317-0.

Lucas, S. M. (2015). The history of venomous spider identification, venom extraction methods and antivenom production: a long journey at the Butantan Institute, São Paulo, Brazil. *J Venom Anim Toxins Incl Trop Dis, 21*, 21. https://doi.org/10.1186/s40409-015-0020-0.

Lucas, S. M., Da Silva Júnior, P. I., Bertani, R., & Cardoso, J. L. (1994, Oct). Mygalomorph spider bites: a report on 91 cases in the state of São Paulo, Brazil. *Toxicon, 32*(10), 1211-1215. https://doi.org/10.1016/0041-0101(94)90350-6.

Malaque, C. M., Santoro, M. L., Cardoso, J. L., Conde, M. R., Novaes, C. T., Risk, J. Y., França, F. O., de Medeiros, C. R., & Fan, H. W. (2011, Dec 1). Clinical picture and laboratorial evaluation in human loxoscelism. *Toxicon, 58*(8), 664-671. https://doi.org/10.1016/j.toxicon.2011.09.011.

McKeown, N., Vetter, R. S., & Hendrickson, R. G. (2014, Jun). Verified spider bites in Oregon (USA) with the intent to assess hobo spider venom toxicity. *Toxicon, 84*, 51-55. https://doi.org/10.1016/j.toxicon.2014.03.009.

Miller, M., O'Leary, M. A., & Isbister, G. K. (2016, Mar). Towards rationalisation of antivenom use in funnel-web spider envenoming: enzyme immunoassays for venom concentrations. *Clin Toxicol (Phila), 54*(3), 245-251. https://doi.org/10.3109/15563650.2015.1122794.

Mold, J. W., & Thompson, D. M. (2004, Sep-Oct). Management of brown recluse spider bites in primary care. *J Am Board Fam Pract, 17*(5), 347-352. https://doi.org/10.3122/jabfm.17.5.347.

Monte, A. A., Bucher-Bartelson, B., & Heard, K. J. (2011, Dec). A US perspective of symptomatic Latrodectus spp. envenomation and treatment: a National Poison Data System review. *Ann Pharmacother, 45*(12), 1491-1498. https://doi.org/10.1345/aph.1Q424.

Müller, G. J. (1993, Jun). Black and brown widow spider bites in South Africa. A series of 45 cases. *S Afr Med J, 83*(6), 399-405.

Nicholson, G. M., & Graudins, A. (2002, Sep). Spiders of medical importance in the Asia-Pacific: atracotoxin, latrotoxin and related spider neurotoxins. *Clin Exp Pharmacol Physiol, 29*(9), 785-794. https://doi.org/10.1046/j.1440-1681.2002.03741.x.

Niruntarai, S., Rueanpingwang, K., & Othong, R. (2021, Aug). Patients with centipede bites presenting to a university hospital in Bangkok: a 10-year retrospective study. *Clin Toxicol (Phila), 59*(8), 721-726. https://doi.org/10.1080/15563650.2020.1865543.

Oliveira-Mendes, B. B. R., Chatzaki, M., Sales-Medina, D. F., Leal, H. G., van der Veer, R., Biscoto, G. L., Gonçalves, P. M., Soares da Silva, T., Guerra-Duarte, C., Kalapothakis, E., & Horta, C. C. R. (2020, Jan 15). From taxonomy to molecular characterization of brown spider venom: An overview focused on Loxosceles similis. *Toxicon, 173*, 5-19. https://doi.org/10.1016/j.toxicon.2019.11.002.

Ross, E. J., Jamal, Z., & Yee, J. (2021). Centipede Envenomation. In *StatPearls*. StatPearls Publishing Copyright © 2021, StatPearls Publishing LLC.

Russell, F. E., & Gertsch, W. J. (1983). For those who treat spider or suspected spider bites. *Toxicon, 21*(3), 337-339. https://doi.org/10.1016/0041-0101(83)90089-2.

Sams, H. H., Dunnick, C. A., Smith, M. L., & King, L. E., Jr. (2001, Apr). Necrotic arachnidism. *J Am Acad Dermatol, 44*(4), 561-573; quiz 573-566. https://doi.org/10.1067/mjd.2001.112385.

Shackleford, R., Veillon, D., Maxwell, N., LaChance, L., Jusino, T., Cotelingam, J., & Carrington, P. (2015, Mar-Apr). The black widow spider bite: differential diagnosis, clinical manifestations, and treatment options. *J La State Med Soc, 167*(2), 74-78.

Swanson, D. L., & Vetter, R. S. (2005, Feb 17). Bites of brown recluse spiders and suspected necrotic arachnidism. *N Engl J Med, 352*(7), 700-707. https://doi.org/10.1056/NEJMra041184.

Tambourgi, D. V., de, F. F. P. M., van den Berg, C. W., Gonçalves-de-Andrade, R. M., Ferracini, M., Paixão-Cavalcante, D., Morgan, B. P., & Rushmere, N. K. (2004, Jul). Molecular cloning, expression, function and immunoreactivities of members of a gene family of sphingomyelinases from Loxosceles venom glands. *Mol Immunol, 41*(8), 831-840. https://doi.org/10.1016/j.molimm.2004.03.027.

Van Den Berg, C. W., De Andrade, R. M., Magnoli, F. C., Marchbank, K. J., & Tambourgi, D. V. (2002, Sep). Loxosceles spider venom induces metalloproteinase mediated cleavage of MCP/CD46 and MHCI and induces protection against C-mediated lysis. *Immunology, 107*(1), 102-110. https://doi.org/10.1046/j.1365-2567.2002.01468.x.

Vetter, R. S., & Bush, S. P. (2002, Aug 15). Reports of presumptive brown recluse spider bites reinforce improbable diagnosis in regions of North America where the spider is not endemic. *Clin Infect Dis, 35*(4), 442-445. https://doi.org/10.1086/341244.

Vetter, R. S., & Isbister, G. K. (2008). Medical aspects of spider bites. *Annu Rev Entomol, 53*, 409-429. https://doi.org/10.1146/annurev.ento.53.103106.093503.

Vetter, R. S., Isbister, G. K., Bush, S. P., & Boutin, L. J. (2006, Jun). Verified bites by yellow sac spiders (genus Cheiracanthium) in the United States and Australia: where is the necrosis? *Am J Trop Med Hyg, 74*(6), 1043-1048.

Vetter, R. S., Vincent, L. S., Danielsen, D. W., Reinker, K. I., Clarke, D. E., Itnyre, A. A., Kabashima, J. N., & Rust, M. K. (2012, Jul). The prevalence of brown widow and black widow spiders (Araneae: Theridiidae) in urban southern California. *J Med Entomol, 49*(4), 947-951. https://doi.org/10.1603/me11285.

Walther, G. R., Roques, A., Hulme, P. E., Sykes, M. T., Pysek, P., Kühn, I., Zobel, M., Bacher, S., Botta-Dukát, Z., Bugmann, H., Czúcz, B., Dauber, J., Hickler, T., Jarosík, V., Kenis, M., Klotz, S., Minchin, D., Moora, M., Nentwig, W., Ott, J., Panov, V. E., Reineking, B., Robinet, C., Semenchenko, V., Solarz, W., Thuiller, W., Vilà, M., Vohland, K., & Settele, J. (2009, Dec). Alien species in a warmer world: risks and opportunities. *Trends Ecol Evol, 24*(12), 686-693. https://doi.org/10.1016/j.tree.2009.06.008.

Wendell, R. P. (2003, May). Brown recluse spiders: a review to help guide physicians in nonendemic areas. *South Med J, 96*(5), 486-490. https://doi.org/10.1097/01.Smj.0000066761.59212.22.

White, J. (1998, Nov). Envenoming and antivenom use in Australia. *Toxicon, 36*(11), 1483-1492. https://doi.org/10.1016/s0041-0101(98)00138-x.

White, J., & Harbord, M. (1985, Jan 7). Latrodectism as mimic. *Med J Aust, 142*(1), 75. https://doi.org/10.5694/j.1326-5377.1985.tb113300.x.

Wood, D. L., Miljenović, T., Cai, S., Raven, R. J., Kaas, Q., Escoubas, P., Herzig, V., Wilson, D., & King, G. F. (2009, Aug 13). ArachnoServer: a database of protein toxins from spiders. *BMC Genomics, 10*, 375. https://doi.org/10.1186/1471-2164-10-375.

Yildiz, A., Biçeroglu, S., Yakut, N., Bilir, C., Akdemir, R., & Akilli, A. (2006, Apr). Acute myocardial infarction in a young man caused by centipede sting. *Emerg Med J, 23*(4), e30. https://doi.org/10.1136/emj.2005.030007.

Chapter 14

Scorpion Stings

Halil Ibrahim Çikriklar[1,*], MD and Bilge Güner[2]

[1]Department of Emergency Medicine, School of Medicine, Bursa Uludag University, Bursa, Turkey
[2]Department of Emergency Medicine, Sakarya Training and Research Hospital, Sakarya, Turkey

Abstract

Scorpion sting is a life-threatening and endemic toxicological emergency. This review aims to discuss the important species in terms of human poisoning among the known scorpion species and present the diagnosis and treatment of poisonings caused by these scorpions. Scorpion poisoning can cause multiorgan failure, neurotoxicity, and cardiotoxicity in affected individuals. There is no specific test for diagnosis, but history and epidemiological information help to diagnose. Its treatment consists of early recognition of the sting, application of the specific antivenom, and cardiorespiratory and systemic support. Management is determined by the degree of poisoning. The bite areas of patients with scorpion stings should be cleaned, and tetanus prophylaxis should be provided when necessary. Symptomatic treatment aims to relieve pain using standard analgesics and anti-inflammatory drugs. While adults may appear to be poisoned more often, children are more likely to develop serious illnesses that require intensive supportive care. The effectiveness of the antivenom has not been convincingly proven. Recommendations for using scorpion-specific antidotes vary with specific scorpion species. The dose of antivenom depends on the type of scorpion, the estimated amount of venom entering the body, and the severity of the poisoning. Clinicians should follow the guidelines of their local experts and the manufacturer's instructions when determining the antivenom dose. Scorpions often hide among stones, on roofs, or in clothing. Keeping the house's surroundings clean; It is recommended to disinfect the places where scorpions settle periodically and not to walk barefoot, especially at night, to prevent scorpion poisoning.

Keywords: scorpion, poisoning, antivenom, emergency

---

* Corresponding Author's Email: halilcikriklar@gmail.com.

In: Environmental Emergencies and Injuries in Nature
Editors: Murat Yücel, Murat Güzel and İbrahim İkizceli
ISBN: 978-1-68507-833-1
© 2022 Nova Science Publishers, Inc.

Introduction

A scorpion sting is a life-threatening and endemic toxicological emergency (Santos et al., 2016). More than one million scorpion bites are reported worldwide each year, with a prevalence of 20 per 100,000 people. About 5% of reported cases are severe, and about 0.3% of severe cases are fatal (Binorkar and Parlikar, 2016). Scorpion poisoning can be fatal, especially for children (Isbister and Bawaskar, 2014).

This review aims to discuss the important species in terms of human poisoning among the known scorpion species and present the diagnosis and treatment of poisonings caused by these scorpions.

Scorpion Venom

Scorpion venom is produced in glands located in the distal part of the tail. It consists of polypeptides with enzymatic and proinflammatory properties (Abroug et al., 2020). Scorpion venoms are complex mixtures containing mucopolysaccharides, hyaluronidase, phospholipase, acetylcholinesterase, serotonin, histamine, protease inhibitors, histamine releasers, and neurotoxins (Isbister and Bawaskar, 2014).

Alpha-toxins, which are important factors in human poisoning, bind to sodium channels in cell membranes and cause excessive catecholamine (epinephrine, norepinephrine) and acetylcholine release (Isbister and Bawaskar, 2014).

This excessive release of neurotransmitters causes an autonomic storm. It manifests as cholinergic excess, marked bronchorea, salivation, bronchospasm, sweating, priapism, lacrimation, vomiting, diarrhea, and bradycardia. These effects usually last only a few hours after a scorpion sting (Isbister and Bawaskar, 2014). Sympathetic stimulation typically persists and results in hypertension, tachycardia, and agitation. Severe poisoning may cause myocardial damage and progress with arrhythmias, myocarditis, pulmonary edema, cardiogenic shock, and multisystem organ failure (Isbister and Bawaskar, 2014).

Tityus or Leiurus poisoning may cause acute pancreatitis (Santos et al., 2016).

Distribution

Until the end of the nineteenth century (1899-1900), there were about 250 known scorpion species. By 1975, this number had reached 700 species. Today, there are about 2200 known species of scorpions (Sousa et al., 2017). Of the total of 18 families, 11 release a potentially deadly venom (Godoy et al., 2021). Almost all species harmful to humans belong to the Buthidae family (Isbister and Bawaskar, 2014).

Scorpion poisoning can cause multiple organ failure, neurotoxicity, and cardiotoxicity in affected individuals (Bahloul et al., 2010, Isbister and Bawaskar, 2014). In general, all species produce cardiovascular toxicity (Cupo, 2015). Some species, such as Centruroides and Parabuthus, predominantly affect the neuromuscular system (Isbister and Bawaskar, 2014; Torabi et al., 2017). Hemiscorpius lepturus toxin causes tissue and organ necrosis. Diffuse intravascular coagulation (DIC) causes a picture characterized by hemolysis, hemoglobinuria, and acute kidney injury (Torabi et al., 2017). The geographical distributions of the dangerous scorpion species that cause serious poisoning among the known scorpions of today and the specific appearance of some of them are presented below.

Causes of Autonomic Dysfunction or "Autonomous Storm"

Tityus (Latin America): 5-6 cm long and of various colors (brown, yellow, and black). Tityus serrulatus lives in the tropical climates of Brazil (Cupo, 2015).

Androctonus (North Africa, Middle East, Israel, India, Pakistan, and Southeast Asia): Androctonus crassicauda is a black scorpion reaching 12 cm in length (Sucard, 2017).

Buthus (Mediterranean Spain, North Africa, Middle East): (Aboumaad et al., 2014).

Leiurus (North Africa, Middle East, Israel, Lebanon, Turkey, and Iran): (Bawaskar and Bawaskar, 2012).

Hottentotta (Asia, especially India): Hottentotta tamulus (red scorpion) is about 9 cm in size and red. It is the most dangerous scorpion native to India, living in tropical and subtropical plains (Nagaraj et al., 2015).

Causes of Neuromuscular Toxicity

Centruroides (United States, Mexico, and Central America): Centruroides exilicauda is 4 to 7 cm long. It ranges from yellow to brown or tan. The presence of a subacular tooth, a tubercle at the base of the needle, is unique to C. exilicauda and helps to distinguish this highly neurotoxic scorpion from other species (LoVecchio and McBride, 2003).

Parabuthus transvaalicus (South Africa) is a large species in the Buthidae family. It can reach up to 150 mm in length. Intoxication causes neurotoxic effects. Symptoms include abnormal reflexes, bladder symptoms, dysphagia, sweating, and hypersalivation (Bergman, 1997).

Causes of Skin and Tissue Necrosis, Hemolysis, DIC, Acute Kidney Injury, and Non-Infectious Hemolytic Uremic Syndrome (HUS)

Hemiscorpius lepturus (Middle East) is a yellow, thin-tailed scorpion 5 to 8 cm long (Dehghani et al., 2018). It has a bead-shaped and articulated tail. Stings are most common at night while the victim sleeps and often in spring and summer. Children and adolescents younger than five are most commonly affected (Pipelzadeh et al., 2007).

Clinical Findings

Scorpions often hide among stones, on roofs, or in clothing. They usually avoid people. That is why scorpion stings often happen when someone accidentally steps on them or, for example, while putting on their clothes. Therefore, scorpion stings often occur in the extremities (Santos et al., 2016). Scorpion poisoning can cause cardiovascular, respiratory, hematological, renal, and neurological clinical manifestations. Clinical manifestations vary in a wide spectrum depending on the scorpion species and the plasma concentration of the toxin (Cupo, 2015).

Local Symptoms

In 66-90% of scorpion stings that cause autonomic dysfunction, skin changes such as local pain, paresthesia, erythema, and edema are seen without systemic effects (Cupo, 2015). Most scorpion (Centruroides, Parabuthus) poisonings that cause neuromuscular toxicity do not cause pain (O'Connor et al., 2018). Hemiscorpius lepturus causes a relatively painless sting. In addition, stings often occur at night while the patient is asleep and are usually not noticed until the morning (Dehghani and Fathi, 2012). Stings most often involve the lower extremities. Patients come to medical attention for signs of cutaneous manifestations, hemolysis, hemoglobinuria, or hematuria. Initial skin manifestations typically consist of a sting site with a central spot and a mildly painful and pruritic erythematous or purpuric macule or papule. It may be difficult to see the sting site. Other cutaneous manifestations include concentric pruritic plaques, sterile lymphangitis, cellulitis, local or generalized erythematous rash, and purpuric plaques, or purpuric bullae up to 5 cm in diameter at or near the sting, may develop within 24 hours of the sting (Dehghani et al., 2018).

One to two days after the poisoning, patients may develop systemic symptoms such as fever, pallor, fatigue, general edema, and/or red urine (Valavi et al., 2016). These findings are most likely to develop in children younger than five years of age and indicate the presence of acute hemolysis. Petechiae, easy bruising and bleeding indicate DIC (Radmanesh, 1998).

Cardiovascular Symptoms

Alpha receptor stimulation by scorpion toxin causes hypertension, tachycardia, myocardial dysfunction, and pulmonary edema (Petricevich, 2010). Hypoxia and hypoperfusion resulting from pulmonary edema or cardiogenic shock can cause multiorgan failure (Abroug et al., 2020).

Neurological Findings

Central nervous system findings

Central nervous system involvement is rare in adults but common in children (85%). The most common neurological symptoms were irritability (83.4%), sweating (81.5%), hyperthermia (33.6%), and priapism (48.2%) in men. In addition, 14.7% of the children had seizures and 11% had coma (Bahloul, 2010).

Embolism secondary to myocarditis and arrhythmia, an acute increase in blood pressure following an autonomic storm, excessive catecholamine-induced cerebral vasospasm, toxin-mediated endothelial damage, and vasculitis may cause an ischemic stroke (Dube et al., 2011). Generalized tonic-clonic seizures, motor weakness, hemiplegia, dizziness, visual field defects, blindness, and dysarthria are possible stroke symptoms (Gupta et al., 2012). Seizures and coma may develop in severe cases (Sandoval and Lebrun, 2002).

Autonomous Changes
Depending on the scorpion species, the systemic effects of the autonomous storm occur within four hours of its sting (Sucard, 2017). Initially, cholinergic symptoms resulting from parasympathetic activation predominate, such as nausea, vomiting, diarrhea, sweating, increased salivation, tears, and respiratory secretions. In severe cases, the increase in sympathetic activity predominates, such as hypertension, arrhythmias, and heart failure (Abroug et al., 2020).

Neuromuscular Toxicity
About 10 to 30 per cent of patients stung by scorpions of the Centruroides or Parabuthus species develop neuromuscular toxicity, which can be life-threatening. Symptoms can begin immediately after poisoning and typically progress to maximum severity within 5 hours. Symptoms decrease at a rate that varies with the victim's age and the degree of poisoning. Symptomatic improvement usually occurs within 9 to 30 hours (O'Connor et al., 2018).

Peripheral Nervous System Findings
Guillain-Barre-like syndrome, myelitis, abnormal eye movements, facial and eye paralysis, fasciculations, and muscle contractions simulating seizures have been reported. Neuromuscular activation syndromes contribute to respiratory failure (Isbister and Bawaskar, 2014).

Pancreatitis
Pancreatitis may accompany systemic toxicity from Tityus and Leiurus species (Sucard, 2017).

Mortality

Stings are rarely fatal in developed countries but are still a significant cause of death in developing countries (Chippaux and Goyffon, 2008). Complications such as respiratory and cardiac shock, acute pulmonary edema, and progressive high blood pressure are generally listed among the causes of death in the first 24 hours (Boşnak et al., 2009).

Diagnosis

There are no specific diagnostic tests for scorpion poisoning (Abroug et al., 2020). Therefore, it is essential to ask questions about the event itself, investigate different epidemiological aspects, and identify dangerous species (Godoy et al., 2021).

Laboratory

Although laboratory findings are not essential for diagnosing scorpion poisoning, they help classification (Cupo, 2015). Lactic acidosis with leukocytosis, hyperglycemia, and hypokalemia may be seen in patients with systemic findings (Santos et al., 2016).

If cardiotoxicity develops in scorpion poisoning, troponin or CK-MB elevation is observed (Chakroun-Walha et al., 2018). If obtained, BNP or NT-proBNP is typically elevated (Cupo, 2015).

Hemolysis in adults is usually mild and resolves spontaneously within two to three weeks without treatment. However, hemolysis is severe in children and may progress with a rapid decrease in hemoglobin. DIC, microangiopathic anemia, acute pigment-related kidney damage, and, rarely, non-infectious HUS may develop (Dehghani et al., 2018). If DIC develops, thrombocytopenia, prolonged PT/INR, aPTT, increased D-dimer, and decreased fibrinogen levels may occur. If acute kidney injury develops, creatinine increase, uremia, hyperkalemia, and severe metabolic acidosis may be observed (Valavi et al., 2016).

Pancreatitis may accompany systemic toxicity from stings of the Tityus and Leiurus species. Elevated lipase or amylase indicates pancreatitis (Sucard, 2017).

Electrocardiogram

If cardiotoxicity has developed in scorpion poisoning, Q waves, ST-segment elevation or depression, T elevation or inversion, U waves, and/or prolonged QTc intervals may be seen (Chakroun-Walha et al., 2018).

Radiology

Pulmonary edema and cardiac enlargement on chest X-ray are important indicators of heart failure (Bawaskar and Bawaskar, 2012).

In patients with heart failure, echocardiography typically shows an acute, decreased ejection fraction with decreased left ventricular systolic function (Cupo and Hering S. E., 2002).

If neurological findings are present, imaging should include computerized tomography (CT) scan or magnetic resonance imaging (MRI) (Mosquera et al., 2003).

Management

The foundations of the specific therapeutic approach are early recognition of the sting, specific antivenom administration, and cardiorespiratory and systemic support (Abroug et al., 2020; Santos et al., 2016; Cupo, 2015).

Studies have shown that scorpion venom spreads very quickly throughout the body, so the time between the sting and application is very critical (Santana et al., 1996). The first precaution is to thoroughly wash the sting site to prevent the venom from spreading into the intravascular flow. Local ice or pressure dressing may be applied. If possible, the scorpion can be caught by taking the necessary safety precautions (Godoy et al., 2021).

Staging

Management is determined by the degree of poisoning. Various classification systems have been described for scorpion poisoning (Cupo, 2015; Isbister and Bawaskar, 2014; Bawaskar and Bawaskar, 2012; Khattabi et al., 2011). A current three-stage staging arranged according to the severity of signs and symptoms is presented below (Abroug et al., 2020; Santos et al., 2016; Cupo, 2015).

- Stage I (mild): Pain and erythema at the sting site; agitation, tachycardia.
- Stage II (moderate): In addition to the above symptoms, sweating, nausea, vomiting, tachypnea, and hypertension.
- Stage III (severe): Severe systemic and multiorgan life-threatening involvement.
- Stage III corresponds to being potentially fatal. At this stage, the risk of cardiovascular collapse is highest, associated with major respiratory complications: pulmonary edema, bronchospasm, and cyanosis (Bahloul, 2010).

General Principles

Wound Care

The bite areas of patients with scorpion stings should be cleaned, and tetanus prophylaxis should be provided when necessary (Isbister and Bawaskar, 2014). Tourniquet and local incision are not recommended (Bawaskar and Bawaskar, 2012). Excision of the area should be avoided as it does not prevent systemic toxicity and may create a larger and deeper wound. If extensive ulceration occurs, surgical debridement and skin grafting may be necessary (Dehghani et al., 2018).

Some patients with local effects after a scorpion sting may develop cardiotoxicity and autonomic dysfunction. Therefore, patients with local findings should be observed for up to 24 hours in an environment that can provide intensive care (Cupo, 2015).

Symptomatic Treatment

Symptomatic treatment aims to relieve pain using standard analgesics and anti-inflammatory drugs (Abroug et al., 2020; Santos et al., 2016; Cupo, 2015). The pain of patients with scorpion stings should be controlled. Oral nonsteroidal anti-inflammatory agents (e.g., ibuprofen or acetaminophen) are sufficient for pain management in many patients (Isbister and Bawaskar, 2014). In patients presenting with more severe pain, regional anesthesia can be applied using topical anesthetics (for example, lidocaine or tetracaine) or a long-acting agent (for example, bupivacaine) (Aksel et al., 2015).

Antiemetics (metoclopramide, ondansetron) are required in severe and recurrent vomiting cases (Godoy et al., 2021).

Atropine can potentiate sympathomimetic effects after poisoning. Therefore, it should be avoided unless severe bradycardia (hypotension and/or bradycardia with somnolence) or third-degree atrioventricular block develops (Isbister and Bawaskar, 2014).

Routine use of antihistamines, corticosteroids, and antibiotics is not recommended unless administered to reduce the severity of a possible allergic reaction to antivenom (Abroug et al., 2020; Santos et al., 2016; Cupo, 2015).

Neurological Symptoms

There is no specific treatment for neurological involvement in scorpion poisonings. Benzodiazepines (clonazepam) can be used in the presence of myoclonus. Seizures should be managed with antiepileptic drugs. Standard treatment is applied in stroke cases (Godoy et al., 2021).

Intensive Care Support

Although adults seem to be poisoned more often, children are more likely to develop serious illnesses that require intensive supportive care (LoVecchio and McBride, 2003). Elderly patients with systemic manifestations of Hemiscorpius lepturus poisoning and all children, regardless of the severity of the poisoning, should receive care in the intensive care unit (Dehghani et al., 2018). The first step in treatment is assessing and ensuring cardiorespiratory stability (Abroug et al., 2020; Santos et al., 2016; Cupo, 2015; Isbister and Bawaskar, 2014).

Heart Failure

Excessive release of catecholamines after scorpion poisoning can lead to heart failure. Prazosin acts as a vasodilator by preventing excessive catecholamine release. Thus, it provides treatment for heart failure and acute pulmonary edema and is more effective when given with antivenom (Rodrigo and Gnanathasan, 2017).

The combination of continuous introvenous nitroglycerin infusion and dobutamine has been used successfully to treat pulmonary edema and decompensated shock in critically ill patients (Isbister and Bawaskar, 2014). A different study comparing intravenous dobutamine with prazosin concluded that recovery is faster with prazosin in treating pulmonary edema in pediatric patients (Gupta et al., 2010).

Shock

In cases of cardiogenic shock (heart failure, myocarditis, neurogenic cardiomyopathy), measures to alleviate pulmonary edema and low cardiac output, including diuretics, inotropic drugs (dobutamine, milrinone), and in some cases alpha and beta-blockers, should be used. Furthermore, it is necessary to correct and stabilize the acute increase in hypertension with vasodilators (Abroug et al., 2020; Santos et al., 2016; Cupo, 2015; Isbister and Bawaskar, 2014).

In cases of distribution shock, appropriate use of isotonic fluids (0.9% saline) is required to correct the hypovolemic state and hypoperfusion due to intense vasodilation. If the mean arterial pressure does not improve despite volume expansion, the use of vasopressors (norepinephrine) is mandatory (Abroug et al., 2020; Santos et al., 2016; Cupo, 2015; Isbister and Bawaskar, 2014).

Respiratory Failure
Oxygen therapy can correct hypoxemia in mild to moderate cases of respiratory failure. If this is not enough, high-flow nasal cannulas or the initiation of non-invasive mechanical ventilation techniques is necessary (Abroug et al., 2020; Santos et al., 2016; Cupo, 2015; Isbister and Bawaskar, 2014).

When ARDS develops, deep sedoanalgesia and protective mechanical ventilation are required (Abroug et al., 2020). In severe cases, the prone (prone) position and neuromuscular blockers (vecuronium, atracurium) can be used (Godoy et al., 2021).

Sympathetic Toxicity
Prazosin, a postganglionic alpha 1-adrenergic receptor blocker, is the primary treatment for sympathetic storm due to excessive catecholamine release. Prazosin has also been shown to reduce the risk of progression to cardiotoxicity (Pandi et al., 2014). Studies have shown that prazosin reduces mortality (Bawaskar and Bawaskar, 2012; Gupta, 2006). The recommended dose of prazosin for scorpion poisoning is 0.5 mg (30 micrograms/kg, maximum dose 0.5 mg) orally or via gastric tube every three hours until systemic toxicity resolves (Gupta, 2006).

Hemolysis
The hemoglobin or hematocrit values of patients with laboratory findings consistent with hemolysis should be monitored frequently. Patients with symptomatic anemia should receive a blood transfusion (Valavi et al., 2016).

Antivenom

Antivenom treatment is recommended for patients after scorpion bites (Bahloul et al., 2013, Cupo, 2015). Intravenous administration of scorpion antivenom is intended to block the action of the venom. The dosage depends on the severity of the condition and the type of serum present (Abroug et al., 2020; Santos et al., 2016).

Duration
The time between the bite and administration of the antivenom is critical (Godoy et al., 2021). Pharmacokinetic studies have shown that the subcutaneous absorption of the venom is rapid and reaches its lowest value in 60 minutes (Cupo, 2015). Therefore, administration of the antivenom within one hour significantly reduces the venom concentration (Godoy et al., 2021).

Discussions
The effectiveness of the antivenom has not been convincingly proven. The antidote only neutralizes the circulating and absorbed toxin at the sting site. It does not neutralize the toxin or the released mediators attached to the nerve endings. Therefore, its use is controversial, especially in cases with severe systemic disorders (Abroug et al., 2020; Santos et al., 2016; Cupo, 2015; Isbister and Bawaskar, 2014).

A study on children showed that using antidotes for scorpion stings such as Centruroides sculpturatus in the USA is beneficial. This study showed that neurotoxic symptoms improved 4 hours after antivenom infusion, and the total midazolam requirement required for the treatment of agitation decreased (Boyer et al., 2009). Similarly, LoVecchio et al., have been shown that recovery time is shortened in children younger than two years of age who use anti-Centruroides sp. antivenom for stings (2003). Rodrigo et al.,'s meta-analysis of Centruroides sculpturatus has shown that antidote administration is beneficial for scorpion stings (2017).

Two randomized trials using serum plus prazosin specific to Mesobuthus species (red scorpion) in children in India showed greater efficacy when antivenom was added to the treatment compared to the use of prazosin alone (Pandi et al., 2014).

Since scorpion species are heterogeneous, the effectiveness of the antidote cannot be generalized (Foex, 2011).

Antivenom Indications

Recommendations for using scorpion-specific antidotes vary with specific scorpion species. Intravenous scorpion-specific antivenom is recommended for patients stung by Hottentotta species. Antivenom administered to patients with stage II poisoning also significantly reduces the amount of medication needed to control hypertension and prevents progression to cardiotoxicity (Pandi et al., 2014; Rodrigo and Gnanathasan, 2017).

There are no studies of intravenous scorpion-specific antivenom efficacy for patients stung by Tityus or Leiurus species. However, although the evidence for antivenom to Leiurus species is inconsistent, small observational studies suggest potential benefits in patients with cardiotoxicity (De Rezende et al., 1995).

For patients with systemic toxicity after Hemiscorpius lepturus stings, it is recommended that Razi polyvalent scorpion antidote (Karaj, Iran) be administered intravenously as soon as possible, ideally within two hours after the sting (Seyedian et al., 2012).

Evidence does not support the administration of a scorpion-specific antidote to patients with Grade II or higher poisoning after being stung by Androctonus or Buthus species (Rodrigo and Gnanathasan, 2017).

Dose of Antivenom

The dose of antivenom depends on the type of scorpion that stings, the estimated amount of venom entering the body at the time of the sting, and the severity of the poisoning (Cupo, 2015); e.g., in South Africa, antivenom is available in 5 mL ampoules. The standard dose is one to two ampoules intravenously for adults and children. An additional 5 mL dose may be administered if the clinical response is inadequate. The efficacy of one or three doses of antivenom for Centruroides spp. is similar in the United States (Quan et al., 2019). Clinicians should follow the directions of their local experts and the manufacturer's instructions when determining the antivenom dose (Isbister and Bawaskar, 2014).

Allergy

Except for antidotes produced in Iran and Egypt, scorpion antidotes consist of equine derivative F(ab')2 fragments. Limited evidence from small studies suggests a low risk of anaphylaxis or serum sickness after scorpion-specific F(ab')2 equine antivenom. Allergic reactions should be managed by immediately stopping the IV infusion of the antidote and treating symptoms appropriately (Pandi et al., 2014; Rodrigo and Gnanathasan, 2017).

Conclusion

Scorpion stings are a life-threatening medical emergency, especially in underdeveloped countries. The number of known scorpion species is increasing day by day. Today, the number of scorpions that can be fatal to humans is small. However, scorpion poisoning can cause cardiotoxicity, neurotoxicity, and multiorgan failure, especially in children.

As scorpion venom spreads very quickly throughout the body, early diagnosis and treatment are important. There is no specific test for diagnosing scorpion poisoning: the patient's history and knowledge of the venomous species common in the area aid in the diagnosis.

The treatment consists of local wound care, pain control, specific antivenom administration, symptomatic treatment in patients with systemic findings, and intensive care support in severe cases.

Precautions such as environmental cleaning and not walking barefoot protect against scorpion stings.

References

Aboumaâd, B., Lahssaini, M., Tiger, A. and Benhassain, S. M. (2014). Clinical comparison of scorpion envenomation by Androctonus mauritanicus and Buthus occitanus in children. *Toxicon*, 90, 337-43.

Abroug, F., Ouanes-Besbes, L., Ouanes, I., Dachraoui, F., Hassen, MF., Haguiga, H., ... Brun-Buisson, C. (2011). Meta-analysis of controlled studies on immunotherapy in severe scorpion envenomation. *Emerg Med J*, 28, 963-9.

Abroug, F., Ouanes-Besbes, L., Tilouche, N. and Elatrous S. (2020). Scorpion envenomation: state of the art. *Intensive Care Med*, 46, 401-10.

Aksel, G., Güler, S., Doğan, N. Ö. and Çorbacioğlu, Ş. K. (2015). A randomized trial comparing intravenous paracetamol, topical lidocaine, and ice application for treatment of pain associated with scorpion stings. *Hum Exp Toxicol*, 34:662-70.

Bahloul, M., Chaari, A., Dammak, H., Samet, M., Chtara, K., Chelly, H., ... Bouaziz, M. (2013). Pulmonary edema following scorpion envenomation: mechanisms, clinical manifestations, diagnosis and treatment. *Int J Cardiol*, 162, 86-91.

Bahloul, M., Chabchoub, I., Chaari, A., Chtara, K., Kallel, H., Dammak, H., ... Bouaziz, M. (2010). Scorpion envenomation among children: clinical manifestations and outcome (analysis of 685 cases). *Am J Trop Med Hyg*, 83, 1084-92.

Bawaskar, H. S. and Bawaskar P. H. (2012). Scorpion sting: update. *J Assoc Physicians India*, 60:46-55.

Bergman, N. J. (1997). Clinical description of Parabuthus transvaalicus scorpionism in Zimbabwe. *Toxicon*, 35, 759-771.

Binorkar, S. and Parlikar R. (2016). Epidemiology, presentation and integrated management of scorpion sting envenomation. *Int J Pharmacol Toxicol*, 4, 33-9.

Boşnak, M., Ece, A., Yolbaş, İ., Boşnak V., Kaplan, M. and Gürkan, F. (2009). Scorpion sting envenomation in children in southeast Turkey. *Wilderness Environ Med*, 20(2), 118-24.

Boyer, L. V., Theodorou, A. A., Berg, R. A., Mallie, J., Chávez-Méndez, A., García-Ubbelohde, W., ... Alagón, A. (2009). Antivenom for critically ill children with neurotoxicity from scorpion stings. *N Engl J Med*, 360, 2090-8.

Chakroun-Walha, O., Karray, R., Jerbi, M., Nasri, A., Issaoui, F., Amine, B. R., ... and Rekik, N. (2018). Update on the Epidemiology of Scorpion Envenomation in the South of Tunisia. *Wilderness Environ Med*, 29(1), 29-35.

Chippaux, J. P. and Goyffon, M. (2008). Epidemiology of scorpionism: a global appraisal. *Acta Trop*, 107, 71-9.

Cupo, P and Hering, S. E. (2002). Cardiac troponin I release after severe scorpion envenoming by Tityus serrulatus. *Toxicon*, 40:823-30.

Cupo, P. (2015). Clinical update on scorpion envenoming. *Rev Soc Bras Med Trop*, 48, 642-9.

De Rezende, N. A., Dias, M. B., Campolina, D., Chavez-Olortegui, C., Diniz, C. R. and Amaral, C. F. (1995). Efficacy of antivenom therapy for neutralizing circulating venom antigens in patients stung by Tityus serrulatus scorpions. *Am J Trop Med Hyg*, 1995, 52:277-80.

Dehghani, R. and Fathi, B. (2012). Scorpion sting in Iran: a review. *Toxicon*, 60, 919-33.

Dehghani, R., Kamiabi, F. and Mohammadi, M. (2018). Scorpionism by Hemiscorpius spp. in Iran: a review. *J Venom Anim Toxins Incl Trop Dis*, 24, 8.

Dube, S., Sharma, V. K., Dubey, T. N., Gouda, N. B. and Shrivastava, V. (2011). Fatal intracerebral haemorrhage following scorpion sting. *J Indian Med Assoc*, 109, 194-5.

Foex, B. A. (2011). Meta-analysis of controlled studies on immunotherapy in severe scorpion envenomation: a commentary. *Emerg Med J*, 28(11), 915-6.

Godoy, D. A., Badenes, R., Seifi, S., Salehi, S. and Seifi, A. (2021). Neurological and Systemic Manifestations of Severe Scorpion Envenomation. *Cureus*, 13(4), e14715.

Gupta, B. D., Parakh, M. and Purohit, A. (2010). Management of scorpion sting: prazosin or dobutamine. *J Trop Pediatr*, 56(2), 115-8.

Gupta, S., Tewari, A. and Nair, V. (2012). Cerebellar infarct with neurogenic pulmonary edema following viper bite. *J Neurosci Rural Pract*, 3, 74-6.

Gupta, V. (2006). Prazosin: a pharmacological antidote for scorpion envenomation. *J Trop Pediatr*, 52(2), 150-1.

Isbister, G. K. and Bawaskar, H. S. (2014). Scorpion envenomation. *N Engl J Med*, 371, 457-63.

Jalali, A., Bavarsad-Omidian, N., Babaei, M., Najafzadeh, H. and Rezaei, S. (2012). The pharmacokinetics of Hemiscorpius lepturus scorpion venom and Razi antivenom following intramuscular administration in rat. *J Venom Res*, 3:1-6.

Khattabi, A., Soulaymani-Bencheikh, R., Achour, S. and Salmi, LR. (2011). Classification of clinical consequences of scorpion stings: consensus development. *Trans R Soc Trop Med Hyg*, 105, 364-369.

Lourenço, W. R. (2016). Scorpion incidents, misidentification cases and possible implications for the final interpretation of results. *J Venom Anim Toxins incl Trop Dis*, 22, 1.

LoVecchio, F. and McBride, C. (2003). Scorpion envenomations in young children in central Arizona. *J Toxicol Clin Toxicol*, 41(7), 937-40.

Mosquera, A., Idrovo, L. A., Tafur, A. and Del Brutto, O. H. (2003). Stroke following Bothrops spp. snakebite. *Neurology*, 60, 1577-80.

Nagaraj, S. K., Dattatreya, P. and Boramuthi, T. N. (2015). Indian scorpions collected in Karnataka: maintenance in captivity, venom extraction and toxicity studies. *J Venom Anim Toxins Incl Trop Dis*, 4, 21, 51.

O'Connor, A. D., Padilla-Jones, A. and Ruha A. M. (2018). Severe bark scorpion envenomation in adults. *Clin Toxicol (Phila)*, 56(3), 170-174.

Pandi, K., Krishnamurthy, S., Srinivasaraghavan, R. and Mahadevan, S. (2014). Efficacy of scorpion antivenom plus prazosin versus prazosin alone for Mesobuthus tamulus scorpion sting envenomation in children: a randomised controlled trial. *Arch Dis Child*, 99, 575-80.

Petricevich, V. L. (2010). Scorpion venom and the inflammatory response. *Mediators Inflamm*, 2010, 903295.

Quan, D., LoVecchio, F., Bhattarai, B., Flores, M., Frechette, A. and Sinha, M. (2019). Comparing clinical outcomes between two scorpion antivenom dosing strategies in children. *Clin Toxicol (Phila)*, 57, 760-4.

Radmanesh, M. (1998). Cutaneous manifestations of the Hemiscorpius lepturus sting: a clinical study. *Int J Dermatol*, 37, 500-7.

Rodrigo, C. and Gnanathasan, A. (2017). Management of scorpion envenoming: a systematic review and meta-analysis of controlled clinical trials. *Syst Rev*, 6(1), 74.

Sandoval, M. R. and Lebrun, I. (2002). TsTx toxin isolated from Tityus serrulatus scorpion venom-induced spontaneous recurrent seizures and mossy fiber sprouting. *Epilepsia*, 43:36.

Santos, M. S., Silva, C. G., Neto, B. S., Grangeiro Júnior, C. R., Lopes, V. H., Teixeira Júnior, A. G., ... and Lima, MA. (2016). Clinical and Epidemiological Aspects of Scorpionism in the World: A Systematic Review. *Wilderness Environ Med*, 27, 504-518.

Seyedian, R., Jalali, A., Babaee, M. H., Pipelzadeh, M. H. and Rezaee, S. (2012). A biodistribution study of Hemiscorpius lepturus scorpion venom and available polyclonal antivenom in rats. *J Venom Anim Toxins Incl Trop Dis*, 18(4).

Sousa, P., Arnedo M. and Harris D. J. (2017). Updated catalogue and taxonomic notes on the old-world scorpion genus Buthus leach, 1815 (Scorpiones, Buthidae). *ZooKeys*, 686, 15-84.

Sucard, J. R. (2017). Scorpion envenomation. In: *Auerbach's Wilderness Medicine*, 7th edition, Auerback, P. S., Cushing, T. A., Harris, N. S. (Eds), Elsevier, Philadelphia. Vol 1, p. 1017.

Torabi, E., Behdani, M., Chafi, M. H., Moazzami, R., Sabatier, J. M., Khalaj, V., … and lethality of a novel recombinant dermonecrotic venom phospholipase D from Hemiscorpius lepturus. *Toxins*, 9, 102-118.

Valavi, E., Amuri, P., Ahmadzadeh, A., Bahman Cheraghian, B. and Ahankoob, E. (2016). Acute kidney injury in Hemiscorpius lepturus scorpion stung children: Risk factors and clinical features. *Saudi J Kidney Dis Transpl*, 27:936-41.

Chapter 15

Snakebites

Şener Cindoruk*, MD and İremgül Güngör, MD

Samsun Training and Research Hospital, Department of Emergency Medicine, Samsun, Turkey

Abstract

Snakebites or stings are seen in almost all continents of the world. Venomous snakes are responsible for approximately 1.5-3 million snakebites and possibly over 100,000 deaths annually worldwide. Venomous snakes are usually species with triangular, elliptical pupils in head shapes, pits in front of their pupils to detect heat, and single rowed tail scales. Sharp teeth marks on the bite mark suggest that the snake bite is poisonous. Non-venomous snakes generally have an oval head structure, round pupils, no sharp teeth, and double-rowed tail scales. There are many teeth marks in the bite mark. Snake venom mainly causes neurotoxicity and hematotoxicity. Although snakebite causes severe intoxication, the mortality rate is low with appropriate first aid intervention and effective treatment. Tourniquets should not be used; compression bands or elastic bandages can prevent edema and delay poison absorption without disturbing the circulation. The first 6-8 hours after a snake bite are critical. Antivenom is the most crucial step in the treatment of venomous snake bites. If there are clear clinical findings or laboratory abnormalities of systemic poisoning, such as neurotoxic action, consumption coagulopathy, rhabdomyolysis, cardiogenic shock, renal failure or significant local tissue injury, the patient should be given antivenom. If there are no signs of systemic poisoning, the changes should be monitored for at least 12 hours, or even longer for some snake species.

Keywords: snakebite, poisoning, environmental emergencies

Introduction

Snakebites or stings can cause problems for people in almost all continents of the world. They are more common in countries with tropical and subtropical climates. About 600 of the 3000 snake species known to live on Earth are venomous. Venomous snakes are responsible for approximately 1.5-3 million bites and possibly more than 100,000 deaths annually worldwide

---

* Corresponding Author's Email: drsener06@gmail.com.

In: Environmental Emergencies and Injuries in Nature
Editors: Murat Yücel, Murat Güzel and İbrahim İkizceli
ISBN: 978-1-68507-833-1

(Tintinalli, 2019). Snake bites are responsible for significant mortality and morbidity worldwide, especially in the south and southeast of the Asian continent, Africa, and Latin America (Aziz et al., 2015). Venomous snakes usually bite their prey and rarely bite people they see as a threat. Snake bites are a condition that can cause more than 120,000 deaths each year (Bhaumik et al., 2020). Although snakebites cause severe intoxication, the mortality rate is low with appropriate first aid intervention and effective treatment (Açikalin et al., 2008). Due to the availability of antivenom, ease of access, and improvements in emergency and intensive care, mortality rates are below 0.5% today (Mowry et al., 2016).

According to some characteristics of the snake and the bite, it can be predicted whether it is poisonous or non-poisonous. Venomous snakes are usually species with triangular, elliptical pupils in head shapes, pits in front of their pupils to detect heat, and single-rowed tail scales. Sharp teeth marks on the bite mark suggest that the snake bite is poisonous. Non-venomous snakes generally have an oval head structure, round pupils, no sharp teeth, and double-rowed tail scales. There are many teeth marks in the bite mark (Kundanati et al., 2020; Walls, 2017). The four venomous snake families are Colubridae (representing 70% of all snake species), Elapidae, Viperidae, and Atractaspididae. In regard to Colubridae, this family has very little risk for venomous bites in humans as they are posterior-toothed snakes. The Elapidae family includes cobras, kraits, mambas, and coral snakes and these are more prevalent than other snake families. The Hydrophiidae family includes sea snakes. The Viperidae family includes the Gaboon viper, the Russell viper represented by the puff adder, the saw-scale and the European viper. The Crotalidae (pit vipers) are occasionally accepted as a separate family and occasionally as a subfamily of the Viperidae (Walls, 2017). Snake bites caused by the Viperidae (like pit vipers) and Elapidae (like kraits and cobras) families are particularly dangerous to humans (Kasturiratne et al., 2008; Walls, 2017).

Snake venom mainly causes neurotoxicity and hematotoxicity. The venoms in the more common usage of the toxic components include enzymes, glycoproteins, polypeptides, and low molecular weight organic compounds The proteins that manufacture the most toxic expressions make up 90 to 95% of the venom. Polypeptides are structurally smaller than proteins and absorbed more rapidly, which may explain the effects of venom on neuro-neuronal junctional and neuromuscular junctional membranes and also other organ systems. Phospholipase A may inhibit electron transfer at the cytochrome c level and hydrolyzed mitochondrial enzymes. Correspondingly, phospholipids at the myeline in nerve axons might hydrolyze, acetylcholine at the myoneural junction might separate, and this acetylcholine leads to myonecrosis and causes destruction of erythrocyte membranes. This single enzyme has been recognized in all venoms from the Hydrophiidae, Elapidae, Viperidae and Crotalinae spp. investigated so far (Walls, 2017). Symptoms can typically be classified as local findings or systemic findings. Local findings are usually originated by the enzymatic effect on the cellular and non-cellular structures in the patient's tissues at the bite site. These enzymes can provoke coagulopathy, cell damage, bleeding, hemolysis, and devastation of organelles (Casewell et al., 2020). In some venomous snakes like Elapidae and Hydrophiidae venoms have predominantly systemic findings, and in some venomous snakes like Colubridae, Viperidae, and Crotalinae venoms have predominantly local findings (Walls, 2017).

Crotalin/Pit Viper Snakes

Crotalin snakes belong to the Viperidae family. They are named pit vipers due to the pits located at the middle level between the eye and nostril. Crotalin or pit viper snakes are also discriminated by the presence of two poisoned fangs that fold towards the upper part of the mouth. The rattle distinguishes the rattlesnake from other Crotalin snakes. Rattlesnakes do not always rattle before attacking; many attacks occur without a warning rattle (Tintinalli, 2019). Up to 25% of Crotalin snake bites are dry bites: no local or systemic venom effects develop. The poisoning process is determined by the snake's type and size, the victim's age and size, the time passing after the bite and the characteristics of the snakebite, for example, the location, depth, width and number, and the amount of venom. Therefore, the severity of poisoning after a Crotalin bite is variable (Gold et al., 2002). Initially minor and unimportant damage might develop into a more severe bite. This kind of bite could require large amounts of antivenom.

Elapidae Snakes

Cobras and coral snakes make up a significant portion. In coral snakes, there are Mojave rattlesnakes, many exotic snakes, an eastern coral snake named "Micrurus fulvius," a Texas coral snake named "Micrurus tener," and an Arizona or Sonoran coral snake named "Micruroides euryxanthus." Coral snakes cause about 25 bites every year. All coral snakes have shiny red, yellow and black rings (Tednes and Slesinger, 2021). With the bite of their elapids, signs and symptoms can vary significantly. It can cause a wide range of responses ranging from mild pain and swelling to death. The effects of the venom can even begin hours later, have irreversible consequences, and often require antivenom.

Clinical Features

The signs and symptoms of snakebite are highly variable; the way to assess the severity of the bite is through the patient's clinic. Local poisoning, if left untreated, can cause serious systemic problems as toxic products are absorbed. Victims of a previous snake bite may develop an immunoglobulin E (IgE)-mediated anaphylactic-type reaction upon re-exposure to the venom, and enzymes that stimulated the release of some neurotransmitter such as bradykinin, histamine, and serotonin from the patient's cells determine the severity of anaphylaxis. The effects vary from minimal pain to multiple system failures and also death can be seen within a few days (Walls, 2017).

The signs of crotalin poisoning are tooth scarring, pain at the bite site, and the presence of progressive edema. In general, local swelling occurs within 15-30 minutes after bites. However, in some cases, swelling might not begin within a few hours. In serious cases, edema can impress the whole limb inside an hour (Anz et al., 2010). In milder cases, edema may progress within 1-2 days. The edema in a muscle caused by head and neck bites progresses to compartment syndrome. These kinds of bites can be life-threatening without causing systemic effects. Leakage of blood into the subcutaneous tissue may cause progressive ecchymosis. Ecchymoses might occur in minutes, and hemorrhagic bullae might appear within a few hours (Levine et al.,

2014). Other accompanying findings: Systemic findings such as nausea, vomiting, weakness, numbness in the mouth and tongue, dizziness, muscle fasciculation, cranial nerve weakness due to neuromuscular conduction blockade, ptosis, tachypnea, increased vascular permeability, hypotension, tachycardia, angioedema, and altered consciousness may also be seen. It can cause coagulopathy by activating and depleting fibrinogen and platelets. Hemoconcentration often develops due to fluid extravasation into the subcutaneous tissue; when intravascular volume is restored, the hemoglobin level can be decreased within a few days (Tintinalli, 2019; Walls, 2017). Mortality is rarer in distal bites and significantly increases in intravenous (IV) bites. Death after Crotalin bites is clinically relevant with consumption coagulopathy and increased vascular permeability. Essentially, it leads to pulmonary edema, shock, and death. Secondary to these mechanisms, heart and kidney damage occurs. Certain toxins can act directly on organs, such as the heart, vessels, kidneys, lungs, brain or skeletal muscle (Walls, 2017).

Dry bites are thought to occur frequently in the members of the Elapidae family, namely coral snakes. The poisons of the elapids have an inhibitory effect on the heart and skeletal muscle, blocking neuromuscular transmission through acetylcholine receptors. This often causes descending symmetric flaccid paralysis. Symptoms usually develop 2 to 12 hours after the bite happens. Other symptoms include agitation, ptosis, diplopia, myotic pupils, facial asymmetry, dysarthria, vertigo, paresthesias, fasciculations, seizure, rhabdomyolysis, coagulopathy, intracranial hemorrhage, dyspnea, dysphagia, hypersalivation, nausea, respiratory distress, hypoventilation, loss of airway control, and respiratory paralysis. Procoagulant toxins can cause consumptive coagulopathy. After a snakebite hypotension, myoglobinuria, rhabdomyolysis, and direct renal toxicity may occur (Tintinalli, 2019; Walls, 2017). Some cobras in Africa and Asia can spit venom several meters away. If spit in the eye, it is poison; it can cause a painful acute corneal injury, poison ophthalmopathy, and transient blindness, but systemic poisoning does not occur (Tintinalli, 2019).

In general, the bite of a spitting cobra causes moderate to severe local effects, including necrosis, with rare paralytic effects in most species (Tintinalli, 2019). The bite mark gives a risk of bacterial contamination related with gram-negative organisms, and microorganisms which predominate in the snake venom and mouth are cultured. However, many studies show that prophylactic antibiotics for these microorganisms are not indicated for snake bites. Besides, these snake bites cause tetanus, osteomyelitis, cellulitis, or gas gangrene accompanied with or without poisoning cases. This often happens significantly when extensive local tissue destruction has occurred, treatment is delayed, or the primary examination is not performed correctly and at the site (Greene et al., 2021).

Diagnosis

Snakebite diagnoses with presence of teeth sings and a history such a disclosure to snake in a field. Snake poisoning is diagnosed by demonstrating the presence of a snake bite and tissue damage. Clinically, damage may present in three ways: local injury (like edema, pain, ecchymosis), hematological abnormality (like thrombocytopenia, increased prothrombin time, hypofibrinogenemia), or systemic findings (paresthesias at the rim of the mouth, mucosal edema around the mouth, hypotension, tachycardia, metallic body or rubbery taste). Abnormalities in these areas show that the toxic effects are developing. If there are none of these symptoms for 8 to 12 hours after the snakebite, this means a dry bite (Tintinalli, 2019).

Essential findings, electrocardiogram, hemoglobin level, platelet count, electrolyte levels, kidney function tests (blood urea nitrogen and creatine), creatine kinase, fibrinogen, fibrin breakdown products, electrolytes, prothrombin time (PT), INR (international normalized ratio), activated partial thromboplastin time (aPTT), d-dimer, and urinalysis should be evaluated. For plasma replacement, erythrocyte suspension, whole blood, blood group, and a cross match sample should be taken (Walls, 2017). Enzyme-linked immunosorbent assay (ELISA) testing can be done for specific rattlesnake species. Still, the emergency department's turnaround time is too long and will not yield any treatment change (Gilliam et al., 2013). Laboratory tests usually determine whether a patient needs antivenom therapy. These tests should be done at admission and 6 and 12 hours after the bite (earlier if clinical abnormalities develop). Coagulopathy, rhabdomyolysis, kidney damage, hyponatremia, and a syndrome similar to hemolytic-uremic syndrome (thrombocytopenia, anemia, intravascular hemolysis) may be observed. The Snake Venom Detection Kit® "SVDK; bioCSL, Parkville, Victoria, Australia" can be used to classify snake venom at the bite location or in the urine (Tintinalli, 2019). Ultrasonography can be used to assess the extent and depth of the dermatological involvement of a snake bite (Vohra et al., 2014). Differential diagnosis of venomous snake bites includes dry bites, non-venomous snake bites, spider and tick bites, scorpion and Hymenoptera stings, dermatological diseases such as toxic epidermal necrolysis (TEN), Stevens-Johnson syndrome, and methicillin-resistant staphylococcus aureus (MRSA) infection (Walls, 2017).

Treatment

First-aid measures should never replace definitive therapy and should not delay antivenom administration. If possible, separate the victim from the snake to avoid more bites. Use a big stick, or another object longer than the snake to push the snake away from the victim. If necessary, kill the snake by striking the back of its head. If possible, the snake species should be identified with safety in mind. All patients bitten by Crotalin snakes should be taken to the healthcare center or hospital. Threatening first aid practices like aspiration and incision should be avoided. Electrotherapy of the bite location is difficult and useless; it could be causing electrical injuries. Submergence in icy water worsens the injury. Using ice will not help to slow the spread of the venom, but an icepack covered by a towel and put on the bitten area will help to reduce pain. The tourniquet should not be used; it obstructs the arterial flow and causes ischemia. Compression bands or elastic bandages can be instrumental in the absence of emergency medical care, being wrapped circumferentially over the bite, and applied with tension to restrict superficial venous and lymphatic flow while preserving distal pulses and capillary filling. The aim is to prevent edema and delay venom absorption. The excitement and physical activity of the patient, movement of the bitten area, alcohol consumption, and a deeper bite may increase the spread of the venom. This situation can be somewhat reduced by calming the victim, immobilizing the bitten area, and not giving the victim anything by mouth. The compression immobilization bandage is a compression pad placed over the bite site combined with a tight elastic bandage wrap and limb immobilization. This technique is recommended for coral snakes and other elapid snake bites but is generally not recommended for Crotalin bites as it can increase pain in the area (Tintinalli, 2019; Walls, 2017). Limb immobilization and neutral positioning are provided in the prehospital phase to reduce venom absorption and pain. Do not loosen tourniquets or constrictor bands so far as the antivenom is available, except for overtightened tourniquets that impair arterial circulation, which may cause limb ischemia. It is anticipated that systemic poisoning may progress rapidly upon local injury, and advanced life support measures should be taken. An IV route should be established from an area other than the bite area, and oxygen support should be started. If feasible, extra medical treatments should be initiated, such as cardiac monitoring, IV fluids, and drugs like adrenaline and analgesics. If the patient is hypotensive, quickly give IV isotonic fluids. He should be transferred to a center where snake poisoning is managed (Tintinalli, 2019; Walls, 2017).

In the emergency room, the patient's anamnesis by the clinician should include the time since the bite, the number of bites, whether first aid was given, and the type, location, and symptoms of the bite (e.g., pain, numbness, nausea, tingling around the mouth, metallic taste in the mouth, muscle cramps, shortness of breath, and dizziness). A brief medical history should include recent tetanus vaccination, medications, and any cardiovascular, hematological, renal, and respiratory problems. A history of allergies to wool-containing materials, papaya, papain, chymopapain, or pineapple should be taken, emphasizing symptoms after horse or sheep product exposure. All snake bites should be evaluated and monitored to provide advanced life support. The first 6-8 hours after a snake bite are very important. During this time, medical treatment can help to prevent the morbidity and mortality associated with severe poisoning.

Antivenom is the most crucial step in the treatment of venomous snake bites. It should be given when there is clarity of clinical findings or a laboratory abnormality of systemic poisoning. Clinical indications to antivenom treatment include neurotoxic impacts like ptosis, cranial nerve damage, progressive muscle fragility or diaphragm paralysis, respiratory insufficiency, cardiogenic shock, consumption coagulopathy, rhabdomyolysis, acute renal failure, critical local tissue damage, or vomiting recalcitrant to antiemetics. In the non-presence of systemic poisoning evidence, the patient should be observed for at least 12 hours or longer for some species (Hall, 2001).

Poisoning can be divided into five grades according to its severity, from grade 0 (no signs of intoxication) to grade IV (very serious poisoning), and the amount of antidote can be correlated with the degree of poisoning:

- *Grade 0*: There is no evidence of poisoning, but a suspected snakebite. It could be a bite mark. There is pain, a less than one-inch circumferential edema, and minimal erythema. Systemic signs and laboratory changes are not seen in the first 12 hours after the bite. Antivenom is not used; wound care, tetanus prophylaxis, and the IV route are followed, for 8-12 hours.
- *Grade I*: There is mild poisoning, and snakebite is suspicious. A tooth mark is usually present. The pain is mild or moderate, and throbbing. This injury has 1 to 5 inches of edema and is surrounded by erythema. Systemic symptoms and laboratory changes are not seen within 12 hours. Antivenom is usually not used, but one vial can be used if edema progresses. This is followed by routine wound care, tetanus prophylaxis and the IV route, for 12-24 hours.
- *Grade II*: Moderate intoxication, there is more serious and widespread pain, swelling spreads to the limb and also ecchymoses and petechiae in the edema area. Nausea, vomiting, and subfebrile fever are present. Depending on the severity of the poisoning, 2-4 vials of antivenom can be used. Routine wound care, tetanus prophylaxis, the IV

route, monitoring, antibiotherapy, analgesics, and hydration are recommended. Depending on the clinical situation, service/intensive care follow-up is required.

- *Grade III*: Intoxication is serious. These cases may be initially similar to grade I or II poisonings but may progress rapidly. Inside 12 hours, swelling spreads to the extremities and may affect part of the limb and also petechiae and ecchymoses may spread. Systemic involvement and laboratory abnormalities occur. Depending on the severity of poisoning, 4-6 vials or more of antivenom can be used depending on the response. Routine wound care, tetanus prophylaxis, the IV route, monitoring, antibiotherapy, analgesics, and hydration are recommended. A fasciotomy is required if compartment syndrome develops. The patient needs intensive care follow-up.

- *Grade IV*: Intoxication is very serious and most commonly seen after the bite of a giant rattle snake. It is characterized by sudden, searing pain, rapidly progressive edema that can reach and involve the limb inside a few hours, ecchymosis, a hemorrhagic bullae pattern, and necrosis. Systemic symptoms, which usually begin 15 minutes after the bite, can be seen. An intravenous bite can result in death because of cardiopulmonary arrest immediately after the bite (Walls, 2017).

Dart et al., proposed different rating systems and higher doses of antidotes: Grades 0 and I represent minimal poisoning, grade II represents moderate poisoning, and grades III and IV serious poisoning. Both systems can be used interchangeably. Grade II-III-IV poisonings are candidates for antivenom (Dart et al., 2001).

Antivenom consists of heterologic antibodies produced from the serum of animals that are immunized with the proper snake venom. The immune serum is collected from host animals (e.g., horse, sheep) and then digested with papain (FabAV) or pepsin (Fab2AV) to produce antibody fragments. Antibodies bind and neutralize poison molecules. All snakebite patients who develop progressive symptoms should be treated with antivenom. Progression is defined as worsening local damage, abnormal laboratory results, or systemic manifestations. The antivenom should be diluted intravenously to create a "first control." Skin testing is not recommended before application and should be prepared for the treatment of anaphylaxis. The first control goal is to stop the progression of clinical worsening. Documentation of the initial control is critical because the most common error in management is underdosing early in treatment. There is no definite dose for the initial antivenom dose. Dilute the determined dose of antivenom to approximately 1:10 in saline (reduced dilution may be considered in children and adults with heart or renal failure), start the infusion slowly in case of an allergic reaction; step by step, increase the speed to deliver the total dose in about 20-30 minutes. Give children the same dose as adults. A child who has been bitten usually takes in more venom per body weight, so more antivenom is needed to neutralize it. After the initial control is achieved, two vials of maintenance doses are recommended for FabAV. Fab2AV dosing schedules differ, and the healthcare provider should consider using antivenom according to product labeling and in consultation with a poison center (Lavonas et al., 2004). The whole volume may be reduced in children but the same number of vials should be given. The intraosseous (IO) path can be used if IV path access is not available; nevertheless, antivenom should not be injected intramuscularly. Venom-induced hypovolemia may delay the absorption of the antidote and therefore, an antivenom injection must be given at a critical care unit like the emergency room or intensive care unit with direct physician oversight and presenting resuscitative drugs (including epinephrine) and equipment. If an anaphylaxis or the other acute allergic reaction to the antivenom occurs, immediately pause the infusion and use antihistamines (histamine-1 or/and histamine-2 receptor blockers). For anaphylaxis, epinephrine must be readily applicable. Continue to monitor for the progression and increasing of edema and findings of systemic poisoning and later on antivenom infusion. Evaluate limb circumference at various sites of the upper and lower bite and draw the progressive margin of swelling with a pencil every 30 minutes. These various measures are an objective indicator of progress and management for antivenom implementation – recount the laboratory tests every 4 hours or/and later each antivenom treatment. Recall doses of antivenom might be required if the patient's clinical status rapidly declines. Perform isotonic fluid infusion followed by vasopressor agents like norepinephrine or epinephrine, for hypotension. Antivenom is the first treatment for hematological abnormalities, but if active hemorrhage occurs, plasmapheresis may be required after antivenom administration. Compartment syndrome is another complication of snake bites. When the venom is injected or spreads to a muscle compartment, the pressure may increase, manifested by severe pain, usually localized and resistant to opiate analgesics. The use of fasciotomy is doubtful, as there is not enough conclusive evidence to support its use. Clean up the bite site and determine the necessity for tetanus vaccination. Take wound samples for culture and assess antibiotics if there are findings of infection. Despite the fact that some authors recommend antibiotic prophylaxis, available data do not defend its use. Using steroids is not essential; routine use is not recommended. However, they should be used to treat allergic reactions or serum sickness. Although serum sickness is rare after antivenom treatment, it should be considered in the presence of fever, rash, and arthralgia (Tintinalli, 2019; Walls, 2017). Most patients acquire over ten vials of equine serum-derived antivenom, and roughly 15% of patients receiving FabAV develop serum sickness up to one week later. It can be used to administer diphenhydramine and cimetidine and, in severe cases, for corticosteroid therapy (Walls, 2017).

Antivenom cannot preserve toxic findings, such as descending symmetric flaccid paralysis, rhabdomyolysis and acute renal failure. Therefore, it is essential to anticipate and implement antivenom early. If this is impossible, support respiratory and renal function as necessary for the clinical status. Developing descending symmetric flaccid paralysis commonly requires airway passage protection and also respiratory support for days or even months. Pregnancy is not a contraindication for antivenom therapy.

There is no high standard for case series and definitive conclusions about the dose of antivenom to be given depending on the ratio of the neutralization capacity of the antivenoms. While one bottle may clear the poison from the blood, the evidence to suggest that one bottle is sufficient and neutralizes all the effects of the poison is weak. For safety, the starting dose should be two vials of appropriate antivenom. Fewer antidotes may be sufficient for minor poisonings, but more may be indicated clinically based on the snake involved (species, size, location), the number of bites, and the severity of patient effects. While undertreatment can be fatal or lead to morbidity with expensive long-term hospitalizations, overtreatment is probably not harmful. The antivenom cost is insignificant compared to other issues (Tibballs, 2020).

Local injury care includes daily cleaning with soap and water and applying a sterile gauze patch to open wounds. A plastic and reconstructive surgery consultation might be required for debridement or skin grafting. Debridement should doubtlessly not be performed three days after the snakebite till the coagulopathy has resolved. Surgical investigation of the bite injury is not necessary and may be harmful. Skin grafts are sometimes required after bites by pit vipers that create large necrotic areas. Fasciotomy is occasionally indicated unless compartment pressures rise above 30 mm Hg and there are signs of true compartment syndrome. Adequate doses of antivenom are recommended to reduce intracompartmental pressures before any fasciotomy is considered. In the case of infection, the use of broad-spectrum antibiotics should be considered. Physical therapy is often required and must begin soon after the acute phase of poisoning is complete.

Alternative ways are being investigated to prevent the inadequacy of antivenom therapy and related complications. Methods such as bioactive elements obtained from herbal sources, peptides and also small molecule inhibitors are being studied. However, these alternative approaches have many disadvantages that need to be developed with further in-vitro and in-vivo experiments (Alangode et al., 2020). The World Health Organization suggests that for snakebite treatment in the Asia and Africa regions there is a valuable online resource for diagnosis and treatment (Tintinalli, 2019).

Discharge and Follow-Up

The absence of bite marks and symptoms or faint signs does not mean there is no poisoning. Routine physical examination and laboratory findings do not reliably exclude significant poisoning. Patients should be observed in the emergency room for a minimum of 6 or 8 hours before the discharge decision. Patients with dry bite oversight for 6 to 8 hours can be discharged by telling them to apply again if pain, swelling, or bleeding develops. These patients should be offered tetanus vaccination, instructions for wound care, and a check-up within 24 to 48 hours when indicated. Patients with severe bites who receive antivenom should be followed up in the intensive care unit for 24-48 hours. If necessary, resuscitation equipment, ventilators, vasopressor support, invasive monitoring, and dialysis equipment should be available. Service admission may be considered for patients with minor or moderate toxicity who have completed or do not necessitate more antivenom therapy. When swelling begins to improve, patients are ready to be discharged from the hospital when the coagulopathy has resolved. Physical therapy for the bite site (especially the hand) is suggested after edema has subsided, and the coagulopathy has resolved. Patients should return if symptoms recur, or bruising, or other signs of recurrent coagulation disorder develop. Discharged patient follow-up is required to monitor local infection and serum sickness. The patient must be informed about the findings of serum sickness and should be told to apply again if these symptoms develop (Tintinalli, 2019; Walls, 2017).

Conclusion

Snake bites or stings are seen in many places around the world. Venomous snakes are responsible for approximately 1.5-3 million snakebites and possibly more than 100,000 deaths annually worldwide. Snake venom mainly causes neurotoxicity and hematotoxicity. It can show local and systemic effects. Although snakebite causes severe intoxication, the mortality rate is low with appropriate first aid intervention and effective treatment. Antivenom is the most crucial step in the treatment of venomous snake bites. Antivenom treatment must be given only in cases where there is clarity of clinical or laboratory evidence of systemic poisoning, neurotoxic effects, consumption coagulopathy, rhabdomyolysis, acute renal failure, cardiogenic shock, or critical local tissue damage. Pregnancy is not a contraindication for antivenom therapy, and no dose adjustment is required in children.

References

Açikalin, A., Gökel, Y., Kuvandik, G., Duru, M., Köseoğlu, Z., & Satar, S. (2008). The efficacy of low-dose antivenom therapy on morbidity and mortality in snakebite cases. *Am J Emerg Med*, *26*(4), 402-407. https://doi.org/10.1016/j.ajem.2007.06.017.

Alangode, A., Rajan, K., & Nair, B. G. (2020). Snake antivenom: Challenges and alternate approaches. *Biochem Pharmacol*, *181*, 114135. https://doi.org/10.1016/j.bcp.2020.114135.

Anz, A. W., Schweppe, M., Halvorson, J., Bushnell, B., Sternberg, M., & Andrew Koman, L. (2010). Management of venomous snakebite injury to the extremities. *J Am Acad Orthop Surg*, *18*(12), 749-759. https://doi.org/10.5435/00124635-201012000-00005.

Aziz, H., Rhee, P., Pandit, V., Tang, A., Gries, L., & Joseph, B. (2015). The current concepts in management of animal (dog, cat, snake, scorpion) and human bite wounds. *J Trauma Acute Care Surg*, *78*(3), 641-648. https://doi.org/10.1097/ta.0000000000000531.

Bhaumik, S., Beri, D., Lassi, Z. S., & Jagnoor, J. (2020). Interventions for the management of snakebite envenoming: An overview of systematic reviews. *PLoS Negl Trop Dis*, *14*(10), e0008727. https://doi.org/10.1371/journal.pntd.0008727.

Casewell, N. R., Jackson, T. N. W., Laustsen, A. H., & Sunagar, K. (2020). Causes and Consequences of Snake Venom Variation. *Trends Pharmacol Sci*, *41*(8), 570-581. https://doi.org/10.1016/j.tips. 2020.05.006.

Dart, R. C., Seifert, S. A., Boyer, L. V., Clark, R. F., Hall, E., McKinney, P., ... Porter, R. S. (2001). A randomized multicenter trial of crotalinae polyvalent immune Fab (ovine) antivenom for the treatment for crotaline snakebite in the United States. *Arch Intern Med*, *161*(16), 2030-2036. https://doi.org/10.1001/archinte.161.16.2030.

Gilliam, L. L., Ownby, C. L., McFarlane, D., Canida, A., Holbrook, T. C., Payton, M. E., & Krehbiel, C. R. (2013). Development of a double sandwich fluorescent ELISA to detect rattlesnake venom in biological samples from horses with a clinical diagnosis of rattlesnake bite. *Toxicon*, *73*, 63-68. https://doi.org/10.1016/j.toxicon.2013.06.022.

Gold, B. S., Dart, R. C., & Barish, R. A. (2002). Bites of venomous snakes. *N Engl J Med*, *347*(5), 347-356. https://doi.org/10.1056/NEJMra013477.

Greene, S., Ruha, A. M., Campleman, S., Brent, J., & Wax, P. (2021). Epidemiology, Clinical Features, and Management of Texas Coral Snake (Micrurus tener) Envenomations Reported to the North American Snakebite Registry. *J Med Toxicol*, *17*(1), 51-56. https://doi.org/10.1007/s13181-020-00806-3.

Hall, E. L. (2001). Role of surgical intervention in the management of crotaline snake envenomation. *Ann Emerg Med*, *37*(2), 175-180. https://doi.org/10.1067/mem.2001.113373.

Kasturiratne, A., Wickremasinghe, A. R., de Silva, N., Gunawardena, N. K., Pathmeswaran, A., Premaratna, R., ... de Silva, H. J. (2008). The global burden of snakebite: a literature analysis and modelling based on regional estimates of envenoming and deaths. *PLoS Med*, *5*(11), e218. https://doi.org/10.1371/journal.pmed.0050218.

Kundanati, L., Guarino, R., Menegon, M., & Pugno, N. M. (2020). Mechanics of snake biting: Experiments and modelling. *J Mech Behav Biomed Mater*, *112*, 104020. https://doi.org/10.1016/j.jmbbm.2020.104020.

Lavonas, E. J., Gerardo, C. J., O'Malley, G., Arnold, T. C., Bush, S. P., Banner, W., Jr., ... Kerns, W. P., 2nd. (2004). Initial experience with Crotalidae polyvalent immune Fab (ovine) antivenom in the treatment of copperhead snakebite. *Ann Emerg Med*, *43*(2), 200-206. https://doi.org/10.1016/j.annemergmed.2003.08.009.

Levine, M., Ruha, A. M., Padilla-Jones, A., Gerkin, R., & Thomas, S. H. (2014). Bleeding following rattlesnake envenomation in patients with preenvenomation use of antiplatelet or anticoagulant medications. *Acad Emerg Med*, *21*(3), 301-307. https://doi.org/10.1111/acem.12333.

Mowry, J. B., Spyker, D. A., Brooks, D. E., Zimmerman, A., & Schauben, J. L. (2016). 2015 Annual Report of the American Association of Poison Control Centers' National Poison Data System (NPDS): 33rd Annual Report. *Clin Toxicol (Phila)*, *54*(10), 924-1109. https://doi.org/10.1080/15563650.2016.1245421.

Tednes, M., & Slesinger, T. L. (2021). Evaluation and Treatment of Snake Envenomations. In *StatPearls*. StatPearls Publishing. Copyright © 2021, StatPearls Publishing LLC.

Tibballs, J. (2020). Australian snake antivenom dosing: What is scientific and safe? *Anaesth Intensive Care*, *48*(2), 129-133. https://doi.org/10.1177/0310057x19865268.

Tintinalli, M., Yealy, Meckler, Stapczynski, Cline, and Thomas. (2019). *Tintinalli's Emergency Medicine A Comprehensive Study Guide* (J. E. Tintinalli, Ed. 9th Edition ed.). McGraw Hill Medical Books.

Vohra, R., Rangan, C., & Bengiamin, R. (2014). Sonographic signs of snakebite. *Clin Toxicol (Phila)*, *52*(9), 948-951. https://doi.org/10.3109/15563650.2014.958613.

Walls, H. G.-H. (2017). *Rosen's Emergency Medicine Concepts and Clinical Practice* (M. Ron M. Walls, Ed. Vol. 9 th). Elsevier.

Chapter 16

Pet Bites

Ali Duman*, MD and Yunus Emre Özlüer, MD

Department of Emergency Medicine, Aydın Adnan Menderes University, Aydın, Turkey

Abstract

Pet bites may commonly cause severe complications across the globe. Approximately 2% of the population in the world experience pet bites each year. Dogs are responsible in 85% to 90% of the cases, whereas cat bites occur in 5% to 10%. Pet bites are more common in the male gender. The features of the injury site may vary depending on age, sex, and the biting animal. Injuries are classified into three groups: puncture injuries, lacerations, and avulsions (where tissue loss occurs). Even though they are less common, the risk of infection is higher in cat bites. The risk is also higher in crushing and puncture injuries of the tendons, joints, and bones, injuries affecting vessels, and injuries of the hands, face, feet, and genitals. The initial evaluation should prioritize hemodynamical stabilization before obtaining a history and a physical examination. Early aggressive and meticulous irrigation is recommended in pet bites due to gross contamination. Suturing these bite wounds is controversial. In patients with uncompromised immunity, non-extending bite wounds, wounds in the scalp and the face, and superficial wounds affecting only one layer of the skin may be suitable for suturing. Leaving the wound for secondary healing is recommended in crushing and puncture injuries, cat bites, bite wounds in the hands and feet, wounds 12 hours after the incident, patients with decreased immunity and patients with venous stasis. Post-exposure antibiotic prophylaxis with an appropriate antibiotic is one of the most controversial topics. Amoxicillin-clavulanate is the first-line agent in prophylaxis. An additional boost for tetanus and rabies should also be considered.

Keywords: emergency, pet, bite, wound

Introduction

Animal bites are common and may be associated with significant morbidity. Wounds due to pet bites can be classified as puncture wounds, lacerations, and crushing or avulsion wounds.

---

* Corresponding Author's Email: aliduman3489@gmail.com.

In: Environmental Emergencies and Injuries in Nature
Editors: Murat Yücel, Murat Güzel and İbrahim İkizceli
ISBN: 978-1-68507-833-1

Serious complications including infections, deformities, zoonotic diseases, and death may occur due to pet bites (Benson et al., 2006).

Epidemiology

The annual incidence of pet bites is approximately 2% in the world. Two to five million pet bites occur in North America, representing 1% of ED presentations and 10.000 admissions in a year. Also, representing 1% of the ED presentations in the USA, the annual cost of health care for pet bites is more than 50 million USD (Ellis, 2014). The incidence is reported as 50-60 per 100.000 in two regions (Bologna and South Tirol) of Italy. Each year, 20 to 35 people, most of them children, die in the USA because of dog attacks. The mortality rate of cat bites is reported as around 0.5% to 1.2% in the literature (Morosetti, 2013). According to the studies, responsibility for the bites falls as follows: 85% to 90% dogs, 5% to 10% cats, 2% to 3% humans and, 2% to 3% rodents. Most dog and cat bites are caused by either people's pets or the familiar animals around them (MacBean, 2007). Pet bites are more frequent in male adults and children. Cat bites are more frequent in women and girls, whereas dog bites are more frequent in boys (Murphy, 2021). In particular, most dog bite victims are boys between the ages of five and nine (Aziz et al., 2015).

Classification of the Wounds

The wound site varies according to the age and sex of the victim, and the type of animal that bites. The extremities and face are more frequently affected in dog bites. Animal bites to the face are much more common in children than adults, with about 10% of bites involving the head and neck in adults compared to about 75% in children (Chhabra, 2015). Sixty-six per cent of cat bites are typically seen in the upper extremities, particularly the hands (Aziz et al., 2015). Bite wounds are classified as puncture wounds, avulsions (with tissue loss) and lacerations. Dog bites tend to be mostly lacerations and avulsions, while cat bites usually cause puncture wounds. Most cat bites end up as small wounds, and the victims do not usually seek medical help (Murphy, 2021).

Microbiology

Although cat bites are less frequent than dog bites, they pose a higher risk for infections (Hurt, 2018). For instance, in a retrospective case series of more than 2500 dog bites and around 1000 cat bites, infection rates were reported as 7% and 49%, respectively (Jaindl et al., 2012; Jakeman, 2020). There is an increased risk of infections in puncture and crushing wounds to the tendons, joints, bones, and vessels and injuries to the face, hands, feet, and genital area. Also, the presence of prosthetic joints and heart valves, delayed admission (> 8 hours) to a medical center, and the presence of diabetes, asplenia, lymphedema, systemic lupus erythematosus, renal insufficiency, and immune compromisation are other risk factors for infections (Rothe, 2015). The risk for infections may differ according to the type of pathogens in an animal's mouth flora. Most of the infections that develop are polymicrobial. The most common isolated bacteria are Pasteurella (P. multocida, P. canis), Staphylococci, Streptococci, Corynebacterium, Moraxella and Neisseria spp. Capnocytophaga spp. and Bergeyella zoohelcum are other aerobic pathogens that spread into deeper tissues (Murphy, 2021). Pasteurella spp. can be isolated in 50% of the dog and 75% of the cat bite wounds. Capnocytophaga canimorsus may cause bacteremia and severe sepsis, particularly in patients with asplenia, underlying liver disease, and alcoholism. Bartonella henselae can be transmitted by the bite of an infected cat. Contact with cat saliva through a scratch, disintegrated skin and mucosa, and exposure to fleas are other routes for transmission (Butler, 2015). Infection may develop due to pathogens in the oral flora of the bitten animal and pathogens in the skin flora of the bitten person (Murphy, 2021). Both aerobic and anaerobic pathogens are isolated in 60% of the wound infections, while the skin flora is isolated in 40% of the cases. The average incubation period in pet bites is 12 to 24 hours (Savu, 2021).

Initial Evaluation

The initial evaluation should follow advanced trauma life support (ATLS) guidelines. History taking and physical examination should be performed following the confirmation of hemodynamic stability. History should include the species of the biting animal, the time of injury, the presence of underlying diseases, the vaccination status of the biting animal if known, and information about whether the biting animal was provoked. The patient's vaccination status for tetanus, medications, and allergies should also be noted (Hurt, 2018). Physical examination should carefully focus on extensive deep puncture wounds in the adjacent areas of the head, neck, torso, and joints. Bite wounds should be evaluated for foreign bodies in the wound. Also, a detailed neurovascular examination should be performed distal to the wound. Drawing on a diagram or taking a photo may be helpful when recording the features of irregularly shaped wounds (Rothe, 2015). Infection due to a bite wound may be superficial (e.g., cellulitis with or without abscess) or deep (e.g., abscess, septic arthritis, osteomyelitis, tenosynovitis, or necrotizing soft tissue infections). The classical features of cellulitis are fever, tenderness, erythema, swelling, and warmth, and purulent discharge or lymphangitis may be associated. Permanent or progressive pain following the injury, pain with passive movements, discordant pain in physical examination, the presence of crepitus, swelling of the neighboring joint, and clinical features indicating systemic inflammation (fever, hemodynamical instability) should raise suspicion of an infection in deeper tissues (Aziz et al., 2015).

Laboratory and Imaging

A laboratory evaluation should be performed in patients with infected wounds. However, it should be kept in mind that there are no specific tests. For example, leukocytosis and elevated serum inflammatory markers may not be present (Oehler, 2009). Imaging is mostly unnecessary in superficial, uninfected wounds. However, imaging with X-ray or computed tomography is mandatory in deep bite wounds, including those near joints, to investigate any presence of foreign bodies (e.g., teeth), fractures, or disruption of a joint (Steen, 2015).

Wound Management

Early and aggressive irrigation of the wounds is recommended due to gross contamination, as well as for acquiring a bloodless and clean area for further evaluation of the wound and preventing secondary infections in pet bites. 0.9% saline is safe, effective, and cheap, and widely accessible for irrigation. More significantly, complicated wounds involving joints, tendons, or muscles may require an aggressive pulse irrigation and surgical evaluation. Aggressive pulse irrigation uses solutions under pressure to reduce bacterial colonization, remove debris and prevent infection. Surgical debridement is recommended for the wound edges and nonviable, dead tissues (Murphy, 2021).

The suturing of bite wounds is controversial. The infection rates are similar in superficial wounds with adequate irrigation and sutured wounds either primarily or secondarily (Jakeman, 2020). However, superficial and simple wounds to the head and face in patients with adequate immunity may be sutured. Primary suturing of dog bites with aggressive pulse irrigation and wound debridement and administration of antibiotics results in a better cosmetic appearance without significant risk of infection. Subcutaneous suturing should be avoided or done with caution. Bite wounds should not be fixed using tissue adhesives (Hurt, 2018).

For crush and puncture wounds, cat bite wounds (excluding wounds on the face), wounds on the hands and feet, and those where 12 hours ($\geq$ 24 hours for wounds on the face) have passed since the bite, it is recommended to leave the wounds to secondary healing in immunocompromised (including diabetes) patients and patients with venous stasis. Wounds left open for secondary healing should be debrided, copiously irrigated, dressed, and evaluated daily for signs of infection (Hurt, 2018).

There is a clinical consensus that facial wounds first require primary suturing because of cosmetic reasons and a lower infection rate than other sites. Dog bite wounds, especially on the face, may be sutured even if they are a few days old. It is generally accepted that the time limit for primary suturing is 12 hours, while it can be extended to 24 hours for facial injury. For complex face lacerations, deep wounds involving bones, tendons, and joints, or other important tissues, and wounds with neurovascular deficits there should be consultation with a surgeon (Rothe, 2015).

Medical Management

Post-exposure antibiotic prophylaxis for most bites is controversial. There is consensus on the initiation of prophylactic antibiotic therapy in wounds requiring surgical repair and primary sutured lacerations, wounds on the hand, face, or genitals, wounds near bone or joints (including prosthetic joints), wounds with underlying venous or lymphatic insufficiency (including vascular grafts), wounds in immunocompromised patients (diabetes) and deep punctures or lacerations (particularly cat bites) (Aziz et al., 2015). On the other hand, prophylactic antibiotic therapy is not necessary for wounds with delayed presentations for more than 24 hours if there are no signs of infection (Rothe, 2015).

The choice of antibiotics for prophylaxis is another controversial topic. The primary purpose of the initial antibiotic therapy is to cover anaerobes and Staphylococci, Streptococci, and Pasteurella spp. (Aziz et al., 2015). The first choice for prophylaxis is amoxicillin-clavulanate. In patients with high-risk infections, the first dose of the antibiotic can be given intravenously (e.g., ampicillin-sulbactam, piperacillin-tazobactam, carbapenem, or ticarcillin-clavulanate). A combination of doxycycline or clindamycin with a fluoroquinolone is a good option for patients with allergies to penicillin. The duration for prophylaxis is 3 to 5 days (Aziz et al., 2015).

Tetanus prophylaxis should not be overlooked in the care of an animal and even human bite injury. Tetanus toxoid should be administered according to the vaccination status of the patient. Rabies virus may be transmitted via bites, abrasions, or scratches, or contact with the infected animal saliva through disintegrated skin or mucosa. In the bites of potentially rabid animals, in addition to timely application, early and vigorous cleaning with soap and water and the use of an antiseptic with activity against the rabies virus are important methods to reduce the risk of transmission (Aziz et al., 2015).

Conclusion

Pet bites remain a significant public health problem. Pet bites can cause serious infections and complications. These complications can be prevented with a detailed evaluation, timely wound irrigation, wound care, prophylactic antibiotics in high-risk patients, and close follow-up.

References

Aziz, H., Rhee, P., Pandit, V., Tang, A., Gries, L., Joseph, B. (2015). The current concepts in management of animals (dog, cat, snake, scorpion) and human bite wounds. *J. Trauma Acute Care Surg.*, 78 (3), 641-648.
Benson, L. S., Edwards, S. L., Schiff, A., P., Williams, C., S., Visotsky, J., L. (2006). Dog and cat bites to the hand: treatment and cost assessment. *J. Hand Surg. Am.*, 31 (3), 468-73.
Butler, T. (2015). Capnocytophaga canimorsus: an emerging cause of sepsis, meningitis, and post-splenectomy infection after dog bites. *Eur. J. Clin. Microbiol. Infect. Dis.*, 34, 1271-1281.
Chhabra, S., Chhabra, N., Gaba, S. (2015). Maxillofacial injuries due to animal bites. *J. Maxillofac. Oral. Surg.*, 14, 142–53.
Ellis, R., Ellis, C. (2014). Dog and cat bites. *Am. Fam. Physician.*, 90(4), 239-243.
Hurt, J. B., Maday, K. R. (2018). Management and treatment of animal bites. *JAAPA Off J. Am. Acad. Physician Assist.*, 31, 27–31.
Jaindl, M., Grünauer, J., Platzer, P., Endler, G., Thallinger, C., Leitgeb, J., Kovar, F. M. (2012). The management of bite wounds in children--a retrospective analysis at a level I trauma centre. *Injury*, 43, 2117-2121.
Jakeman, M., Oxley, J. A., Owczarczak-Garstecka, S. C., Westgarth, C. (2020). Pet dog bites in children: management and prevention. *BMJ Paediatrics*, 4 (1):e000726. doi: 10.1136/bmjpo-2020-000726. PMID: 32821860; PMCID: PMC7422634.
MacBean, C., E., Taylor, M. D. D., Ashby, Karen. (2007). Animal and human bite injuries in Victoria, 1998-2004. *Med. J. Aust.*, 186 (1), 38-40.
Morosetti, G., Torson, M., Pier, C. (2013). Lesions caused by animals in the autonomous province of South Tyrol in 2010: Fact-inding for prevention. *Veterinaria Italiana.* 49, 37–50.
Murphy, J., Qaisi, M. (2021). Management of Human and Animal Bites. *Oral Maxillofacial Surg. Clin. N. Am.*, 33, 373–380.
Oehler, R. L., Velez, A. P., Mizrachi, M., Lamarche, J., Gompfet, S. (2009). Bite-related and septic syndromes caused by cats and dogs. *Lancet Infect. Dis.*, 9, 439-447.

Rothe, K., Tsokos, M., Handrick, W. (2015). Animal and human bite wounds. *Dtsch. Arztebl. Int.,* 112, 433–43.

Savu, A. N., Schoenbrunner, A. R., Politi, R., Janis, J. E. (2021). Practical Review of the Management of Animal Bites. *Plast Reconstr. Surg. Glob.,* 9, e3778.

Steen, T, Ravin, K., Timmons, S., Kershenovich, A. (2015). Intracranial Injuries from Dog Bites in Children. *Pediatr. Neurosurg.,* 50, 187-195.

Chapter 17

Wild Animal Injuries

Serkan Emre Eroglu[1,*] and Murat Cetin[2]

[1]Department of Emergency Medicine, University of Health Sciences, Istanbul, Turkey
[2]Department of Emergency Medicine, Manisa Merkezefendi State Hospital, Manisa, Turkey

Abstract

Not all injuries from wild animals want support for treatment unless there is an infection and other complication or there is a fear of rabies. If their injuries are minor, patients are quickly discharged from the emergency room. Biting predominates in injuries by bear and especially wolf, while deer and wild boar do not seem to bite their victims. The bear uses both its claws to strike, resulting in crush injuries and fractures. Crush injuries and fractures are rare in wolf and boar attacks.

Keywords: wild, animal, injury, bite, trauma

Introduction

The management of patients presenting with wild animal bites and injuries requires a different evaluation from routine trauma cases. The bites and injuries of patients from wild animals can transmit systemic diseases that can cause significant morbidity and mortality. In order to reduce the consequences of trauma injury after an animal encounter, treatment management should be done with strong scientific evidence. Injuries from pets are more common in developed countries, but their incidence is increasing. The impact on the entire health economy is also much greater. As human population growth and the establishment of non-urban areas continue, the frequency of human-wild animal encounters will increase. There are no published reports characterizing the typical wild animal attack victim.

When human injuries caused by animals were evaluated, it was seen that the majority of bites or injuries caused by pets and animals were often provoked. Again, men have an injury rate of 150% to 250% compared to women of all ages. Understanding animal bite injury patterns will also be the first step towards improved treatment and prevention. It requires detailed and up-to-date information about the prevention of such animal behavior patterns and

---

* Corresponding Author's Email: drseroglu@gmail.com.

In: Environmental Emergencies and Injuries in Nature
Editors: Murat Yücel, Murat Güzel and İbrahim İkizceli
ISBN: 978-1-68507-833-1

their personalities. Animals become aggressive when they feel threatened, and reducing the risk of injury often relies on composure and an understanding of animal behavior (Sinclair CL and Zhou C 1995).

Evaluation and Management of Injury

Attacks by wild animals can cause blunt or penetrating trauma, with possible hypovolemic shock due to blood loss, airway injury, and thoracic and intra-abdominal trauma. It is important to carry out rapid transport according to the patient's condition and to start the treatment early by performing all physical examinations (Wroe and McHenry 2005). Serious complications and prolonged infections after animal bites often result from inadequate first aid and medical care delays. If the patient cannot get early treatment in a short time, simple first aid measures should be taken immediately. In many cases of bleeding and shock, even a simple tourniquet application can be life-saving. If necessary, prehospital resuscitation is initiated and completed, and important wounds should be cleaned with plenty of water at the scene. Early wound cleaning reduces the possibility of bacterial infection. It is also effective against the risk of infection from rabies and other viruses.

In general, covering the area of contaminated bites and claw wounds is not recommended. Preferably, boiled drinking water will be sufficient for wound irrigation. Ordinary hand soap can add some bactericidal, antiviral and cleansing properties. If the normal saline solution contains 1% to 5% povidone-iodine, it can be used as an irrigant for contaminated wounds. After cleaning the wound, it should be covered with a sterile dressing or dry cloth. Hand or foot wounds may require immobilization. If the attacked patient continues to be treated, consideration should also be given to capturing the animal for examination, if possible. Behaviors such as an unprovoked animal attack will increase the suspicion of rabies. If there are signs of hypovolemic shock, rapid and targeted resuscitation with blood products and intravenous volume expanders may be required.

Wound Treatment

All bites should be considered as contaminated and dirty wounds. Animal bites should be evaluated for blunt trauma and visceral injuries that are less hidden outside the wound. Especially in children, animal bites can progress quickly to vital structures such as joints or the skull (Drobatz and Smith 2003). Except for the most minor and isolated bite injuries, trauma patients require a head-to-toe whole-body assessment. When removing dead tissue with debridement, the aim is to create clean surgical wound edges to create a wound that heals faster. Again, topical antiseptic ointments are highly effective for promoting the healing of minor skin wounds. Three main considerations determine whether a wound should be sutured: cosmetic reasons, functional reasons, and risk factors. Although all facial wounds are low risk, almost all are sutured. Risk factors are mixed and multifactorial (Rhea and Weber 2014).

The time after injury is critical; for some mammalian bites, the longer the interval, the greater is the chance of infection. In developed countries, infection occurs hours after injury and the results are generally very good. Dog bites may be a lower risk, while some species, including wild boars and large wild carnivores, are a higher risk of infection (Gunduz and Turedi 2007). If wound closure is risky, surgical consultation should be considered for other options, including delayed closure or vacuum assisted closure.

Face and Hand Injuries

Face and hand wounds are the most common injuries because people often use their hands in the defense of an aggressive animal. Such wounds require special follow-up and treatment. In addition, they have anatomically complex and functionally very important tasks. Because of the high morbidity and persistent residual deterioration that occur with facial and hand infections, it is necessary to treat them aggressively (Wiggins and Akelman 1994). Small and uncomplicated lacerations can be repaired within 12-24 hours. Patients with severe infections require specialist consultation and hospitalization should be considered within the indication.

Prophylactic Antibiotics

Many case studies do not support the use of prophylactic antibiotics for low-risk wounds or bites. To be most effective, prophylactic antibiotics should be administered early. Injuries requiring early antibiotic therapy should be identified promptly during triage, preferably upon entry to the treatment facility. Oral antibiotics with high bioavailability are acceptable for the treatment of limited infections. IV administration is definitely preferred for serious infections. Treatment should be tailored to the widest variety of pathogens that are most likely for a particular bite type (Cummings 1994). The choice of antibiotics for most land mammals is based on experience with human, dog and cat bites. After an animal bite is contaminated, the prompt administration of antibiotic therapy is important. Organisms typically found in bite wounds are source-specific (Table 1). If antibiotic treatment is to be given, antibiotics associated with the attacking animal species should be preferred. Otherwise, broad-spectrum antibiotics may be the first choice.

Table 1. Source-specific microorganisms in bite injuries

Bear	Aeromonas and Streptococcus
Horse	Actinobacillus equuli-like bacterium
Cat	Pasteurella and Pseudomonas
Pig	Actinobacillus suis
Ungulates	Pasteurella and Acinetobacillus
Crocodiles	Aeromonas

Tetanus Prophylaxis

Tetanus-producing organisms are ubiquitous, and infections can result from minor wounds. The mortality rate is high because tetanus treatment is not effective. In the United States, cases of human tetanus from animal bites exceed cases of rabies infection by 2:1 each year (Centers for

Disease Control and Prevention 2007). Clostridium tetani spores are ubiquitous in soil, and the teeth, and saliva of animals; therefore, a risk of tetanus may exist from any animal injury to the skin.

Tetanus vaccination rates are highest in developed countries and fall dramatically in developing countries (World Health Organization 2013). Tetanus can be prevented but many people still do not receive tetanus immunoprophylaxis in accordance with guidelines. Appropriate emergency prophylaxis against tetanus remains critical but there is often inadequate intervention.

Rabies

The risk of rabies depends on factors such as the type of animal and whether rabies is native to that region. It is important to know the incidence of rabies in local species. It is useful to monitor the behavior of the animal. The appearance of a fox or bat in an urban setting that is not afraid of humans within other atypical behavior should raise the suspicion of rabies. The comprehensive and prompt early treatment of wounds in animals with suspected rabies can reduce the viral load. Clean all bite wounds immediately with soap and plenty of water (Smith and Fishbein 1991).

Complications

A wound infection is usually diagnosed on the basis of erythema, swelling, and tenderness accompanying the wound, which eventually progresses to cellulitis, lymphangitis, and local lymphadenopathy. Signs and symptoms of systemic infection are rare. In addition, victims of trauma or fatal events may develop post-traumatic stress disorder (PTSD). Severe and multiple attacks or those associated with deep bites are more likely to cause PTSD symptoms.

Wild Animal Attacks

Lions

Lions are the second largest of the big cats. They are primarily scavengers and attack with fewer kills. In their deadly attack, they often kill instantly with a bite to the head or neck, or a claw blow that can snap an ox neck. As they are so strong, many who survive the initial blow are later found to die of infection. When attacked, the most protective behavior has not been determined. Some survivors noted that allowing the lion to chew on an arm or leg protected them from an attack of the individual's entire body (Packer and Ikanda 2005).

Coyotes and Hyenas

Coyotes typically display an increasing array of bold behaviors before attacking. A coyote bite should be treated like a dog bite in terms of antibiotic selection and wound closure problems;

If the animal cannot be caught and examined, rabies prophylaxis should be done. Hyenas have extremely powerful jaws and biting power (Seimenis and Tabbaa 2014). They can cut off the limbs and heads of children. It is common for hyenas to drag their victims. After the attack, most people usually survive, but their facial and bodily integrity is greatly impaired.

Wolves

The differences in bite mark between wolves and dogs can be attributed to differences in genetics, breeding, socialization and attack momentum. When wolves squeeze, trap, or burrow, they are provoked and carry out many attacks against humans. No other animal can be as ferocious as wolves when rabid. Wild wolf bites contain a characteristic crushed and softened texture. They should be carefully debrided.

Foxes

Foxes usually attack most of their own rabid foxes. Fox bites have caused eyelid tears in children sleeping in tents, and perforations in the toes and legs of adults. Foxes typically inflict more puncture wounds than other dogs, making their bites more prone to infection (Metro West Daily News 2014).

Camels

Bite injuries are quite common in areas where camels are used for daily or agricultural purposes. They are herbivores. Although they are generally adaptable, camels are much more likely to bite during the rutting season and bite fatalities have been reported (Lazarus and Price 2001). Almost all camel bites are unique. The movements of the animal's head during biting cause severe tissue damage and limb avulsion. Rarely, a camel can break its victim's neck.

Deers

Deer attacks are reported less frequently. Although typically docile, they can be aggressive, especially during the fall and spring seasons. As a reservoir of disease-hosting vector ticks, deer contribute to the increased incidence of human Lyme disease. Deer bites are rarely serious, and there are bites to the arm or back that are usually well covered by clothing (Haikonen and Summala 2001).

Bears

Bear injuries require a broad range of outpatient management, often ranging from major treatments that typically result in significant functional disability, to hospitalization and surgical intervention. The teeth of bears, especially the canines, are large and robust. Although the teeth are not particularly sharp, the strength of the jaw muscles allows the teeth to penetrate deep into the soft tissues and fracture the facial bones, hand and forearm bones with ease. Trauma typically results from punctures caused by shearing, tearing, and crushing forces. Claws are another major source of trauma. Bear claws give injuries that result in significant blunt trauma, particularly to the head and neck, thorax and abdominal cavity. For this reason, people attacked by bears should be evaluated repeatedly for hidden blunt trauma (Rasool and Wani 2010).

The best way to avoid bear-related injuries is to avoid surprising the bear. If we are attacked by a bear, we can take several important steps to minimize injury.

1) Let the bear understand that you are human and not a prey species. Move away from any visual obstructions to allow the bear to see clearly.
2) While staying calm is the hardest part, don't make sudden movements or shout, especially in encounters with a grizzly bear. The bear may see this as an aggressive act and respond to you with aggression.
3) Do not look directly at the bear. Looking sideways at it can provide you with an opportunity to determine the bear's reaction. Don't think about climbing a tree or running away. It is impossible to cross a bear, and running can prevent the bear from accurately identifying a human. As a result, it can launch an attack.
4) If he starts an attack, clasp your hands behind your head, and bend your head forward to protect your head and neck in a fetal or prone position. Never try to look at the bear during the attack.
5) After the attack, stay on the ground until you are sure the bear has gone. It may not have completely left the area. Victims who stood up after the first attack before the bear left were often more severely injured during the second attack.
6) When you think that the bear has left the area, look around, moving as little as possible, and try to determine which way the bear has gone.

All victims of bear attacks should be considered as having major trauma and should be transferred to the most appropriate center after stabilization (Norwood and McAuley 2000). Bear-borne injuries are usually occult and produce more deep tissue necrosis than initially expected. It should be borne in mind that internal injuries from direct penetration (claws, teeth) or blunt trauma may be common (Table 2).

Table 2. Risk factors for infection from bear bites

High risk	Low risk
50 years and older	Under 50 years
Hand, wrist or foot injuries	Injuries to the face, scalp, ears or mouth
Scalp or facial injuries in infants	Self-biting of the buccal mucosa
Cheek bite	Removable lacerations and abrasions
Bites on the artery and nerve	
Bites on the large joint	
Chronic alcoholism	
Diabetes mellitus	
Chronic corticosteroid therapy	

In some studies, almost 50% of patients developed an infection after a bear attack. Shortly after injury, the wound should be examined for high-low risk before infection is suspected (Table 2). Victims of bear attacks who fall into the high-risk category should be treated with broad-spectrum agents to include Staphylococcus aureus and gram-negative rods, in addition to anaerobes. Although rare, rabies has been documented in black bears. All bear attack victims should be evaluated for the risk of rabies vaccination and its benefits.

Crocodiles

The crocodile has serious gripping power and locks its grip by placing the two lower teeth into the holes in the upper jaw. Most attacks take place in water. When a crocodile is unable to completely drag its attacker under water, it may grasp a limb or then turn over and over again until the limb separates. All attacks are predatory and crocodile teeth often cause large lacerations in the trunk (Forrester and Holstege 2012). In order to avoid crocodile attacks, individuals should not swim at dusk when crocodiles are active, should not swim with a dog that will attract the attention of crocodiles, and should not swim alone.

Elephants

The elephant is the largest land animal and may be one of the most dangerous wild animals. Elephants kill by trampling with their feet, strangling with their tusks, or hitting with a proboscis. Elephants often dismember the victim's body and scatter the pieces, then cover them with grass and twigs. Early warning signs before an attack are the sound made by the lifting of the head and trunk, the opening of the ears, the swaying of the trunk and the wagging of the tail (Lazarus and Price 2001).

Conclusion

Simple and serious animal bites are common and responsible for 4.7 million emergency room visits (about 1% of all visits) in the United States each year. Treatment of animal bites is determined by the species involved and the location and severity of the bite. Children are at greater risk for serious bites and more likely than adults to be seen for medical care. Preventing animal attacks requires extensive knowledge of the behavior patterns and personalities of animals. A person who wishes to avoid the bite of a particular species can usually only learn about the behavior of that species from those who work with it on a regular basis.

References

Centers for Disease Control and Prevention (2007). *Vaccination coverage among U.S. adults: National immunization survey, Adult.*

Cummings P. (1994) Antibiotics to prevent infection in patients with dog bite wounds: A meta-analysis of randomized trials. *Ann. Emerg. Med.*; 23:535

D'Amore D C and Moreno K (2011). The effects of biting and pulling on the forces generated during feeding in the Komodo dragon (Varanuskomodoensis). *PLoS ONE.*

Drobatz K and Smith G (2003). Evaluation of risk factors for bite wounds inlicted on caregivers by dogs and cats in a veterinary teaching hospital. *J. Am.Vet. Med. Assoc.;* 223:312.

Forrester J A and Holstege C P (2012). Fatalities from venomous and non venomous animals in the United States (1999-2007). *Wilderness Environ. Med.;* 23:146–52.

Gilbert AT and Petersen BW (2012) Evidence of rabies virus exposure among humans in the Peruvian Amazon. *Am. J. Trop. Med. Hyg.;* 87:206–15.

Gunduz A and Turedi S (2007) Wild boar attacks. *Wilderness Environ. Med.;* 18:117–19.

Haikonen H and Summala H (2001). Deer-vehiclecrashes: Extensive peak at 1 hour after sunset. *Am. J. Prev Med.;* 21:209.

Lazarus H M an dPrice R S (2001). Dangers of large exoticpets from foreign lands. *J. Trauma* 2001; 51:1014.

Lazarus H M and Price R S (2001). Dangers of large exotic pets from foreign lands. *J. Trauma;* 51:1014

Metro West Daily News (FraminghamMass) (2014). *Rabid fox killed after attacks in Framingham.*

Norwood S and McAuley C (2000). Mechanisms and patterns of injuries related to large animals. *J. Trauma;* 48:740.

Packer C and Ikanda D (2005) Conservation biology: Lion attacks on humans in Tanzania. *Nature* 2005;436:927.

Rasool A and Wani A H (2010). Incidence and pattern of bear maul injuries in Kashmir. *Injury;*41:116.

Rhea S K and Weber D J (2014) Use of state wide emergency department surveillance data to assess incidence of animal bite injuries among humans in North Carolina. *J. Am.Vet. Med. Assoc.* 2014; 244:597–603.

Seimenis A and Tabbaa D (2014). Stray animal populations and public health in the South Mediterranean and the Middle East regions. *Vet. Ital.;* 50:131–6.

Sinclair C L and Zhou C (1995) Descriptive epidemiology of animalbites in Indiana, 1990-92: A rationale for intervention. *Public Health Rep.;* 110:64.

Smith J S and Fishbein D B (1991) Unexplained rabies in three immigrants in the United States: A virologic investigation. *N. Engl. J. Med.* 1991; 324:205.

Wiggins ME, Akelman E. (1994) The management of dog bites and dog bite infections to the hand. *Orthopedics;* 17:617.

World Health Organization (2013). *Immunization, vaccines and biologicals: Immunization coverage.*

Wroe S and Mc Henry C (2005) Bite club: Comparative bite force in big biting mammals and the prediction of predatory behaviour in fosil taxa. *Proc. Biol. Sci.;* 272:619–25.

Chapter 18

Tick Emergencies

Metin Yadigaroğlu[1,*], MD and Nurçin Öğreten Yadigaroğlu[2], MD

[1]Samsun University Faculty of Medicine, Department of Emergency Medicine, Samsun, Turkey
[2]Karadeniz Technical University Faculty of Medicine, Department of Internal Medicine, Trabzon, Turkey

Abstract

Ticks are ectoparasites commonly found all over the world. Tick-borne diseases find their place under the heading of "environmental emergencies" because they are ectoparasites and can transmit the many diseases that they carry to humans. Many microorganisms such as bacteria, viruses, spirochetes, rickettsia, protozoa, and nematodes are among the disease agents transmitted by ticks. In addition, toxins can also be transferred. With the contact of ticks with humans, a wide variety of microorganisms and various diseases and clinical pictures can occur in various geographies. Among these diseases, some situations are life-threatening and require urgent intervention. In this context, the management of tick emergencies is critical. In order to properly manage the disease and the patient, it is necessary to know the diseases transmitted by ticks and the emergencies of these diseases.

Keywords: tick, emergency, environment, infectious disease

Introduction

While ticks live underground in cold weather, they begin to emerge when the weather starts to warm up. When this mobility of ticks and people's commitment to nature coincide, tick contact is inevitable. A humid climate, vegetation consisting of trees and bushes, being on the migration routes of animals, the global warming trend, and spring and summer seasons are particularly seen as geographical risk factors for tick contact. Occupations (such as farmer, veterinarian) and hobbies (such as hunting, outdoor sports) also constitute the personal risk group of tick contact (Hayney et al., 1999). The primary hosts are animals, but humans become hosts by accident. Ticks pierce the host skin with a projection called a hypostome and stick there. They secrete anticoagulant, anesthetic, and anti-inflammatory substances to the area where they are

---

* Corresponding Author's Email: metin.yadigaroglu@samsun.edu.tr.

In: Environmental Emergencies and Injuries in Nature
Editors: Murat Yücel, Murat Güzel and İbrahim İkizceli
ISBN: 978-1-68507-833-1

attached and then begin to suck blood. In this way, the host either does not notice the tick or realizes it too late. Until that stage, the pathogens listed above are transferred to the host. After a variable incubation period, signs of disease may appear. With the passage of toxins or similar substances to the host, sudden fatal complications such as anaphylaxis may occur without an incubation period.

Ticks that cause these negativities; are living things with hundreds of known species that can feed on the blood of all known vertebrates except fish, which cannot be eradicated from the world for now (Nuhoglu et al., 2008). When this is the case, diseases transmitted by tick contact are seen as an important environmental public health problem worldwide.

A Review of Ticks and Tick-Borne Diseases in the World

About 900 known tick species are divided into two groups as hard ticks (Ixodidae) and soft ticks (Argasidae) (Boulanger et al., 2019). More than 700 species are in the group of hard ticks, while the rest are in the group of soft ticks. There are different tick species in these two groups (Table 1). So many different types of ticks show themselves by creating various diseases in various geographies worldwide. In this context, states have set out various guidelines for recognizing and managing the most common tick-borne diseases. For example, while Lyme Disease and tick-borne bacterial diseases are given priority in the European guidelines, Lyme disease/Borieliosis is found to be alone in the Australian and Canadian guidelines. While the guidelines in India were created based on rickettsial diseases alone, in Turkey, they focused on Crimean-Congo Hemorrhagic Fever (CCHF). The guidelines in which tick-borne diseases are presented with the widest variety of diseases are the American guidelines. The Centers for Disease Control and Prevention (CDC): Tick-borne diseases of the United States guidelines divide tick-borne diseases into two groups, those seen in and outside the United States. Anaplasmosis, babesiosis, Colorado tick fever, ehrlichiosis, Lyme disease, Powassan disease, rocky mountain spotted fever, tick-borne relapsing fever, and tularemia are seen as diseases caused by tick contact in America. In contrast, Crimean Congo hemorrhagic fever, Kyasanur forest disease, Lyme disease, Omsk hemorrhagic fever, and tick-borne encephalitis are listed among the tick-borne diseases seen outside the United States in the guidelines. However, in the globalizing world, the importance of geographical borders for all these diseases is gradually decreasing.

Table 1. Classification of ticks

Hard ticks (Ixodidae family)	
	Amblyomma
	Dermacentor
	Haemaphysalis
	Hyalomma
	Ixodes
	Rhipicephalus
Soft ticks (Argasidae family)	
	Argas
	Ornithodoros

Perhaps the most critical step in managing tick-borne emergencies is to detect the tick attached to the skin and remove it from the body as soon as possible. This approach will reduce the possibility of potential disease transmission (Republic of Turkey Ministry of Health, 2019). At this point, the most important thing to note is that a health worker should complete the tick-removal process, if possible, because health workers' success in the tick removal process was found to be high (Sahin et al., 2020). If it is impossible for the health worker to reach, it is necessary to remove the tick from the closest place where the tick comes into contact with the skin without using any chemicals.

Many methods that are not superior to each other can be used for tick removal in patients admitted to the emergency department. Perhaps the most used method is the extraction method with forceps or rope for ease of transportation. Whichever way is used, aggressive approaches that will cause the tick to empty its stomach contents should be avoided. It should be gently pulled by holding the tick close to the skin and constant force. After the tick is removed, the lesion site should be cleaned with antiseptic solutions, and the whole body should be scanned for possible additional tick exposure.

The most feared clinical situation in the acute phase of tick exposure is anaphylaxis. IgE-type antibodies developed against anticoagulants, anesthetic, and anti-inflammatory proteins in tick saliva can cause anaphylaxis in the host (Commins & Platts-Mills, 2013). It can even be triggered by pulling the tick from the skin (Takayama & Takagaki, 2020). In the treatment of anaphylaxis, the first thing to do is to ensure the patient's airway safety and to support their breathing and circulation. Simultaneously with these, intramuscular epinephrine is administered immediately. After epinephrine, H1 and H2 receptor antagonists, corticosteroids, beta2 agonists, and glucagon therapy are recommended if needed. The patient should be observed for possible biphasic reactions, and an allergist should be consulted if necessary (Pflipsen & Vega Colon, 2020). In addition, sensitivity to Galactose-α-1,3-galactose (α-Gal) found in the intestines of some ticks after tick exposure has also been shown to cause anaphylaxis, especially in endemic tick regions in North America, Europe, Asia, Central America, and Africa (van Nunen, 2015).

Another clinical pathology in patients with ticks on their bodies is tick paralysis. Neurotoxins in the saliva of ticks cause this condition. It is especially seen in North America and Australia. The patient does not notice the tick in contact with their skin, and neurological symptoms such as diplopia, dysphagia, speech disorder, and ataxia develop, followed by vague symptoms such as weakness. With ascending paralysis, it is often included in the differential diagnosis with Guillain-Barre syndrome. In the case of newly developing ataxia, tick paralysis should definitely be included in the differential diagnosis, especially for the pediatric age group. The most crucial step for managing tick paralysis is to suspect the disease and terminate the exposure to the tick. In untreated cases, respiratory failure and death may occur with the progression of ascending paralysis (Simon, 2021).

Patients with tick contact can apply to health institutions in various ways:

- Those who have contact with ticks and apply for the removal of the tick on their body;
- Those who have contact with ticks and apply after removing the tick themselves;
- Those who have contact with ticks and apply with symptoms after removing the tick from their body; and

- Those who do not have a history of tick contact but who present with various symptoms and are diagnosed with a disease that may develop after tick exposure as a result of clinical evaluations.

The rate of development of severe symptoms in patients after tick exposure is usually shallow (Jahfari et al., 2016; Boulanger et al., 2019). Except for symptoms that develop early after exposure (such as anaphylaxis, allergic reaction, urticaria), symptoms generally begin to occur after an incubation period of two weeks. Patients applying to the hospital after tick contact who are not symptomatic should be informed about the symptoms that may develop, considering this incubation period.

Patients mainly present with weakness, joint pain, headache, nausea, vomiting, fever, nontraumatic skin and subcutaneous hemorrhages, epistaxis, hematuria, and altered consciousness. From the first contact stage between patients and healthcare professionals, it is essential to take personal protective measures to prevent possible contamination. Complete blood count, liver and kidney function tests, and coagulation parameters should be requested at the initial stage from symptomatic patients, and then necessary treatments should be started immediately. During the diagnosis and treatment process, necessary consultations with infectious diseases should be made.

Perhaps the most common tick-borne bacterial infection is Lyme Disease, the most common vector-borne disease in the northern hemisphere. The causative agent is Borrelia burgdorferi. The most common clinical presentation is skin involvement (erythema cronicum migrans). When this lesion(s) is seen in a patient with no history of ticks, exposure to ticks should be considered, and antibiotic treatment (amoxicillin and doxycycline) should be started. In untreated cases, the lesions begin to spread throughout the body. The patient's clinic may worsen with accompanying joint involvement, and cardiac and neurological symptoms (Stanek et al., 2012).

The presence of small, pink, non-fading, and non-pruritic rashes in the extremities (forearm, hand, and ankle) in the follow-up period in patients with fever should suggest rickettsial diseases, especially in the spotted fever group, and antibiotic treatment (tetracycline or doxycycline) should be started immediately, just like in Lyme disease.

Ulceroglandular tularemia should be considered in patients with swelling and painful skin lesions in the cervical, occipital and inguinal skin regions, especially in the cervical region, after tick exposure. The causative agent of the disease is Francisella tularensis. In addition, ocular findings (such as painful conjunctivitis, chemosis, eyelid edema) should also suggest oculoglandular tularemia (Nuhoglu et al., 2008). Appropriate antibiotic therapy for the disease should be started immediately (such as tetracycline/streptomycin).

Crimean-Congo Hemorrhagic Fever should be considered in the presence of hemorrhagic symptoms following tick contact, fever, malaise, and joint pain. It is common among tick-borne disease agents in Africa, Europe, and Western Asia. Bleeding can reach profound dimensions and progress to life-threatening disseminated intravascular coagulation (DIC). Consultation on infectious diseases should be made for the patient, and supportive treatment should be started immediately (Camp et al., 2020).

Tick-borne encephalitis (TBE) should be considered in the case of loss of cognitive functions after nonspecific symptoms such as fever, nausea, and vomiting that develop after tick contact. The causative agent of the disease is the virus of the same name, and its fatality is high. Europe, Russia, Far East Asia, and Japan are considered as endemic areas for the disease (Yoshii, 2019).

One of the tick-borne diseases is babesiosis, which is a parasitic disease. Babesiosis is also called piroplasmosis because of the similarity of the causative agent with plasmodium. It is rare, but death occurs in nearly half of the patients. Fever, anemia, jaundice, and hemoglobinuria are the most common symptoms and signs after tick exposure. While azithromycin is recommended as the initial therapy, clindamycin or quinines can be used in severe cases (Vannier & Krause, 2012).

Conclusion

Tick-borne emergent pathologies can lead to outcomes such as DIC, acute respiratory distress syndrome (ARDS), multiple organ failure (MODs), coma, and death. Diagnosing all these clinical presentations may also be accessible for patients with a history of tick exposure. However, the most challenging situation for the clinician is the management of patients who do not have a history of tick contact or are unable to give a history (elderly, pediatric, uncommunicative, unconscious, etc.). In all cases where tick contact is suspected, the anamnesis should be detailed, and the infectious diseases department should be contacted for further examination and treatment management.

References

Boulanger, N., Boyer, P., Talagrand-Reboul, E., & Hansmann, Y. (2019). Ticks and tick-borne diseases. *Medecine et maladies infectieuses*, *49*(2), 87–97. https://doi.org/10.1016/j.medmal.2019.01.007

Camp, J. V., Kannan, D. O., Osman, B. M., Shah, M. S., Howarth, B., Khafaga, T., Weidinger, P., Karuvantevida, N., Kolodziejek, J., Mazrooei, H., Wolf, N., Loney, T., & Nowotny, N. (2020). Crimean-Congo Hemorrhagic Fever Virus Endemicity in United Arab Emirates, 2019. *Emerging infectious diseases*, *26*(5), 1019–1021. https://doi.org/10.3201/eid2605.191414.

Commins, S. P., & Platts-Mills, T. A. (2013). Tick bites and red meat allergy. *Current opinion in allergy and clinical immunology*, *13*(4), 354–359. https://doi.org/10.1097/ACI.0b013e3283624560.

Hayney, M. S., Grunske, M. M., & Boh, L. E. (1999). Lyme disease prevention and vaccine prophylaxis. *The Annals of pharmacotherapy*, *33*(6), 723–729. https://doi.org/10.1345/aph.18285.

Jahfari, S., Hofhuis, A., Fonville, M., van der Giessen, J., van Pelt, W., & Sprong, H. (2016). Molecular Detection of Tick-Borne Pathogens in Humans with Tick Bites and Erythema Migrans, in the Netherlands. PLoS neglected tropical diseases, 10(10), e0005042. https://doi.org/10.1371/journal. pntd.0005042.

Nuhoğlu, İ., Aydın, M., Türedi, S., Gündüz, A., Topbaş, M. (2008). Kene İle Bulaşan Hastalıklar. TAF Prev. Med. Bull., 7(5), 461-8. (Diseases Transmitted by Ticks).

Pflipsen, M. C., & Vega Colon, K. M. (2020). Anaphylaxis: Recognition and Management. *American family physician*, *102*(6), 355–362.

Republic of Turkey Ministry of Health Turkey Zoonotic Diseases Action Plan (2019-2023), Crimean-Congo Hemorrhagic Fever, Ankara 2019.

Simon, L. V., West, B., & McKinney, W. P. (2021). Tick Paralysis. In *StatPearls*. StatPearls Publishing.

Stanek, G., Wormser, G. P., Gray, J., & Strle, F. (2012). Lyme borreliosis. *Lancet (London, England)*, *379*(9814), 461–473. https://doi.org/10.1016/S0140-6736(11)60103-7.

Şahin, A. R., Hakkoymaz, H., Taşdoğan, A. M., & Kireçci, E. (2020). Evaluation and comparison of tick detachment techniques and technical mistakes made during tick removal. *Turkish journal of trauma & emergency surgery TJTES*, *26*(3), 405–410. https://doi.org/10.14744/tjtes.2020.59680.

Takayama, N., & Takagaki, Y. (2020). Tick anaphylaxis triggered by pulling out the tick. *Acute medicine & surgery*, *7*(1), e503. https://doi.org/10.1002/ams2.503.

van Nunen S. (2015). Tick-induced allergies: mammalian meat allergy, tick anaphylaxis and their significance. *Asia Pacific allergy*, *5*(1), 3–16. https://doi.org/10.5415/apallergy.2015.5.1.3.

Vannier, E., & Krause, P. J. (2012). Human babesiosis. *The New England journal of medicine*, *366*(25), 2397–2407. https://doi.org/10.1056/NEJMra1202018.

Yoshii K. (2019). Epidemiology and pathological mechanisms of tick-borne encephalitis. *The Journal of veterinary medical science*, *81*(3), 343–347. https://doi.org/10.1292/jvms.18-0373.

Chapter 19

Mosquito-Borne Diseases

Selim Görgün*, MD and Aydan Çevik Varol, MD

Department of Microbiology and Clinical Microbiology, Health Science University,
Samsun Training and Research Hospital, Samsun, Turkey
Department of Family Physicians, Namık Kemal University, Tekirdag, Turkey

Abstract

Among mosquito-borne diseases; malaria, dengue fever, Japanese encephalitis, West Nile disease, yellow fever, chikungunya and Zika virus infection are noteworthy. These diseases, which are spread by mosquitoes, were previously isolated geographically, but have spread globally in the globalizing world.

In order to limit the spread in these patients, who are often given symptomatic and supportive treatment in the clinic, it is important to take a more comprehensive patient history and perform a detailed physical examination. Effective vaccines against the virus remain the front line of defense for these diseases. Although an effective vaccine has been used to prevent yellow fever infection by travelers traveling to endemic areas since the mid-20th century, the agent is still widely seen around the world. For this reason, people who go to risky geographical areas should also use sprays effective against the carrier vector and pay attention to their clothing choices. In addition, a real-time PCR test (RT-PCR) performed with virus-specific primers and probes targeting the causative virus can be used in the diagnosis of vector-borne Zikavirus (ZIKV), dengue fever virus (DENV), chikungunya virus (CHIKV) and yellow fever virus (YFV), which are common all over the world.

Keywords: mosquitoes, mosquito-borne diseases, malaria, West Nile, yellow fever, Zika virus

Introduction

Although mosquito-borne diseases are more frequently seen in tropical and subtropical countries close to the equator, in today's world where travel opportunities are increasing, they have the potential to spread in the community and cause serious public health problems in cases

---

* Corresponding Author's Email: selimgorgun55@gmail.com.

In: Environmental Emergencies and Injuries in Nature
Editors: Murat Yücel, Murat Güzel and İbrahim İkizceli
ISBN: 978-1-68507-833-1

where control and eradication cannot be done effectively. Although we have limited measures to combat these diseases, vaccination and chemoprophylaxis are recommended especially for people who will travel to endemic regions.

Mosquitoes are small insects, which are taxonomically divided into more than 40 genera and about 3500 species. Arbo viruses are mosquito-borne viruses, pathogens that reproduce in mosquitoes and infect vertebrates such as humans and animals during their biological cycle (Xia 2018).

Mosquito-Borne Viral Illnesses

Zika Virus

Zika virus (ZIKV) operates on humans in a large geographical area stretching from the north of the African continent and Southeast-Asia to the Pacific coast of French Polynesia to the countries of South and Central America (Frumence et al., 2016). ZKV infection is spread through mosquito bites or sexual contact with infected people. Aedes aegypti mosquitoes are blamed as the main vector in virus transmission (Javed et al., 2018). The clinical picture is mild and often asymptomatic. However, ZIKV infection, which may occur in the first 6 months of pregnancy, especially in cases with late diagnosis, has a serious intrauterine effect that may lead to a fetal anomaly (Allison et al., 2019; Driggers et al., 2016). ZIKV agent is an Arbo virus and included in the Flaviviridae family in taxonomy. The first epidemic spread occurred in the South Pacific in early 2000. In the last 15 years, there has been evidence of a serious spread, especially in the Western hemisphere (Frumence et al., 2016). In various studies on ZIKV, clinically, fever, conjunctivitis, maculopapular rash, different symptoms and complaints such as headache, arthralgia and myalgia, as well as neurological complications such as congenital microcephaly and Guillain-Barré syndrome (symmetric ascending flaccid paralysis), which are frequently caused by epidemics, take their place in the literature (Ferraris et al., 2019; Frumence et al., 2016).

In recent years, there have been studies reporting that structures called small membrane-associated interferon-inducible transmembrane proteins (IFITM) inhibit flavivirus replication (Bailey et al., 2014; Chesarino et al., 2015).

Dengue Fever

Dengue fever virus (DENV), an arbovirus belonging to the Flavivirus genus of the family Flaviviridae, is frequently seen in tropical countries and can cause serious results ranging from a mild clinical picture like arthralgia to life-threatening hemorrhagic fever and shock. It is transmitted by Aedes mosquitoes such as Aedes aegypti and Aedes albopictus and has 4 sub-serotypes that can cause the disease (Khetarpal & Khanna, 2016).

According to the World Health Organization (WHO), approximately half a billion people are infected with the dengue fever agent, which is detected in more than 100 countries around the world, and approximately 20.000 deaths occur due to the hemorrhagic form that develops due to this infection (Teyssou, 2009).

Since dengue fever is widespread at the global level, its economic impact is undeniable. For this reason, vaccine development studies cannot be ignored. At the vaccination stage, it is aimed to provide broad and robust immunity to all four dengue serotypes at the same time. Recombinant preparations prepared as live, vectored and killed are used (Singhasivanon & Jacobson, 2009; Hombach, 2009).

Chikungunya Virus

Chikungunya virus (CHIKV) is a mosquito-transmitted alpha virus identified in the Togaviridae family. CHIKV, whose main vectors are mosquitoes of the Aedes species, was first described in 1952 in Tanzania (Caglioti et al., 2013). In addition, due to the risk of spreading the disease, it is reported that it has the potential to cause an epidemic in African and Asian countries (Sam et al., 2015). The infection, which is widely diagnosed in the USA, has symptoms similar to dengue fever. However, post-viral chronic inflammatory rheumatism is seen in the post-infective period in approximately 50% of the cases. Joint pain often involves large joints in the extremities and symmetrically (Vu et al., 2017). The infection has no specific treatment. It is important to protect people from mosquito bites in endemic countries (Caglioti et al., 2013).

Yellow Fever

Yellow fever, an RNA virus and a mosquito-borne flavivirus infection is mostly seen in sub-Saharan Africa and South American countries. An effective vaccine is used by the travelers since 1940s (Monath and Vasconcelos 2015). Yellow fever virus (YFV) is reported to be transmitted by using Haemagogus, Sabethes or Aedes aegypti mosquitoes as vectors (Litvoc et al., 2018).

Although yellow fever can be seen to be clinically asymptomatic, it can also lead to serious clinical pictures that lead to renal, hepatic and neurological disorders and bleeding attacks (Litvoc et al., 2018). In yellow fever, acute renal failure (ARF) occurs although the pathophysiology is not fully understood or high mortality is observed when multiple organ involvement occurs, even in intensive care unit conditions. In addition, a real-time PCR test (RT-PCR) performed with virus-specific primers and probes targeting the causative virus can be used in the diagnosis of vector-borne ZIKV, DENV, CHIKV and YFV, which are common all over the world (Mansuy 2018; Wu 2018).

Encephalitis Viruses

Japanese encephalitis virus (JEV), the prototype Nakayama strain found in the 1950s, is a member of the Flaviviridae family and the Flavivirus genus. The first isolation was the brain tissue of a fatal encephalitis case. Culex mosquitoes often act as vectors in JEV (Xia et al., 2018).

West Nile virus (WNV) was first isolated in the West Nile region of the African country of Uganda in the second half of the 1930s. Over the years, it has been included in the literature with new cases detected in Africa, Asia, Europe, Australia and North America. The main disease vector for WNV is mosquitoes of the Culex genus. In febrile cases, diarrhea, vomiting, joint pain, headache, body aches or rash may accompany the clinical picture. In patients with a history of travel to endemic regions, a long-lasting history of weakness and fatigue should be kept in mind (Xia et al., 2018).

St. Louis encephalitis virus (SLEV) is a pathogen, and although it was the cause of the epidemic, which emerged in St. Louis, Missouri, USA, in the early 1930s and reached people vectorial with the Culex genus mosquitoes, it has lost its popularity in recent years (Diaz et al., 2018).

WNV and SLEV are both flaviviruses, which are considered to be serologically related (Maharaj et al., 2018). When various proteins specific to WNV, JEV and SLEV viruses are investigated, methionine-labeled tryptic peptides of these structures are closer to WNV and SLEV agents when studied with a high-performance liquid chromatography (HPLC) device, and JEV has been found to have a different structure (Wright and Warr, 1986). Culex spp. mosquitoes are a frequent vectorial contributor to human encephalitis outbreaks in North America (Reisen, 2003).

Although WNV is frequently seen in the western hemisphere, it is reported that it is not an infectious disease specific to a certain region in the world as a result of numerous studies (Nalca et al., 2003). Research states that effective vaccines against the virus remain the front line of defense for these diseases. In this issue, there are no vaccines approved for human use to prevent SLEV. However, safe and effective vaccines against JEV have been used for a long time (Nalca et al., 2003).

Since West Nile virus causes infections and deaths with long-term viremia in house sparrows and many bird species in nature, preventive measures can be taken with various laboratory scans in this regard (Maharaj et al., 2018).

An important issue is SLEV transmission through blood product transfusion, which is reported in the literature as a case report. This finding emphasizes the need for clinicians to be more careful in evaluating patients for the transmission of SLEV (Venkat, 2015).

The most common clinical syndromes in SLEV are encephalitis, febrile illness, and meningitis. In addition, mortality was higher in patients with neuroinvasive disease and over 45 years of age (Curren et al., 2018).

Like most viral diseases, there is no defined, routinely used and specific treatment method to prevent these diseases in arboviral encephalitis (Nalca et al., 2003). In the prevention of the disease, various measures to reduce mosquito populations in living areas and personal protective measures to prevent disease transmission by mosquitoes are needed (Curren et al., 2018).

Other Mosquito-Associated Viruses

Different pathogen viruses and vectors are isolated by Chinese geography in the Asia region. Batai virus (BATV) is often carried by Anopheles philippinensis and causes infection in humans. Tahyna virus (TAHV) is caused by Aedes vexans, Aedes detritus and Culex spp. transmitted by humans isolated from sporadic cases (Xia, 2018).

A Mosquito-Borne Infectious Disease, Malaria

Malaria is a mosquito-borne infectious disease that begins with clinical symptoms such as fever, fatigue, vomiting and headache. According to WHO data, about half a million people die from malaria each year. Malaria is caused by Plasmodium species named P. falciparum, P. knowlesi, P. vivax, P. malariae, P. ovale curtisi and P. ovale wallikeri (Garrido-Cardenas et al., 2019). Plasmodium species are transmitted by mosquitoes of the genus Anopheles, with nearly 500 species classified into 7 subspecies (Singh et al., 2021). Especially, in sub-Saharan Africa, infections due to Plasmodium falciparum are dominant. Plasmodium vivax, associated with severe morbidity and mortality is also detected in Africa, but mostly in Asian and South American countries. The process of gametocytogenesis is observed within approximately 1-2 weeks after the appearance of parasites in human blood. Vector mosquitoes initiate egg production by feeding on human blood. Male and female gametocytes settle in the midgut lumen of the mosquito during this feeding. Sporozoites, which are then released into the hemolymph in the mosquito, infect the salivary gland of the vector. Sporozoite forms are transmitted to humans by mosquito bites (Singh et al., 2021). In malaria infection, the clinical picture begins with the schizont rupture of the liver and the release of merozoites into the peripheral circulation after the silent infection period. The process continues for 1-2 days when Plasmodium merozoites repeat the dispersal and asexual life cycles such as trophozoite development and a schizont rupture occurs (Milner, 2018).

The determination of some serious complications during malaria is also seen. For example, severe malaria anemia is common in pediatric patients, especially in the first 2 years of life, in highly endemic areas. Acidosis is due to a decrease in pH secondary to the production of Plasmodium lactate dehydrogenase (pLDH) by the malaria parasite. If respiratory distress accompanies this, it should be considered that the clinical picture will turn into severe malaria. With the development of cerebral malaria patients are admitted to the emergency department. Respiratory center suppression secondary to somnolence and/or brain edema during admission may also increase the level of acidosis. The ability of P. falciparum to bind to the endothelium may cause cerebral involvement in all age groups. It is reported that mortality may be higher in the pediatric age group in this situation (Milner, 2018).

In the diagnosis of malaria, in addition to the classical disease history and physical examination, peripheral blood smears presented in the laboratory are also stained with Giemsa. In recent years, new molecular methods have been developed to use these traditional approaches, especially in silent and undiagnosed cases, using the 18S rRNA gene-based Plasmodium species specific dot18S screening (Steenkeste, 2009).

It is important to start anti-malarial treatment early in the hospitalized patient in case of complications such as intense jaundice, cerebral involvement, acidosis, convulsions, shock, and coma in the malaria clinic (Cheng and Yansouni, 2013).

Conclusion

In mosquito-borne diseases, prevention of the disease before it occurs is one of the main methods as well as treatment. The key factors for prevention are avoidance of insects in endemic areas, eradication of mosquitoes and their sources, and the use of mosquito repellents.

References

Allison, J. R., Hogue, A. L., Shafer, C. W., & Huntington, M. K. (2019). Infectious Disease: Mosquito-Borne Viral Illnesses. *FP essentials*, 476, 11–17.

Bailey, C. C., Zhong, G., Huang, I. C., & Farzan, M. (2014). IFITM-Family Proteins: The Cell's First Line of Antiviral Defense. *Annual review of virology*, 1, 261–283. https://doi.org/10.1146/annurev-virology-031413-085537.

Caglioti, C., Lalle, E., Castilletti, C., Carletti, F., Capobianchi, M. R., & Bordi, L. (2013). Chikungunya virus infection: an overview. *The new microbiologica*, 36(3), 211–227.

Cheng, M. P., & Yansouni, C. P. (2013). Management of severe malaria in the intensive care unit. *Critical care clinics*, 29(4), 865–885. https://doi.org/10.1016/j.ccc.2013.06.008.

Chesarino, N. M., McMichael, T. M., & Yount, J. S. (2015). E3 Ubiquitin Ligase NEDD4 Promotes Influenza Virus Infection by Decreasing Levels of the Antiviral Protein IFITM3. *PLoS pathogens*, 11(8), e1005095. https://doi.org/10.1371/journal.ppat.1005095.

Curren, E. J., Lindsey, N. P., Fischer, M., & Hills, S. L. (2018). St. Louis Encephalitis Virus Disease in the United States, 2003-2017. *The American journal of tropical medicine and hygiene*, 99(4), 1074–1079. https://doi.org/10.4269/ajtmh.18-0420.

Diaz, A., Coffey, L. L., Burkett-Cadena, N., & Day, J. F. (2018). Reemergence of St. Louis Encephalitis Virus in the Americas. *Emerging infectious diseases*, 24(12), 2150–2157. https://doi.org/10.3201/eid2412.180372.

Driggers, R. W., Ho, C. Y., Korhonen, E. M., Kuivanen, S., Jääskeläinen, A. J., Smura, T., Rosenberg, A., Hill, D. A., DeBiasi, R. L., Vezina, G., Timofeev, J., Rodriguez, F. J., Levanov, L., Razak, J., Iyengar, P., Hennenfent, A., Kennedy, R., Lanciotti, R., du Plessis, A., & Vapalahti, O. (2016). Zika Virus Infection with Prolonged Maternal Viremia and Fetal Brain Abnormalities. *The New England journal of medicine*, 374(22), 2142–2151. https://doi.org/10.1056/NEJMoa1601824.

Ferraris, P., Yssel, H., & Missé, D. (2019). Zika virus infection: an update. *Microbes and infection*, 21(8-9), 353–360. https://doi.org/10.1016/j.micinf.2019.04.005.

Frumence, E., Roche, M., Krejbich-Trotot, P., El-Kalamouni, C., Nativel, B., Rondeau, P., Missé, D., Gadea, G., Viranaicken, W., & Desprès, P. (2016). The South Pacific epidemic strain of Zika virus replicates efficiently in human epithelial A549 cells leading to IFN-β production and apoptosis induction. *Virology*, 493, 217–226. https://doi.org/10.1016/j.virol.2016.03.006.

Garrido-Cardenas, J. A., González-Cerón, L., Manzano-Agugliaro, F., & Mesa-Valle, C. (2019). Plasmodium genomics: an approach for learning about and ending human malaria. *Parasitology research*, 118(1), 1–27. https://doi.org/10.1007/s00436-018-6127-9.

Hombach J. (2009). Guidelines for clinical trials of dengue vaccine in endemic areas. *Journal of clinical virology : the official publication of the Pan American Society for Clinical Virology*, 46 Suppl. 2, S7–S9. https://doi.org/10.1016/S1386-6532(09)70287-2.

Javed, F., Manzoor, K. N., Ali, M., Haq, I. U., Khan, A. A., Zaib, A., & Manzoor, S. (2018). Zika virus: what we need to know? *Journal of basic microbiology*, 58(1), 3–16. https://doi.org/10.1002/jobm.201700398.

Khetarpal, N., & Khanna, I. (2016). Dengue Fever: Causes, Complications, and Vaccine Strategies. *Journal of immunology research*, 2016, 6803098. https://doi.org/10.1155/2016/6803098.

Litvoc, M. N., Novaes, C., & Lopes, M. (2018). Yellow fever. *Revista da Associacao Medica Brasileira* (1992), 64(2), 106–113. https://doi.org/10.1590/1806-9282.64.02.106.

Maharaj, P. D., Bosco-Lauth, A. M., Langevin, S. A., Anishchenko, M., Bowen, R. A., Reisen, W. K., & Brault, A. C. (2018). West Nile and St. Louis encephalitis viral genetic determinants of avian host competence. *PLoS neglected tropical diseases*, 12(2), e0006302. https://doi.org/10.1371/journal.pntd.0006302.

Mansuy, J. M., Lhomme, S., Cazabat, M., Pasquier, C., Martin-Blondel, G., & Izopet, J. (2018). Detection of Zika, dengue and chikungunya viruses using single-reaction multiplex real-time RT-PCR. *Diagnostic microbiology and infectious disease*, 92(4), 284–287. https://doi.org/10.1016/j.diagmicrobio.2018.06.019.

Milner D. A., Jr (2018). Malaria Pathogenesis. *Cold Spring Harbor perspectives in medicine*, 8(1), a025569. https://doi.org/10.1101/cshperspect.a025569.

Monath, T. P., & Vasconcelos, P. F. (2015). Yellow fever. *Journal of clinical virology : the official publication of the Pan American Society for Clinical Virology*, 64, 160–173. https://doi.org/10.1016/j.jcv.2014. 08.030.

Nalca, A., Fellows, P. F., & Whitehouse, C. A. (2003). Vaccines and animal models for arboviral encephalitides. *Antiviral research*, 60(3), 153–174. https://doi.org/10.1016/j.antiviral.2003.08.001.

Reisen W. K. (2003). Epidemiology of St. Louis encephalitis virus. *Advances in virus research*, 61, 139–183. https://doi.org/10.1016/s0065-3527(03)61004-3.

Sam, I. C., Kümmerer, B. M., Chan, Y. F., Roques, P., Drosten, C., & AbuBakar, S. (2015). Updates on chikungunya epidemiology, clinical disease, and diagnostics. *Vector borne and zoonotic diseases* (Larchmont, N.Y.), 15(4), 223–230. https://doi.org/10.1089/vbz.2014.1680.

Singh, M., Suryanshu, Kanika, Singh, G., Dubey, A., & Chaitanya, R. K. (2021). Plasmodium's journey through the Anopheles mosquito: A comprehensive review. *Biochimie*, 181, 176–190. https://doi.org/10.1016/ j.biochi.2020.12.009.

Singhasivanon, P., & Jacobson, J. (2009). Dengue is a major global health problem. Foreword. *Journal of clinical virology : the official publication of the Pan American Society for Clinical Virology*, 46 Suppl 2, S1–S2. https://doi.org/10.1016/S1386-6532(09)70285-9.

Steenkeste, N., Incardona, S., Chy, S., Duval, L., Ekala, M. T., Lim, P., Hewitt, S., Sochantha, T., Socheat, D., Rogier, C., Mercereau-Puijalon, O., Fandeur, T., & Ariey, F. (2009). Towards high-throughput molecular detection of Plasmodium: new approaches and molecular markers. *Malaria journal*, 8, 86. https://doi.org/10.1186/1475-2875-8-86.

Teyssou R. (2009). La dengue: de la maladie à la vaccination [Dengue fever: from disease to vaccination]. *Medecine tropicale : revue du Corps de sante colonial*, 69(4), 333–334.

Venkat, H., Adams, L., Sunenshine, R., Krow-Lucal, E., Levy, C., Kafenbaum, T., Sylvester, T., Smith, K., Townsend, J., Dosmann, M., Kamel, H., Patron, R., Kuehnert, M., Annambhotla, P., Basavaraju, S. V., Rabe, I. B., & SLEV Transmission Investigation Team (2017). St. Louis encephalitis virus possibly transmitted through blood transfusion-Arizona, 2015. *Transfusion*, 57(12), 2987–2994. https://doi.org/ 10.1111/trf.14314.

Vu, D. M., Jungkind, D., & Angelle Desiree LaBeaud (2017). Chikungunya Virus. *Clinics in laboratory medicine*, 37(2), 371–382. https://doi.org/10.1016/j.cll.2017.01.008.

Wright, P. J., & Warr, H. M. (1986). Comparison of proteins specified by Murray Valley encephalitis, West Nile, Japanese encephalitis and St. Louis encephalitis viruses. *The Australian journal of experimental biology and medical science*, 64 (Pt 5), 485–488. https://doi.org/10.1038/icb.1986.52.

Wu, W., Wang, J., Yu, N., Yan, J., Zhuo, Z., Chen, M., Su, X., Fang, M., He, S., Zhang, S., Zhang, Y., Ge, S., & Xia, N. (2018). Development of multiplex real-time reverse-transcriptase polymerase chain reaction assay for simultaneous detection of Zika, dengue, yellow fever, and chikungunya viruses in a single tube. *Journal of medical virology*, 90(11), 1681–1686. https://doi.org/10.1002/jmv.25253.

Xia, H., Wang, Y., Atoni, E., Zhang, B., & Yuan, Z. (2018). Mosquito-Associated Viruses in China. *Virologica Sinica*, 33(1), 5–20. https://doi.org/10.1007/s12250-018-0002-9.

Chapter 20

Rabies

Ömer Salt*, MD

Department of Emergency Medicine, Faculty of Medicine, University of Trakya, Edirne, Turkey

Abstract

Rabies is almost always a fatal viral infection with two classical types: encephalitic and paralytic. After the onset of the disease, it is infrequent to recover. Most of the cases are related to the bite of an infected animal and especially dogs. Diagnosis depends on a history of suspected exposure and clinical symptoms. The most critical point is prevention. Mass dog vaccination can help to improve this aim. It is also important to perform pre-post exposure prophylaxis.

Keywords: encephalitis, infectious disease, rabies

Introduction

Despite all the improvements in disease prevention, rabies still has poor outcomes and high mortality rates worldwide. There are almost 60.000 deaths related to rabies per year, and it is endemic in Africa and relatively endemic in Asia. It is a neurotropic virus and a member of the Lyssavirus genus of the Rhabdoviridae family (Kuzmin et al., 2005). These viruses are bullet-shaped and contain a single-stranded RNA responsible for encoding structural proteins (Hankins & Rosekrans, 2004). This virus family predates neural structures and spreads to the central nervous system (CNS) via peripheral nerves. Although the certain mechanism of the CNS infection is unknown, it is suggested that Lyssaviruses cause dysfunction of neurons rather than death (Jackson, 2016). Another mechanism is mitochondrial dysfunction of neurons due to oxidative stress. Viral amplification starts in the muscle cells and then the sensorial and motor nerves. After that, viral glycoproteins attack the plasma membrane of the muscle cells (Murphy & Bauer, 1974). After the phase of inoculation, the glycoprotein spikes of the viruses attach to the nicotinic acetylcholine receptors.

---

* Corresponding Author's Email: dromersalt@gmail.com.

In: Environmental Emergencies and Injuries in Nature
Editors: Murat Yücel, Murat Güzel and İbrahim İkizceli
ISBN: 978-1-68507-833-1
© 2022 Nova Science Publishers, Inc.

However, the neurons do not contain these receptors and the mechanism of neuronal inoculation (Lentz et al., 1982). Then, the virus migrates towards the dorsal root ganglia at a speed of 100 mm per day (Warrell & Warrell, 2004). When the virus arrives in the spinal cord, it quickly ascends to the brain. The main targets of the virus are the brainstem and the diencephalon (Hemachudna et al., 2002).

After this step, the virus starts to disseminate towards highly innervated tissues like salivary glands (Wilson et al., 1975). Mononuclear cell infiltration and perivascular cuffing can be detected in the microscopic evaluation of CNS nerves. It is also possible to see oval, dense, intracytoplasmic-located "Negri bodies" in these neurons. But not all rabies virus exposures result in disease. Many factors affect the infection, such as type of virus and wound location. It is believed that all mammals could be theoretically infected by rabies viruses (Fishbein & Robinson, 1993).

Epidemiology

The rabies virus family has been distributed all around the world, and is primarily related to dog bites. Louis Pasteur developed the first vaccine against rabies in 1885 (Krebs et al., 2002). Although this vaccine was used extensively, the World Health Organization reported that almost 59.000 people die annually due to canine rabies virus infection (World Health Organization, 2021). A large number of these deaths occur in developing countries. Most of the cases are related to exposure to saliva from the bite of an animal. There are four main animal reservoirs of infection. They are raccoons, skunks, bats and foxes. However, rabies can develop without bite exposure (contact of the saliva with mucous membranes or open skin or transplantation of organs infected by the rabies virus) (Winkler et al., 1973). Although transmission via aerosols was reported in laboratory studies, there are rare cases in the literature (Davis et al., 2007). Transmission through organ transplantation is mainly related to kidney and liver transplantation (Srinivasan et al., 2005). The incubation period of the infection is variable. It could be seen in several days or years after exposure. But the mean period is four weeks to three months (Rupprecht et al., 2002). This period could be shorter for patients exposed to the virus in richly innervated body parts (especially the face). The average incubation period is 45 days, although latency periods between exposure and onset of disease as long as one to eight years have been reported (Smith et al., 1991).

According to the World Health Organization (WHO), there are three categories of rabies virus infection risk:

- Category I – touching or feeding animals, animal licks on intact skin (no exposure);
- Category II – nibbling of uncovered skin, minor scratches or abrasions without bleeding (exposure);
- Category III – single or multiple transdermal bites or scratches, contamination of the mucous membrane or broken skin with saliva from animal licks, exposures due to direct contact with bats (severe exposure).

Clinical Manifestations

If the rabies disease's clinical findings are seen in a patient, it usually progresses to viral encephalopathy and death. Some prodromal symptoms are non-specific for the disease, such as myalgia, mild fever, malaise and chills (Maier et al., 2010). Classical clinical findings include weakness, anorexia, nausea, vomiting, severe headache and sometimes photophobia. This period can last from a few days to a week. It is suggestive that if the patient describes paresthesia it radiates from the wound area to proximally (Hemachudha et al., 1987). After the prodrome period, two major forms of the disease can be seen. The first one is "encephalitic rabies," and the second one is paralytic rabies. Both conditions could start with non-specific prodromal symptoms (Hankins & Rosekrans, 2004). The most common form in humans is encephalitic rabies (80 per cent). There are some atypical symptoms like sensory deficits, brainstem pathologies and seizures in the prodromal phase.

Encephalitic Rabies

The classic findings of encephalitic rabies are pharyngeal spasm, fever, hydrophobia, and hyperactivity, subsiding to paralysis followed by coma and death (Hankins & Rosekrans, 2004). In the classic form of encephalitic rabies, hydrophobia is the most common sign, and it could be seen in up to 50% of patients. After developing a sore throat or dysphagia, an involuntary pharyngeal muscle spasm occurs if the patient attempts to drink water. Thinking about water can trigger involuntary spasms. Although it is uncommon, aerophobia could be seen in these patients (Petersen & Rupprecht, 2021). Due to the spasm of the diaphragm, aspiration and vomiting may occur. Patients could complain about pharyngeal spasms like an air drift, which could last 5-20 seconds. It is related to coughing, vomiting, asphyxia, and respiratory arrest (Black & Rupprecht, 2005). Grimace is due to the facial muscle spasm, and opisthotonos could be seen because of the hyperextension in neck and back muscles. In one-quarter of the patients, autonomic instability is established (Burton et al., 2005). The physical examination could detect changes in the mental situation, muscular tonus, fasciculations, and abnormal plantar response. After the development of coma, areflexia and flaccid paralysis are common.

Paralytic Rabies

After the prodromal period, patients start to complain about generalized weakness, and flaccid paralysis develops. Fewer than 20% of the patients were admitted with ascending paralysis, which could mimic Guillain-Barré syndrome. Paralysis may be symmetrical or asymmetrical. Pain in the affected muscles is typical, but nuchal rigidity, cranial nerve paralysis, and hydrophobia are uncommon. After this period, paralysis ascends, and the patient starts to lose sphincter tone. The main reason of death is paralysis of the respiratory muscles.

Diagnosis

The most critical points of the diagnosis are patient history and high suspicion of the disease (Venkatesan et al., 2013). If there is paresthesia around the site of an animal bite, it should alert the clinician about rabies. It is helpful to perform virus-specific immunofluorescent staining from a skin biopsy or detect antibodies from serum or cerebrospinal fluid (CSF). At this point, the differential diagnosis should be kept in mind. A diagnosis of rabies must be considered in patients who have acute progressive encephalitis with or without a history of an animal bite. Especially for patients with hydrophobia and aerophobia, encephalitic rabies should be one of the potential diagnoses. One of the most important points is to know that almost half of the rabies patients were diagnosed after death (Blanton et al., 2007).

Laboratory Diagnosis

To diagnose rabies before death, multiple specimens such as skin, CSF, and saliva are needed. The most sensitive test for the diagnosis is the skin polymerase chain reaction (PCR) test because the serum antibody levels could be negative until the late phase of the disease. For the patients who have been previously immunized, a second antibody test should be performed to detect if the antibody level is rising (Warrell & Warrell, 2004). If the rabies antibody is detected in the CSF, the infection must be suggested. For the skin biopsy, the preferred area is the posterior part of the neck especially at the hairline. This specimen should contain cutaneous nerves. If serum or CSF is collected, it should be at least 0.5 mL. All of the laboratory samples for rabies infection should be stored at -80°C. For postmortem testing, brainstem and other neural specimens are used to detect immunofluorescence staining for viral antigens. Although Negri bodies and eosinophilic neuronal cytoplasmic inclusions are pathognomonic for rabies infection, it is impossible to detect them in all patients.

Differential Diagnosis

Due to the non-specific prodromal phase, it is difficult to diagnose a patient with rabies infection. But it makes it easier to diagnose if the patient has a clinical picture suggesting paralytic rabies or encephalitis. Other toxic, metabolic, and infectious reasons for encephalopathy should be ruled out (Rupprecht et al., 2002). Guillain-Barré syndrome, poliomyelitis, and acute transverse myelitis can be confused with paralytic rabies. And also, rigidity can be seen in tetanus and strychnine poisoning.

Treatment

Although it is usually possible to prevent rabies with pre-post exposure prophylaxis, it is not always possible due to difficulty accessing vaccines and immunoglobulins in some areas. And unfortunately, there is no effective treatment method for rabies infection. There are two treatment options for patients with suspected or confirmed rabies: the aggressive and palliative approaches. The risks of the treatment modality and prognostic factors should be taken into consideration before the treatment. For the palliative approach, treatment should be focused on the patient's comfort, and sedatives and analgesics can be used freely (Apanga et al., 2016). For sedation and muscle relaxation, the most commonly used benzodiazepine is diazepam. It can be given intramuscularly or intravenously. Other alternative benzodiazepines are lorazepam and midazolam. For patients with agitation, delirium, aggression, or hallucinations, haloperidol can be used intramuscularly or subcutaneously (Warrell et al., 2017). Morphine can be used subcutaneously or intravenously for analgesia. For some patients, it may be necessary to use two or three drug combinations (e.g., midazolam plus haloperidol plus morphine). Anticholinergics such as glycopyrrolate or scopolamine can be used if the patient has a couple of salivary secretions. For the treatment of fever, ibuprofen/acetaminophen or a combination can be used.

The second treatment modality is the aggressive approach. It contains a combination of supportive care and other therapies. Supportive care should be performed in the intensive care unit. To reduce the spread of the virus, some antiviral agents can be used as a part of aggressive treatment. But there is not enough evidence to support this therapy. For this purpose, ribavirin, alfa interferon, and amantadine are the most commonly used antiviral agents. But these agents have some complications such as hematologic, gastrointestinal, or autoimmune. Favipiravir was also used for the treatment, but it failed. If alfa interferon is used, it should be administered intrathecally or intraventricularly (Appolinario et al., 2012). As a purine analog, ribavirin has an in-vitro activity against the rabies virus. But it was seen that it has no efficacy in mouse models. Another treatment option is amantadine. It is a synthetic antiviral agent and inhibits viral replication. But there is not enough evidence for its effectiveness (Busserau et al., 1988). Neuroprotective therapies could be beneficial for treatment. But there is no known effective agent for the treatment of rabies infection. Intranasal cooling or a cooling helmet could be used for therapeutic brain hypothermia (Roy et al., 2007). As a part of neuroprotective therapy, high-dose anesthetic agents can be used for metabolic suppression.

Some treatment methods should be avoided for the treatment of rabies infection. One of them is corticosteroids. They close the blood-brain barrier, and this results in reducing the entry of other therapeutic agents. The other one is minocycline. Although it has an anti-inflammatory and antioxidant effect, it could be harmful in the treatment of rabies infection (Ledesma et al., 2012). For the treatment of cerebral vasospasm, nimodipine, L-arginine, and vitamin C should not be used because they have no positive effect on cerebral vasospasm (Diringer et al., 2011).

Prophylaxis

Some factors should be considered on deciding on post-exposure prophylaxis; whether the patient was contaminated with a bite or the saliva of an animal with rabies or the patient's open mucous membrane, CSF or central nervous system was exposed to the saliva of the animal. But it is difficult to determine whether an animal has a rabies infection. So generally, prophylaxis is administered empirically. However, it should not be forgotten that any potentially infectious material contact with intact skin does not constitute an exposure. Other factors affect the decision of prophylaxis. The risk of rabies increases if the bites are multiple and close to the CNS (Manning et al., 2009). The transmission of rabies from human to human is sporadic but possible with a bite or non-bite exposure. But there is no report about transmission from a rabies-infected patient to a healthcare provider. It is not possible for the rabies virus to survive outside of the host. It is also affected by sunlight, pH, and other factors. As a result, if the virus contained material that is dry, it could be accepted as non-infectious. It is infrequent for an animal bite to have infectious contact with a human mucous membrane (Sitthi-Amorn et al., 1987). One of the essential points of a risk assessment is whether the exposing animal is likely to have rabies. It is necessary to know whether the animal was vaccinated, and provoked, or unprovoked. In general, animals with a suspicion of rabies are observed for ten days. Mort of the animals with rabies die within ten days. If the animal exhibits any symptoms of rabies in the follow-up period, it should be euthanized, and the animal's brain should be tested for rabies (Niezgoda et al., 1997).

Another vital point is pre-exposure prophylaxis. This is essential for people at high risk for rabies infection due to their occupation or travel. If the patient had pre-exposure prophylaxis, it is not necessary to use rabies immunoglobulin (RIG). It is also helpful to protect laboratory workers from accidental infections (Manning et al., 2008).

Rabies Immune Globulin and Vaccine

Before the administration of the rabies vaccine or RIG it is important to start with wound care. All of the wounds, scratches and other exposures should be washed with soap and water. As a virucidal agent, povidone-iodine can be used for cleaning. Other parts of the treatment are tetanus prophylaxis and antibiotic therapy (Dean et al., 1963). For pre- or post-exposure prophylaxis, rabies vaccine could be administered. It should be administered in the deltoid area intramuscularly (Boland et al., 2014). The dose is 1 mL. The vaccine should never be administered in the gluteal region. There are some studies to develop a less expensive vaccine compared to the human diploid cell vaccine. But they are still not complete. Also, to reduce the dose of vaccine, some experimental studies are working on an intradermal injection. But it is not licensed.

If the patient has not been previously vaccinated, passive and active immunization should always be performed. This should include five doses of HDCV and HRIG prophylaxis. Vaccination should start on the day of exposure (day 0) and continue on days 3, 7, 14, and 28. Rabies immune globulin should be administered with the first dose of vaccine. There is no evidence for fetal abnormality during pregnancy vaccination. Some adverse effects include pain at the injection site, redness, swelling, induration, and outcomes after vaccination. But there is no life-threatening event reported. As a part of post-exposure prophylaxis, rabies immune globulin is used commonly. There are two types of RIG. The first one is derived from the plasma of hyperimmunized donors, and the second one is from the horse (equine RIG). In theory, both of them are equally potent (Manning et al., 2008). The dose of HRIG is 20 IU/kg, and ERIG is 40 IU/kg. Due to the risk of suppressing antibody production, only a single dose of RIG is recommended. A significant part of RIG should be administered around and in the wound. The rest could be administered opposite the deltoid side of the vaccine. But if there is no visible wound, RIG could be administered to the contralateral deltoid or anterolateral thigh of the vaccinated side (Cabasso et al., 1971). For post-exposure rabies management, the WHO recommendations can be used (Table 1).

Table 1. World Health Organization post-exposure rabies management

Category	PEP vaccine regimen	RIG	Comments
Category I – Touching or feeding animals, animal licks on intact skin	Not required	Not required	Exposed skin surfaces should be washed
Category II – Nibbling of uncovered skin, minor scratches or abrasions without bleeding	Patients who have NOT been previously immunized: Immediate vaccination with one of the following regimens: • 2-sites ID on days 0, 3, and 7 • 1-site IM on days 0, 3, 7, and between • days 14 and 28 • 2-sites IM on day 0 and 1-site IM on days 7 and 21	Not required	Exposed skin surfaces should be washed
	Patients who have been previously immunized:* • 1-site ID on days 0 and 3 • 4-sites ID on day 0 • 1-site IM on days 0 and 3	Not required	Exposed skin surfaces should be washed
Category III – Single or multiple transdermal bites or scratches, contamination of mucous membrane or broken skin with saliva from animal licks, exposures due to direct contact with bats	Patients who have NOT been previously immunized: Immediate vaccination with one of the following regimens: • 2-sites ID on days 0, 3, and 7 • 1-site IM on days 0, 3, 7, and between days 14 and 28 • 2-sites IM on day 0 and 1-site IM on days 7 and 21	RIG should be administered	Exposed skin surfaces should be washed
	Patients who have been previously immunized:* • 1-site ID on days 0 and 3 • 4-sites ID on day 0 • 1-site IM on days 0 and 3	Not required	Exposed skin surfaces should be washed

* Previously immunized patients include those who have received pre-exposure prophylaxis and completed a post-exposure vaccine regimen >3 months ago. Post-exposure prophylaxis (except for wound care) is not recommended for individuals who have a rabies exposure <3 months after completing a post-exposure vaccine series.

Conclusion

Compared to all other viral encephalitis etiologies, rabies has the highest fatality rates. This makes it more critical. To develop new diagnostic and treatment modalities, we need to solve the mechanism and neuropathogenesis of infection. There are a lot of diagnostic protocols for human rabies. But most of them could be performed postmortem.

For this reason, the most crucial points are prevention, post-exposure prophylaxis, and treatment. It is essential to control the primary vector of rabies to prevent disease. This is possible with mass dog vaccinations. Pre- and post-exposure prophylaxis must be used, especially for the people who are at high risk.

References

Apanga, P. A., Awoonor-Williams, J. K., Acheampong, M., & Adam, M. A. (2016). A Presumptive Case of Human Rabies: A Rare Survived Case in Rural Ghana. *Frontiers in public health*, *4*, 256. https://doi.org/10.3389/fpubh.2016.00256.

Appolinario, C. M., & Jackson, A. C. (2015). Antiviral therapy for human rabies. *Antiviral therapy*, *20*(1), 1–10. https://doi.org/10.3851/IMP2851.

Blanton, J. D., Hanlon, C. A., & Rupprecht, C. E. (2007). Rabies surveillance in the United States during 2006. *Journal of the American Veterinary Medical Association*, *231*(4), 540–556. https://doi.org/10.2460/javma.231.4.540.

Bleck T P, Rupprecht CE. Rhabdoviruses. In: *Principles and Practice of Infectious Diseases*, Sixth Ed, Mandell GL, Bennett J E, Dolin R (Eds), Churchill Livingstone, Philadelphia 200 5. p.2047.

Boland, T. A., McGuone, D., Jindal, J., Rocha, M., Cumming, M., Rupprecht, C. E., Barbosa, T. F., de Novaes Oliveira, R., Chu, C. J., Cole, A. J., Kotait, I., Kuzmina, N. A., Yager, P. A., Kuzmin, I. V., Hedley-Whyte, E. T., Brown, C. M., & Rosenthal, E. S. (2014). Phylogenetic and epidemiologic evidence of multiyear incubation in human rabies. *Annals of neurology*, *75*(1), 155–160. https://doi.org/10.1002/ana.24016.

Burton, E. C., Burns, D. K., Opatowsky, M. J., El-Feky, W. H., Fischbach, B., Melton, L., Sanchez, E., Randall, H., Watkins, D. L., Chang, J., & Klintmalm, G. (2005). Rabies encephalomyelitis: clinical, neuroradiological, and pathological findings in 4 transplant recipients. *Archives of neurology*, *62*(6), 873–882. https://doi.org/10.1001/archneur.62.6.873.

Bussereau, F., Picard, M., Blancou, J., & Sureau, P. (1988). Treatment of rabies in mice and foxes with antiviral compounds. *Acta virologica*, *32*(1), 33–49.

Cabasso, V. J., Loofbourow, J. C., Roby, R. E., & Anuskiewicz, W. (1971). Rabies immune globulin of human origin: preparation and dosage determination in non-exposed volunteer subjects. *Bulletin of the World Health Organization*, *45*(3), 303–315.

Davis, A. D., Rudd, R. J., & Bowen, R. A. (2007). Effects of aerosolized rabies virus exposure on bats and mice. *The Journal of infectious diseases*, *195*(8), 1144–1150. https://doi.org/10.1086/512616.

Diringer, M. N., Bleck, T. P., Claude Hemphill, J., 3rd, Menon, D., Shutter, L., Vespa, P., Bruder, N., Connolly, E. S., Jr, Citerio, G., Gress, D., Hänggi, D., Hoh, B. L., Lanzino, G., Le Roux, P., Rabinstein, A., Schmutzhard, E., Stocchetti, N., Suarez, J. I., Treggiari, M., Tseng, M. Y., … Neurocritical Care Society (2011). Critical care management of patients following aneurysmal subarachnoid hemorrhage: recommendations from the Neurocritical Care Society's Multidisciplinary Consensus Conference. *Neurocritical care*, *15*(2), 211–240. https://doi.org/10.1007/s12028-011-9605-9.

Dean, D. J., Baer, G. M., & Thompson, W. R. (1963). Studies on the local treatment of rabies-infected wounds. *Bulletin of the World Health Organization*, *28*(4), 477–486.

Fishbein, D. B., & Robinson, L. E. (1993). Rabies. *The New England journal of medicine*, *329*(22), 1632–1638. https://doi.org/10.1056/NEJM199311253292208.

Hankins, D. G., & Rosekrans, J. A. (2004). Overview, prevention, and treatment of rabies. *Mayo Clinic proceedings*, *79*(5), 671–676. https://doi.org/10.4065/79.5.671

Hemachudha, T., Phanthumchinda, K., Phanuphak, P., & Manutsathit, S. (1987). Myoedema as a clinical sign in paralytic rabies. *Lancet (London, England)*, *1*(8543), 1210. https://doi.org/10.1016/s0140-6736(87)92186-6.

Hemachudha, T., Laothamatas, J., & Rupprecht, C. E. (2002). Human rabies: a disease of complex neuropathogenetic mechanisms and diagnostic challenges. *The Lancet. Neurology, 1*(2), 101–109. https://doi.org/10.1016/s1474-4422(02)00041-8.

Jackson A. C. (2016). Diabolical effects of rabies encephalitis. *Journal of neurovirology, 22*(1), 8–13. https://doi.org/10.1007/s13365-015-0351-1

Krebs, J. W., Noll, H. R., Rupprecht, C. E., & Childs, J. E. (2002). Rabies surveillance in the United States during 2001. *Journal of the American Veterinary Medical Association, 221*(12), 1690–1701. https://doi.org/10.2460/javma.2002.221.1690.

Kuzmin, I. V., Hughes, G. J., Botvinkin, A. D., Orciari, L. A., & Rupprecht, C. E. (2005). Phylogenetic relationships of Irkut and West Caucasian bat viruses within the Lyssavirus genus and suggested quantitative criteria based on the N gene sequence for lyssavirus genotype definition. *Virus research, 111*(1), 28–43. https://doi.org/10.1016/j.virusres.2005.03.008.

Ledesma, L. A., Lemos, E., & Horta, M. A. (2020). Comparing clinical protocols for the treatment of human rabies: the Milwaukee protocol and the Brazilian protocol (Recife). *Revista da Sociedade Brasileira de Medicina Tropical, 53*, e20200352. https://doi.org/10.1590/0037-8682-0352-2020.

Lentz, T. L., Burrage, T. G., Smith, A. L., Crick, J., & Tignor, G. H. (1982). Is the acetylcholine receptor a rabies virus receptor? *Science (New York, N.Y.), 215*(4529), 182–184. https://doi.org/10.1126/science.7053569.

Maier, T., Schwarting, A., Mauer, D., Ross, R. S., Martens, A., Kliem, V., Wahl, J., Panning, M., Baumgarte, S., Müller, T., Pfefferle, S., Ebel, H., Schmidt, J., Tenner-Racz, K., Racz, P., Schmid, M., Strüber, M., Wolters, B., Gotthardt, D., Bitz, F., ... Drosten, C. (2010). Management and outcomes after multiple corneal and solid organ transplantations from a donor infected with rabies virus. *Clinical infectious diseases: an official publication of the Infectious Diseases Society of America, 50*(8), 1112–1119. https://doi.org/10.1086/651267.

Manning, S. E., Rupprecht, C. E., Fishbein, D., Hanlon, C. A., Lumlertdacha, B., Guerra, M., Meltzer, M. I., Dhankhar, P., Vaidya, S. A., Jenkins, S. R., Sun, B., Hull, H. F., & Advisory Committee on Immunization Practices Centers for Disease Control and Prevention (CDC) (2008). Human rabies prevention--United States, 2008: recommendations of the Advisory Committee on Immunization Practices. *MMWR. Recommendations and reports: Morbidity and mortality weekly report. Recommendations and reports, 57*(RR-3), 1–28.

Murphy, F. A., & Bauer, S. P. (1974). Early street rabies virus infection in striated muscle and later progression to the central nervous system. *Intervirology, 3*(4), 256–268. https://doi.org/10.1159/000149762.

Niezgoda, M., Briggs, D. J., Shaddock, J., Dreesen, D. W., & Rupprecht, C. E. (1997). Pathogenesis of experimentally induced rabies in domestic ferrets. *American journal of veterinary research, 58*(11), 1327–1331.

Petersen B. W., Rupprecht CE. Human Rabies Epidemiology and Diagnosis. US Centers for Disease Control and Prevention, 2011. https://www.intechopen.com/books/non-flaviviru s-encephalitis/human-rabies-epidemiology-and-diagnosis (Accessed on October 10, 2021).

Roy, A., Phares, T. W., Koprowski, H., & Hooper, D. C. (2007). Failure to open the blood-brain barrier and deliver immune effectors to central nervous system tissues leads to the lethal outcome of silver-haired bat rabies virus infection. *Journal of virology, 81*(3), 1110–1118. https://doi.org/10.1128/JVI.01964-06.

Rupprecht, C. E., Hanlon, C. A., & Hemachudha, T. (2002). Rabies re-examined. *The Lancet. Infectious diseases, 2*(6), 327–343. https://doi.org/10.1016/s1473-3099(02)00287-6.

Sitthi-Amorn, C., Jiratanavattana, V., Keoyoo, J., & Sonpunya, N. (1987). The diagnostic properties of laboratory tests for rabies. *International journal of epidemiology, 16*(4), 602–605. https://doi.org/10.1093/ije/16.4.602

Srinivasan, A., Burton, E. C., Kuehnert, M. J., Rupprecht, C., Sutker, W. L., Ksiazek, T. G., Paddock, C. D., Guarner, J., Shieh, W. J., Goldsmith, C., Hanlon, C. A., Zoretic, J., Fischbach, B., Niezgoda, M., El-Feky, W. H., Orciari, L., Sanchez, E. Q., Likos, A., Klintmalm, G. B., Cardo, D., Rabies in Transplant Recipients Investigation Team (2005). Transmission of rabies virus from an organ donor to four transplant recipients. *The New England journal of medicine, 352*(11), 1103–1111. https://doi.org/10.1056/ NEJMoa043018.

Venkatesan, A., Tunkel, A. R., Bloch, K. C., Lauring, A. S., Sejvar, J., Bitnun, A., Stahl, J. P., Mailles, A., Drebot, M., Rupprecht, C. E., Yoder, J., Cope, J. R., Wilson, M. R., Whitley, R. J., Sullivan, J., Granerod,

J., Jones, C., Eastwood, K., Ward, K. N., Durrheim, D. N., … International Encephalitis Consortium (2013). Case definitions, diagnostic algorithms, and priorities in encephalitis: consensus statement of the international encephalitis consortium. *Clinical infectious diseases: an official publication of the Infectious Diseases Society of America*, *57*(8), 1114–1128. https://doi.org/10.1093/cid/cit458.

Warrell, M. J., & Warrell, D. A. (2004). Rabies and other lyssavirus diseases. *Lancet* (London, England), 363(9413), 959–969. https://doi.org/10.1016/S0140-6736(04)15792-9.

Warrell, M., Warrell, D. A., & Tarantola, A. (2017). The Imperative of Palliation in the Management of Rabies Encephalomyelitis. *Tropical medicine and infectious disease*, *2*(4), 52. https://doi.org/10.3390/tropicalmed2040052.

Wilson, J. M., Hettiarachchi, J., & Wijesuriya, L. M. (1975). Presenting features and diagnosis of rabies. *Lancet (London, England)*, *2*(7945), 1139–1140. https://doi.org/10.1016/s0140-6736(75)91021-1.

Winkler, W. G., Fashinell, T. R., Leffingwell, L., Howard, P., & Conomy, P. (1973). Airborne rabies transmission in a laboratory worker. *JAMA*, *226*(10), 1219–1221.

World Health Organization. *WHO Expert Consultation on Rabies*, Third Report. http://apps.who.int/iris/bitstream/handle/10665/272364/9789241210218-eng.pdf?sequence=1&isAllowed=y (Accessed on October 10, 2021).

Chapter 21

Tetanus

Serhat Atalar*, MD

Infectious Diseases and Clinical Microbiology, Ordu State Hospital, Ordu, Turkey

Abstract

Tetanus is a disease of the neurological system characterized by muscle spasms in which tetanospasmin, produced by the anaerobic bacillus *Clostridium tetani* found in the soil, takes an important place in the pathophysiology. The vaccine has been commonly used for the prevention of the disease since the 1940s. Despite the reduced incidence of the disease due to vaccination in developed countries, it is still a significant cause of morbidity and mortality in countries with limited opportunities for vaccination. Most of the reported cases consist of newborn infants and unvaccinated or incompletely vaccinated adults. Medical practices with an inappropriate aseptic technique and acute traumas constitute the most important risk factors. The spores produced by *C. tetani*, which is the causative agent of the disease, are highly resistant to unfavorable environmental conditions. Most of the cases appear within 8-14 days after transmission, and this duration may range between 3 and 21 days. Two toxins called tetanolysin and tetanospasmin are released by the microorganism. Tetanospasmin enters the nervous system through the lower motor neurons and reaches the central nervous system by spreading retrogradely. It leads to muscle rigidity and autonomic instability by preventing the release of neurotransmitters from inhibitory cells. This disease has four clinical types consisting of generalized, localized, cephalic, and neonatal. The clue findings for tetanus are trismus with rigidity in the jaw or masseter and risus sardonicus that develops with increased tone in the orbicularis oris muscle. It is diagnosed with a history and physical examination. The culture for diagnosis is usually difficult and unbeneficial. Its treatment involves ensuring airway patency, administration of benzodiazepine, administration of tetanus immunoglobulin, and metronidazole. Tetanus is not transmitted from person to person. It is possible to prevent the disease through vaccination. However, individuals who have recovered from tetanus have no natural immunity and can be infected again. For the prevention of the disease, the tetanus vaccine should be administered to patients who present with small, clean wounds and have not received at least three doses of tetanus vaccine or whose last dose was administered more than 10 years ago. Patients with incomplete or unknown tetanus vaccine who present with severe or contaminated wounds should receive the vaccine and human tetanus immunoglobulin.

---

* Corresponding Author's Email: drserhatatalar@gmail.com.

In: Environmental Emergencies and Injuries in Nature
Editors: Murat Yücel, Murat Güzel and İbrahim İkizceli
ISBN: 978-1-68507-833-1
© 2022 Nova Science Publishers, Inc.

Keywords: tetanus, tetanus toxoid, tetanospasmin

Introduction

Tetanus is a disease resulting from tetanospasmin produced by *Clostridium tetani*, an anaerobic bacillus that can be found in soil, dust, and animal feces. It is characterized by muscle spasms and affects the neurological system. Although the relationship between the injury and disease was noticed in the ancient Greek and Egyptian civilizations, the vaccine has been used commonly since the 1940s (Birch & Bleck, 2019).

Epidemiology

Despite the gradual decrease in the number of tetanus cases along with the use of the vaccine in developed countries, the disease is currently endemic due to the difficulty in access to the vaccine in developing countries. Although tetanus may affect people of all ages, it is more common in vaccinated pregnant women and mothers and newborns due to unfavorable birth conditions in developing countries and elderly individuals in relation to the level of antibodies with reduced protection over time in developed countries. On a global scale, it is estimated that 48,000-80,000 deaths occurred due to tetanus in 2016 (Kyu et al., 2017). However, the actual number is unknown since tetanus is not required to be reported in many countries. It was reported that approximately 34,000 newborns died of neonatal tetanus in 2015 (WHO, 2015). These data are still very high, although they decreased by 96% compared to the period during which 787,000 newborn infants died in 1988 (WHO, 2016). Along with the widespread use of vaccination, the number of tetanus cases has decreased significantly in developed countries. Two hundred and sixty-four cases of tetanus and 19 deaths were reported by the United States (USA) Centers for Disease Control and Prevention (CDC) between 2009 and 2017.

Microbiology

Clostridium tetani is an obligate anaerobic bacillus, which is Gram-positive in fresh cultures but has variable staining characteristics in older cultures or tissue samples. In the growth phase, it moves slowly with its flagella and produces tetanospasmin (tetanus toxin) and tetanolysin toxins. The plasmid on which tetanospasmin is encoded is present in all toxigenic strains and has a neurotoxic property held responsible for the clinical picture of the disease (Eisel et al., 1986). The role of tetanolysin in the disease is unclear, although it causes damage to the membranes in the adjacent cells and hemolysis. The matured microorganism loses its flagella and produces spores in the terminal region. This appearance resembles a drumstick or racket. Bacterial spores are quite resistant to unfavorable environmental conditions. Although it is resistant to ethanol, phenol, and formalin, it is possible to prevent infectiousness with glutaraldehyde, iodine, hydrogen peroxide, or autoclaving at 121°C for 15 minutes. Even though it can grow in an obligate anaerobic medium at 37°C in the culture, its culture results have no diagnostic value (Birch & Bleck, 2019).

Pathogenesis

The disease emerges when spores found in soil, especially in heavily fertilized areas, in the intestines and feces of various animals, on the surface of rusty tools such as nails and needles, and in wood chips, infect disintegrated human tissues and turn into vegetative bacteria and begin to produce tetanospasmin. Tetanospasmin, one of the most toxic molecules known, binds to peripheral neuron terminals with the vascular and lymphatic flow and reaches the body of the neurons and the central nervous system by retrograde transport along the axons. During this period, in other words, when the toxin travels along the axon, it cannot be neutralized with antitoxin. After the toxin travels to the brain stem and spinal cord, it reaches the extracellular space and presynaptic inhibitory neurons. As a result of the inhibition of inhibitory neurotransmitters released from there by the toxin, the lower motor neurons are affected, and disinhibition and muscle rigidity occur. Agonist and antagonist muscles respond to any stimulus to the motor system by contracting simultaneously. Thus, severe and long-lasting tetanic spasms take place. Furthermore, tetanospasmin triggers many symptoms such as hypertension, hypotension, and arrhythmia by affecting the autonomic nervous system (Farrar et al., 2000).

There is an increased risk of tetanus after the spores enter the tissue following a trauma that disrupts the integrity of tissues, especially in the presence of conditions under which an anaerobic environment occurs, such as ischemia or necrosis. Injuries causing the transmission of *C. tetani* spores, concomitant bacterial co-infection, a foreign body, localized ischemia, and the presence of necrotic tissue are predisposing factors. The conditions that can be considered risky for transmission are injuries caused by factors such as wood chips, nails or wires, gunshot injuries, fractures, burns and aseptic parenteral applications (intravenous substance abuse), an improperly cut newborn umbilical cord (Thwaites et al., 2015), circumcision, necrotic infections involving post-operative intestinal flora, obstetric patients, etc. (Tucker et al., 2014).

Clinical Manifestations

While the incubation period of tetanus varies between 3 and 21 days, the disease starts within 8-14 days in most cases (WHO, 2021). The disease is examined in four clinical types, including generalized, localized, cephalic, and neonatal forms. It is considered that these clinical types occur according to the host factors, such as the presence of antibodies and the entry site of the agent into the body.

The most common form is generalized tetanus. Trismus is observed in 80% of the cases. The symptoms of autonomic hyperactivity, such as sweating and tachycardia, may occur at the early stage of the disease. However, at the later stages, respiratory symptoms due to chest muscles being affected, dysphagia, nuchal rigidity, risus sardonicus, opisthotonus, abdominal rigidity, unstable hypertension or hypotension, arrhythmia, and fever due to pharyngeal muscle involvement may occur. Tonic contractions and severe spasms are quite painful since the disease does not affect consciousness (Birch & Bleck, 2019).

Localized tetanus manifests itself with tonic and spastic muscle contractions in a limb or body area. When it occurs as localized tetanus at the early stage of the disease and the toxin reaches the central nervous system, it may progress to the actual clinical picture in the form of generalized tetanus. A mild or persistent clinical picture may sometimes be observed due to the partial immune response to tetanospasmin (Callison & Nguyen, 2021).

Cephalic tetanus is a special form of localized disease in which the cranial nervous system is nearly always affected after a head or neck trauma. Generalized tetanus may also occur later in patients with cephalic tetanus as in local tetanus. Facial nerve palsy is most frequently observed in this form. It may be accompanied by the involvement of the VI, III, IV, and XII cranial nerves (Birch & Bleck, 2019. Bae & Bourget, 2021).

Neonatal tetanus is frequently observed in the infants of mothers with non-aseptic delivery conditions or inadequate immunization. It typically occurs 5-7 days after delivery (3-24 days). The most common symptom is the absence of sucking. The disease progresses within hours since the axonal length in children is proportionally shorter compared to adults. Patients are lost due to apnea or sepsis after rigidity and spasms. Its mortality rate exceeds 90%, and developmental retardation is observed in those who can survive (Anlar et al., 1989).

Depending on the amount of tetanus toxin that reaches the central nervous system, the severity and frequency of the clinical features of tetanus may differ among cases. The signs and symptoms may progress up to two weeks after the start of the disease. The clinical features of the disease are reduced along with an increase in the period from the incubation period of the disease and onset of symptoms to the occurrence of spasms. The severity of the disease may increase in deep penetrating injuries (Thwaites et al., 2006). The disease may last for 4-6 weeks. The effects of the toxin on the clinical picture of the disease are considered to decrease with the formation of new axons (Birch & Bleck, 2019).

Diagnosis

Tetanus is diagnosed with a history and physical examination. It is necessary to suspect tetanus if there is a risky injury for tetanus and insufficient immunization against tetanus. Laboratory tests are utilized to exclude intoxications that can be confused with the clinical picture of the disease, rather than confirming the diagnosis. Electromyographic studies may be beneficial in suspicious cases, especially in the case of failure to detect the gateway. It is impossible to measure anti-tetanus antibodies in most patients with tetanus. Antibody titer values of 0.01 IU/mL or higher are usually considered to be protective (Bae et al., 2021). Diseases above this titer were rarely reported (Crone et al., 1992).

The wound cultures of *C. tetani* are not useful for diagnosis due to the following three reasons:

1. Even carefully done anaerobic cultures are frequently negative.
2. Even if there is growth in the culture, this does not indicate that the organism contains the toxin-producing plasmid.
3. The disease does not occur if the person has sufficient immunization while there is growth in the culture.

Differential Diagnosis

Dental infections, pharyngeal and peritonsillar abscess, and temporomandibular diseases may be confused with tetanus due to trismus and dysphagia in the beginning. The definitive diagnosis is established by a physical examination and radiology.

Strychnine intoxication is regarded as a good mimic of tetanus after accidental or suicidal ingestion of rat poison. A definitive diagnosis is made by toxicological examination in serum, urine, and tissue. Similar first-line treatments of tetanus and strychnine intoxication ensure that the treatment is initiated without delay and without waiting for the test results.

It is possible to confuse dystonic reactions to neuroleptic drugs or other central dopamine antagonists with the neck stiffness of tetanus. However, the administration of anticholinergic agents (benztropine or diphenhydramine) to patients with dystonic reactions is rapidly effective against dystonic reactions. Such treatment has no effect on patients with tetanus.

Stiff-person syndrome (SPS) is a rare neurological disorder characterized by severe muscle rigidity associated with autoantibodies against glutamic acid decarboxylase. Spasms of the body and limbs may be triggered by auditory, tactile, or emotional stimuli. A rapid response to diazepam, and the absence of trismus or facial spasms, distinguish SPS from true tetanic spasms (Andreadou et al., 2007).

The lack of consciousness in tetanus is an important clue for distinguishing it from viral encephalitis, meningoencephalitis, and meningitis.

Treatment

Tetanus is ideally treated in the intensive care unit by consulting an anesthesiologist or intensive care specialist trained in the management of complications of the disease.

1. Airway management is the first step in treatment. In case of need, endotracheal intubation should be considered using benzodiazepine sedation and neuromuscular blockade (e.g., vecuronium, 0.1 mg/kg) (Afshar et al., 2004).
2. The level of antitoxin, strychnine and dopamine antagonist tests, electrolytes, blood urea nitrogen, creatinine, creatine kinase and urine myoglobin levels should be included in the collection of samples (Birch & Bleck, 2019).
3. It is necessary to clarify the investigation of traces of trauma that may be associated with tetanus, and the incubation period, time of event and immunization status.
4. The administration of benztropine (1-2 mg, IV) or diphenhydramine (50 mg, IV) may be considered to exclude a dystonic reaction to a dopamine blocking agent (Birch & Bleck, 2019).
5. It is possible to administer diazepam (generally 10-30 mg IV as an initial dose) in increments of 5 mg or lorazepam IV in 2 mg increments at intervals of 1-4 hours for controlling spasms and reducing rigidity (Afshar et al., 2011). The infusion of midazolam is another option.
6. The patient is transferred to a quiet and dark area of the intensive care unit.
7. It is necessary to perform wound debridement for all patients as a way to remove necrotic tissue for stopping the production of toxins and wound site management.

8. Due to the irreversible binding of tetanus toxin to tissues, only the unbound toxin can be targeted for neutralization. The use of passive immunization for the neutralization of the unbound toxin is associated with better survival and is considered as the standard treatment. Human tetanus immunoglobulin is frequently preferred. The CDC recommends a dose of 500 units, some around the wound and some intramuscularly. It is necessary to administer immunoglobulin to an extremity different from the one vaccinated. In the absence of human tetanus immunoglobulin, standard immunoglobulin can be administered intravenously (IV) as an alternative (CDC, 2021).

9. Antibiotics are universally recommended despite their minor role in the treatment of tetanus. Nevertheless, it is important to highlight that suitable antimicrobial treatment may fail to remove C. tetani unless sufficient wound debridement is performed (Campbell et al., 2009). Metronidazole (500 mg IV every 6-8 hours) is the preferred treatment for tetanus. However, penicillin G (2-4 million units IV every 4-6 hours) is a safe and effective alternative. One hundred mg of doxycycline every 12 hours is another option. Macrolides, clindamycin, vancomycin, and chloramphenicol are other agents with activity against *C. tetani*. The efficacy of these agents was not evaluated. However, they are likely to be effective based on in-vitro susceptibility data (Afshar et al., 2011). The recommended duration of antimicrobial treatment is 7-10 days.

10. With the purposes of providing an adrenergic blockade and suppressing autonomic hyperactivity, magnesium sulfate can be preferred since it blocks the release of catecholamines by acting as a presynaptic neuromuscular blocker and reduces the receptor response to catecholamines (Thwaites et al., 2006). Labetalol (0.25 to 1 mg/min) can be used instead of propranolol (Buchanan et al., 1978) with reports of sudden death for the beta-receptor blockade.

11. All patients with tetanus should receive complete active immunization (for example, three doses in adults and children over 7 years old) since tetanus is one of the few bacterial diseases that do not provide immunity after acute disease. Vaccines containing tetanus and diphtheria toxoids are initiated immediately after the diagnosis. Such vaccines should be administered at a different site than the tetanus immune globulin.

12. Since patients with tetanus usually become disabled due to long-term muscle loss and contractures, it is necessary to initiate physical treatment as soon as the spasms are over (Trung et al., 2019).

Table 1. Post-exposure prophylaxis in injuries suspected of tetanus (Liang et al., 2018)

Immunization	Type of Wound			
	Clean and Small Wound		Other Wounds *	
	Vaccine	Immunoglobulin	Vaccine	Immunoglobulin
<3 doses of vaccine or Unknown	Yes	No	Yes	No
≥3 doses of vaccine administered	If ≥10 years have passed since the last dose	No	If ≥5 years have passed since the last dose	No

* Injuries in contact with dirt, feces, and saliva, incisional wounds, burns, puncture wounds, bites, frostbite, and gunshot wounds.

Prophylaxis

Tetanus is a disease that can be prevented by vaccination. It is included in the routine vaccination program in many countries. The tetanus vaccine, which is a toxoid vaccine, has different formulations combined with diphtheria and pertussis. Pediatric diphtheria-tetanus (DT) or the adult diphtheria-tetanus (Td) form with a combination of tetanus and diphtheria, the pediatric diphtheria-pertussis-tetanus (DPT) form including tetanus-diphtheria and whole-cell pertussis vaccine, and pediatric diphtheria-tetanus-acellular pertussis (DTaP) or the adult tetanus-diphtheria-acellular pertussis (Tdap) form including acellular pertussis vaccine are available.

The Advisory Committee on Immunization Practices (ACIP) recommends DTaP at 2, 4, 6, and 15-18 months and 4-6 years of age for children and Tdap at 11-12 years of age. In the following years, a booster dose with the Td vaccine is recommended every 10 years. A booster dose is important due to the decreased level of antibodies, especially at advanced ages. It is recommended that one of the booster doses should be selected as Tdap during pregnancy (Rabadi & Brady, 2021).

It is necessary to review the tetanus vaccination history of all patients presenting with injury. The tetanus vaccine should be administered to patients who present with small, clean wounds and have not received at least three doses of tetanus vaccine or whose last dose was administered more than 10 years ago. Patients with an incomplete or unknown tetanus vaccine history who have more severe or contaminated wounds should receive the vaccine and human tetanus immunoglobulin (see Table 1).

Since tetanus disease does not leave immunity, it is necessary not to neglect vaccination for people who have recovered from this disease.

Some patients with humoral immunodeficiency may not respond sufficiently to toxoid injection, and such patients should receive passive immunization for tetanus-prone injuries without considering the period of time since the last booster. Approximately half of the patients lose tetanus immunity after chemotherapy for leukemia or lymphoma. The patients undergoing bone marrow or stem cell transplantation should be revaccinated after the procedure.

Conclusion

Tetanus is a disease that may lead to high mortality and a long hospital stay. It is possible to encounter difficulties in its management since there is no gold standard method for diagnosis; it is based on history and examination, and the trauma focus cannot be found in some of the patients. There is a limited number of randomized controlled studies investigating the treatment. Therefore, prevention and post-exposure prophylaxis are the most important points. Although it can be prevented by vaccination, it is still observed in mothers and their newborns in countries with difficulty in accessing the vaccine and those over the age of 65, when the antibody level starts to decrease, in developed countries. It is necessary to make prophylaxis protocols widespread for the prevention of the disease.

References

Afshar, M., Raju, M., Ansell, D., & Bleck, T. P. (2011). Narrative review: tetanus - a health threat after natural disasters in developing countries. *Annals of internal medicine,* 154(5), 329-335.

Andreadou, E., Kattoulas, E., Sfagos, C., & Vassilopoulos, D. (2007). Stiff person syndrome: avoiding misdiagnosis. *Neurological Sciences,* 28(1), 35-37.

Anlar, B., Yalaz, K., & Dizme, R. (1989). Long-Term Prognosis After Neonatal Tetanus. *Developmental Medicine & Child Neurology,* 31(1), 76-80.

Bae, C., & Bourget, D. (2021). Tetanus. In *StatPearls.* StatPearls Publishing.

Birch, T. B., Bleck T. B. (2019). Tetanus (Clostridium tetani) Chapter 244 In: Bennett, J. E., Dolin, R., & Blaser, M. J. (2019). Mandell, Douglas, and Bennett's Principles and Practice of Infectious Diseases E-Book. *Elsevier Health Sciences*; 2948-53.

Buchanan, N., Smit, L., Cane, R. D., & De Andrade, M. (1978). Sympathetic overactivity in tetanus: fatality associated with propranolol. *British medical journal,* 2(6132), 254.

Callison, C., & Nguyen, H. (2021). Tetanus Prophylaxis. In *StatPearls.* StatPearls Publishing.

Campbell, J. I., Yen, L. T. M., Loan, H. T., Diep, T. S., Nga, T. T. T., Hoang, N. V. M., & Baker, S. (2009). Microbiologic characterization and antimicrobial susceptibility of Clostridium tetani isolated from wounds of patients with clinically diagnosed tetanus. *The American journal of tropical medicine and hygiene*, 80(5), 827-831.

Centers for Disease Control and Prevention. *Tetanus.* https://www.cdc.gov/vaccines/pubs/surv-manual/chpt 16-tetanus.html (Accessed on December 9, 2021).

Crone, N. E., & Reder, A. T. (1992). Severe tetanus in immunized patients with high anti-tetanus titers. *Neurology,* 42(4), 761-761.

Eisel, U., Jarausch, W., Goretzki, K., Henschen, A., Engels, J., Weller, U., ... & Niemann, H. (1986). Tetanus toxin: primary structure, expression in E. coli, and homology with botulinum toxins. *The EMBO journal,* 5(10), 2495-2502.

Farrar, J., & Newton, C. (2000). Neurological aspects of tropical disease. *Journal of Neurology, Neurosurgery & Psychiatry,* 68(2), 135-136.

Gonzales y Tucker, R. D., & Frazee, B. (2014). View from the front lines: an emergency medicine perspective on clostridial infections in injection drug users. *Anaerobe,* 30, 108-115.

Kyu, H. H., Mumford, J. E., Stanaway, J. D., Barber, R. M., Hancock, J. R., Vos, T., & Naghavi, M. (2017). Mortality from tetanus between 1990 and 2015: findings from the global burden of disease study 2015. *BMC Public Health,* 17(1), 1-17.

Liang, J. L., Tiwari, T., Moro, P., Messonnier, N. E., Reingold, A., Sawyer, M., & Clark, T. A. (2018). Prevention of pertussis, tetanus, and diphtheria with vaccines in the United States: recommendations of the Advisory Committee on Immunization Practices (ACIP). *MMWR Recommendations and Reports,* 67(2), 1.

Rabadi, T., & Brady, M. F. (2021). Tetanus Toxoid. *StatPearls* [Internet].

Thwaites, C. L., Beeching, N. J., & Newton, C. R. (2015). Maternal and neonatal tetanus. *The lancet,* 385(9965), 362-370.

Thwaites, C. L., Yen, L. M., Glover, C., Tuan, P. Q., Nga, N. T. N., Parry, J., ... & Farrar, J. J. (2006). Predicting the clinical outcome of tetanus: the tetanus severity score. *Tropical Medicine & International Health,* 11(3), 279-287.

Thwaites, C. L., Yen, L. M., Loan, H. T., Thuy, T. T. D., Thwaites, G. E., Stepniewska, K., ... & Farrar, J. J. (2006). Magnesium sulphate for treatment of severe tetanus: a randomised controlled trial. *The Lancet,* 368(9545), 1436-1443.

Trung, T. N., Duoc, N. V., Nhat, L. T., Yen, L. M., Hao, N. V., Truong, N. T., ... & Thwaites, C. L. (2019). Functional outcome and muscle wasting in adults with tetanus. *Transactions of the Royal Society of Tropical Medicine and Hygiene,* 113(11), 706-713.

World Health Organization. *Tetanos.* https://www.who.int/news-room/fact-sheets/detail/tetanus (Accessed on December 9, 2021).

Chapter 22

Poisonous Plants

Emre Özgen*, MD

Department of Emergency Medicine, Merzifon Karamustafapasa State Hospital Amasya,
Merzifon/Amasya, Turkey

Abstract

Plants are the most important actors of life on earth. On the other hand, intentional or
accidental ingestion of or exposure to poisonous weeds in nature is among the reasons for
the increasing number of applications to the hospital emergency department. Many plant
poisoning cases can be missed because they are not considered differential diagnoses. This
section will discuss the most common exposures to poisonous plants and their effects on
the human body.

Keywords: poisoning, plant, emergency, environmental

Introduction

Plants are vital to the continuation of life on earth. In 2016, about 370,000 plant species
recognized by scientists were identified, and new species are being discovered, particularly in
tropical regions of the world (Group et al., 2016). Plants act as a source of life by providing
oxygen to the earth. They are also widely used for nutrition, recreation, regeneration, and
healing functions. On the other hand, some plants have high toxicities that can cause serious
health problems, and they have been used as biological weapons or for suicide purposes. Such
poisonous plants are used around the world. They can be found in forests, agricultural lands,
wetlands, rivers, or roadsides, and in urban areas such as parks and gardens. Some of the
poisonous plants are used as ornaments in residences.

It should be noted that almost all plants contain chemical toxins such as alkaloids,
glycosides, saponins, resinoids, oxalates, nitrites, and poisonous minerals that can be harmful.
These phytoxins protect plants from potential enemies such as insects, microorganisms, and
animals (Howlett, 2006). Concentrations of phytoxins in plants vary within their body. For

---

* Corresponding Author's Email: emreozgen46523@gmail.com.

In: Environmental Emergencies and Injuries in Nature
Editors: Murat Yücel, Murat Güzel and İbrahim İkizceli
ISBN: 978-1-68507-833-1

example, while some plants have localized levels of phytoxins in one region, some parts can be seen to provide beneficial effects to the contrary, while others are quite toxic. Some plants also have homogeneously distributed toxins throughout the plant, so they can cause toxic effects no matter where the body is touched. Depending on the density of the plant toxin, a toxic response may show changes. A chronic response is usually associated with low doses of the toxin, but an acute response occurs when exposed to high concentrations.

Exposure to Poisonous Plants

Normal cell functioning is disrupted when the plant toxin enters the body through ingestion, inhalation, or skin or eye contact, resulting in plant poisoning.

Ingestion exposure: The most common form of poisoning is through the ingestion of poisonous plants, whether intentional or accidental. Some poisonous plants are very difficult to distinguish from edible plants. Some diseases and even death are caused by eating such plants by mistake and not noticing or being overlooked. Some toxic plants are deliberately ingested and taken into the body due to their healing and therapeutic properties. Humans can be affected and even poisoned due to the narrow gap between beneficial effects and toxicity levels. Some phytoxins can also be transported with products such as meat and milk obtained from livestock (Lopes, Riet-Correa, & Medeiros, 2019).

Inhalation exposure: People can take phytotoxins into their bodies with breathing, resulting in burning and allergic reactions that cause serious mucosal damage to the respiratory tract. Inhalation causes toxins to quickly get into the bloodstream and show their effects.

Exposure through the skin or eye contact: A number of abnormal changes such as contact dermatitis may be observed on the body surfaces that come into contact with toxic plants or liquids belonging to plants. When contact is with the eyes, it can cause visual impairments or even loss of vision. Some plants may cause physical damage to the skin layer through their needles, or surface contact may have no effect (Froberg, Ibrahim, & Furbee, 2007).

Toxic Effects of Phytoxins

Toxic substances in plants can be grouped according to their toxicological effects in humans.

Irritants Group (Chemical and Mechanical)

Contacting these toxins can cause reversible inflammation of a body surface, including the eyes, respiratory tract, skin, or mucous membranes. They can cause redness, itching, pain, and rashes. Contact with the eyes can cause conjunctivitis and blindness in severe cases.

Allergens

Exposure to these toxins triggers an immunological response that can cause rash, itching, and swelling in the exposed area. Allergens can also cause vasodilation and increased permeability of the vessels by releasing histamines. In severe cases, histamines can cause vasoconstriction. In severe cases, histamines can cause vascular collapse.

Anticholinergics

These competitively inhibit the transmission of nerve impulses by inhibiting the neurotransmitter acetylcholine in the parasympathetic nervous system and receptor sites in the brain. This can lead to tachycardia, dry and red skin, mydriasis, hyperthermia, urinary retention, heart rhythm disturbances, respiratory failure, heart failure, seizures, coma, and even death.

Calcium Oxalate Crystals

Calcium oxalate is an insoluble salt formed by the combination of calcium and oxalic acid. It plays an active role in plants that perform photosynthesis. Calcium oxalate crystals are found in many plants. Crystals are found in intracellular vacuoles known as idioblasts (Gómez-Espinoza et al., 2021). When chewed, edema and pain appear in the oral mucosa. Numerous calcium oxalate needles (rafts) and protease found in special cells (idioblasts) and protease in the plant are blamed (Gardner D G, 1994).

Cardiac Glycosides

These have been used since the 18th century to treat cardiovascular diseases, especially congestive heart failure. Many plants belonging to this class have been found, but Zakkum (Nerium oleander) is the most intoxicating plant. Sodium-potassium acts on the ATPase pump, increasing peripheral vascular resistance and heart contractions (Fisch C, 1985).

Convulsants

These include agents that cause abnormal electrical activity in the brain, causing rhythmic, forced contractions of muscles.

Mitotic Inhibitors

These agents interfere with cell division by affecting gastrointestinal and bone marrow cells.

Cyanogenic Components

These originate from the seeds of plants rather than the plants themselves. Metabolites produced due to the digestion of apricot kernels can cause cyanide poisonings, such as peach kernels, apricot flowers, and apricots. It is known that cyanide affects aerobic cell metabolism by preventing oxygen depletion in mitochondria and thus inhibits cellular respiration. The toxin also inhibits oxidative phosphorylation, which affects cellular energy production.

Sodium Channel Activators

These cause sodium channels to open more easily and stay open longer, allowing for a persistent sodium influx that causes the usual electrical impulse sequence in the body to change. This often affects the rate of heart muscle contractions leading to heart failure. Vomiting, motor weakness, and paralysis may occur due to signal loss in the central nervous system (Krenzelok & Mrvos, 2011).

Toxic Proteins (Toxalbumins)

These toxins disable ribosomes and disrupt the synthesis of proteins in the body.

Commonly Visible Poisonous Plants

Abrus Precatorius (Rosary Pea)

Abrus precatorius is a plant that is widely distributed in tropical and subtropical forests. Traditionally, it has been used to treat numerous ailments (Sunday et al., 2016). The smooth seeds are used to make rosaries and necklaces. It contains abrin, one of the most toxic substances known in nature. Chewing even a single bean can be fatal. Hemorrhagic gastroenteritis, unconsciousness, seizures, and coma can be seen. It can even result in death (Worbs et al., 2021).

Aconitum Species

Aconitum is an herbal drug species widely seen in places with an altitude of 1500-2000 meters in the northern hemisphere, mostly in China. They are mostly found in forests and flower gardens. In traditional medicine, aconitum types play a useful role in many cases such as musculoskeletal diseases, edema, gastroenteritis, abdominal pains, gynecological problems, and menstruation disorders (Nyirimigabo, E, 2015). Aconitum species are effective in anticancer, anti-inflammatory and cardioactive processes. The plant is highly poisonous and has a narrow therapeutic window (Lim et al., 2016).

Aconitum species contain high amounts of the sodium channel activator aconitin, especially in their root parts. Neurological and cardiac symptoms occur after the consumption of herbal preparations. After swallowing, the patient may hiss with a burning hiss in the mouth, have increased salivation, signs of gastroenteritis and skin rash. As the severity of the cases increases, vision problems, dizziness, unconsciousness, coma and death may occur (El-Shazly et al., 2016).

Atropa Bella-Donna

Bella-donna means "beautiful woman" in Italian. It is a branched, herbaceous plant with showy, vertically growing berries but it is highly poisonous. Atropine is obtained from the leaves of this plant. Since atropine causes mydriasis in the pupils, women used it in ancient times to look beautiful (Spiegl, 1996). In poisoning, findings such as tachycardia, mydriasis, and speech disorders are observed.

Brugmansia Species (Devil's Trumpet, Jimsonweed)

Brugmansia species occur as cheeky and invasive weeds commonly found in the tropics, particularly in Southern and West Africa. They are used in the traditional treatment of various diseases such as asthma and cough, by grinding the leaves of these plant species and turning them into tea. Brugmansia species contain concentrated anticholinergic alkaloids, including atropine and scopolamine (Alves, Sartoratto, & Trigo, 2007). Plant toxins cause abnormal thirst, dry mouth, urinary retention, dry skin, blurred vision, anxiety, headache, confusion and coma. Eye pain and blurred vision may occur if a person touching the plant with their hand scratches their eyes. In severe cases, the condition can worsen sufficiently to result in death (Capasso & de Feo, 2003).

Cerbera Odollam (Pong Pong)

Cerbera odollam is a tree species that grows in swamps. In its seed part, it contains a cardiac glycoside known as cerberin. The tree is mostly used for evil purposes such as suicide or murder. In Madagascar, this tree species has been found to play a role in the deaths of 3000 people a year (Gaillard, Krishnamoorthy, & Bevalot, 2004). The toxin content found in one seed has enough power to kill a human being. Cerberin toxin causes stomach pain, vomiting, diarrhea, headache, cardiac arrhythmias and even death within hours (Misek, Allen, LeComte, & Mazur, 2018).

Conium Maculatum (Poison Hemlock)

Conium maculatum is a common species that resembles a white-rooted parsnip. It can be distinguished from parsnip as it does not contain hairs in its structure. Although the plant grows regionally in northern Europe and western Asia, it has been seen to grow in many places. Due to its very similarity, it can be mistakenly thought of as a parsnip and consumed. The whole plant is poisonous, especially the roots. It contains piperidine alkaloids called coniine. Coniine is a convulsant poison that causes neuronal hyperexcitability, sweating, hypertension, and tremors and negatively affects vital functions. Severe exposure can cause coma, confusion and death from respiratory failure (Vetter, 2004).

Datura Stramonium

This plant is consumed by drinking tea. Although its origin is North America, it is a plant that can be grown anywhere. It grows mainly as an ornamental plant and weed. It is seen with tubular white flowers and pods of fruit. It is a poisonous plant containing very high levels of tropane alkaloids (hyoscyamine, scopolamine, and atropine) with strong anticholinergic properties, mainly concentrated in its seeds. Anticholinergic findings are observed upon exposure (Soler-Rodríguez, Martín, García-Cambero, Oropesa, & Pérez-López, 2006).

Digitalis Purpurea

Digitalis purpurea is a common ornamental plant in Europe and North America. All parts of the plant contain cardiac glycosides such as digitoxin, gitoxin and gilatoxin. The leaves are grown commercially to manufacture a heart medicine called digitalis, which is used to treat chronic cardiac failure. Exposure is usually the improper use of the plant extract for therapeutic management or mixing with edible plants, and misidentification. The toxin causes extreme fatigue in the body, visual impairment, weakness, headache and abdominal pain. Cases of poisoning resulting in death have also been reported (Negroni et al., 2019).

Dieffenbachia Species (Dumbcane)

Dieffenbachia species are among the plants that are usually planted in pots and can survive with little maintenance. They are widely used for decorative purposes indoors and outdoors in shopping malls, hotels, and office areas. The shrub originates from tropical America and Brazil. Almost every part of the plant contains raphids, long pointed crystals of calcium oxalate. When the raphids are stimulated, for instance when chewing, their crystals immediately cause intense pain in the mouth and respiratory distress due to an inability to speak, or even edema (Cumpston, Vogel, Leikin, & Erickson, 2003). Skin and eye irritation may also occur due to contact with the sap obtained from the plant.

Ecbalium Elaterium

This is mostly preferred for the treatment of sinusitis. Depending on its use, angioedema tables are typical. It is most commonly encountered with respiratory distress and uvula edema (Eti et al., 2018).

Hippomane Mancinella

Popularly known as the "beach apple" tree, Manichel says that while Hippomane mancinella can cause serious medical problems, if the milky sap comes into contact with the skin, it will cause burning, rash and inflammation. The fruit of the tree, which draws attention with its resemblance to a green apple, has a nice smell. It has a milky sap with poisonous properties. In case of contact with the sap, contact dermatitis on the skin, and eye inflammation occur. During rain, raindrops carrying diluted sap can also be toxic, so even standing under a tree can cause allergic reactions due to skin contact. Inhalation of smoke due to burning any part of the tree can cause several respiratory ailments such as bronchitis, cough, and rhinitis. The sap from the fallen leaves makes water poisonous. Cases of food poisoning have also been reported of fruit being swallowed by fish in water into which the fruit has fallen (Aluja et al., 2020).

Mandragora Officinarum

For millennia, numerous plants and seeds have been used for medicinal, psychotropic, or aphrodisiac purposes. Mandragora officinarum is from the Solanaceae family, traditionally known as an aphrodisiac. It causes anticholinergic toxidrome (Nikolaou et al., 2012).

Nerium Oleander

This is widely grown, especially in the Mediterranean region, and used for landscaping in garden decoration. This plant, which has flowers in many colors, grows in greenhouses in cold climates as well as in tropical and subtropical regions. The plant has a sap containing cardiac glycosides such as oleandrin, digitoxigenin, neriun, folinerin and rosagenin. These phytoxins can produce a positive inotropic effect on the heart muscle. This feature has made them important agents of suicide. Inhalation of fumes as a result of burning the plant and ingestion of its leaves and other parts for the purpose of preparing herbal medicine, lead to toxins entering the human body and poisoning may occur. The toxin causes nausea, vomiting, diarrhea, abdominal pain, sweating and weakness. Severe cases may result in cardiovascular collapse. In addition to the systemic toxic effect, localized toxic effects such as contact dermatitis are also observed. For example, when the plant is chewed or the tea is drunk, mucosal damage and necrotic lesions can be seen in the oral cavity (Bandara, Weinstein, White, & Eddleston, 2010).

Ricinus Communis

This is a common plant found scattered about the tropics. It is grown for the production of castor oil, which is used in many fields such as the production of biodiesel, motor oil, cosmetics, hair products, and pharmaceuticals. The plant seeds contain the highly toxic substance lectin ricin (a toxalbumin). It is so effective that even ingesting one or two seeds can cause the death of a person. The substance ricin obtained from this plant has high toxicity and is widely ubiquitous. Because of this feature, it is known as a potential biological weapon. The toxin causes symptoms such as nausea, vomiting, abdominal pain, diarrhea and dehydration. As cases worsen, multiple organ failure and death may occur (Worbs et al., 2011).

Rhododendron Species

Rhododendron species are common in temperate climates and widely used for garden decoration. The entire plant is toxic and contains a sodium channel activator called grayanotoxin. Grayanotoxin has adverse effects on all digestive, respiratory, cardiovascular and neurological systems in the body. Generally, mad honey poisoning occurs with the ingestion of honey produced from the nectar of Rhododendron ponticum and Rhododendron luteum species. After entering the body through the mouth, a sharp burning sensation in the mouth is observed, followed by excessive salivation, nausea, vomiting, diarrhea, dizziness, and double vision. In severe poisonings, cardiac complications, seizures and death occur (Koca & Koca, 2007).

Treatment of Poisoning with Plants

Patients should be monitored, and oxygen support should be given. ABC should be evaluated. When poisoning is suspected, arterial blood gas should be taken first for diagnostic purposes. The presence of metabolic acidosis and high lactate should be investigated. Most patients respond to supportive treatment. 50-100 g of activated charcoal (1 gr/kg for children) should be administered to patients admitted in the first 2 hours after exposure. IV hydration should be initiated in patients with hypotension. Inotrope can be started in resistant hypotension. Rapid cooling should be applied at the fever height. Benzodiazepines should be preferred for agitated patients.

Conclusion

Plants usually grow naturally in various places depending on environmental conditions and their biological structures. It is very likely that service personnel working in sectors such as gardening and livestock and military and other paramilitary bodies work in very close proximity to the plants in the field and are exposed to poisonous plants. Therefore, it is important to identify plants correctly. There is no antidote for most herbs. The general principle of poisoning treatments is essentially symptomatic. Employee health needs to use personal protective equipment during their work. Personal protective equipment should be appropriately designed to suit the risk in a particular area and to a particular phytotoxin and its potential effects. As a result, weeds and poisonous plants in the field should be carefully examined and recognized. In addition, poisonous plants should be removed from pastures and agricultural areas.

References

Aluja, M., Pascacio-Villafán, C., Altúzar-Molina, A., Monribot-Villanueva, J., Guerrero-Analco, J. A., Enciso, E., Guillén, L. (2020). Insights into the Interaction between the Monophagous Tephritid Fly Anastrepha acris and its Highly Toxic Host Hippomane mancinella (Euphorbiaceae). *J. Chem. Ecol.,* 46(4), 430-441. doi:10.1007/s10886-020-01164-8.

Alves, M. N., Sartoratto, A., & Trigo, J. R. (2007). Scopolamine in Brugmansia suaveolens (Solanaceae): defense, allocation, costs, and induced response. *J. Chem. Ecol.,* 33(2), 297-309. doi:10.1007/s10886-006-9214-9.

Bandara, V., Weinstein, S. A., White, J., & Eddleston, M. (2010). A review of the natural history, toxinology, diagnosis and clinical management of Nerium oleander (common oleander) and Thevetia peruviana (yellow oleander) poisoning. *Toxicon,* 56(3), 273-281. doi:10.1016/j.toxicon.2010.03.026.

Capasso, A., & de Feo, V. (2003). Alkaloids from Brugmansia arborea (L.) Lagerhein reduce morphine withdrawal in vitro. *Phytother. Res.,* 17(7), 826-829. doi:10.1002/ptr.1218.

Cumpston, K. L., Vogel, S. N., Leikin, J. B., & Erickson, T. B. (2003). Acute airway compromise after brief exposure to a Dieffenbachia plant. *J. Emerg. Med.,* 25(4), 391-397. doi:10.1016/j.jemermed.2003.02.005.

El-Shazly, M., Tai, C. J., Wu, T. Y., Csupor, D., Hohmann, J., Chang, F. R., & Wu, Y. C. (2016). Use, history, and liquid chromatography/mass spectrometry chemical analysis of Aconitum. *J. Food Drug Anal.* 24(1), 29-45. doi:10.1016/j.jfda.2015.09.001.

Eti, C. M., Vayısoğlu, Y., Kardaş, B., Arpacı, R. B., Horasan, E. S., Kanık, A., Talas, D. (2018). Histopathologic evaluation of Ecballium elaterium applied to nasal mucosa in a rat rhinosinusitis model. *Ear Nose Throat J.,* 97(6), E14-e17.

Fisch C. (1985). William Withering: An account of the foxglove and some of its medical uses 1785-1985. *Journal of the American College of Cardiology,* 5(5 Suppl A), 1A-2A. https://doi.org/10.1016/s0735-1097(85)80456-3.

Froberg, B., Ibrahim, D., & Furbee, R. B. (2007). Plant poisoning. *Emerg. Med. Clin. North Am.,* 25(2), 375-433; abstract ix. doi:10.1016/j.emc.2007.02.013.

Gaillard, Y., Krishnamoorthy, A., & Bevalot, F. (2004). Cerbera odollam: a 'suicide tree' and cause of death in the state of Kerala, India. *J. Ethnopharmacol.,* 95(2-3), 123-126. doi:10.1016/j.jep.2004.08.004.

Gardner D. G. (1994). Injury to the oral mucous membranes caused by the common houseplant, dieffenbachia. A review. *Oral surgery, oral medicine, and oral pathology,* 78(5), 631-633. https://doi.org/10.1016/0030-4220(94)90177-5.

Gómez-Espinoza, O., González-Ramírez, D., Méndez-Gómez, J., Guillén-Watson, R., Medaglia-Mata, A., & Bravo, L. A. (2021). Calcium Oxalate Crystals in Leaves of the Extremophile Plant *Colobanthus quitensis* (Kunth) Bartl. (Caryophyllaceae). *Plants (Basel, Switzerland),* 10(9), 1787. https://doi.org/10.3390/plants10091787.

Group, T. A. P., Chase, M. W., Christenhusz, M. J. M., Fay, M. F., Byng, J. W., Judd, W. S., Stevens, P. F. (2016). An update of the Angiosperm Phylogeny Group classification for the orders and families of flowering plants: APG IV. *Botanical Journal of the Linnean Society,* 181(1), 1-20. doi:10.1111/boj.12385.

Howlett, B. J. (2006). Secondary metabolite toxins and nutrition of plant pathogenic fungi. *Curr. Opin. Plant Biol.,* 9(4), 371-375. doi:10.1016/j.pbi.2006.05.004.

Koca, I., & Koca, A. F. (2007). Poisoning by mad honey: a brief review. *Food Chem. Toxicol.,* 45(8), 1315-1318. doi:10.1016/j.fct.2007.04.006.

Krenzelok, E. P., & Mrvos, R. (2011). Friends and foes in the plant world: A profile of plant ingestions and fatalities. *Clinical Toxicology,* 49(3), 142-149. doi:10.3109/15563650.2011.568945.

Lim, C. S., Chhabra, N., Leikin, S., Fischbein, C., Mueller, G. M., & Nelson, M. E. (2016). Atlas of select poisonous plants and mushrooms. *Dis. Mon.,* 62(3), 41-66. doi:10.1016/j.disamonth.2015.12.002.

Lopes, J., Riet-Correa, F., & Medeiros, R. (2019). Phytotoxins eliminated by milk: A review. *Pesquisa Veterinária Brasileira,* 39, 231-237. doi:10.1590/1678-5150-pvb-6058.

Misek, R., Allen, G., LeComte, V., & Mazur, N. (2018). Fatality Following Intentional Ingestion of Cerbera odollam Seeds. *Clin. Pract. Cases Emerg. Med.,* 2(3), 223-226. doi:10.5811/cpcem.2018.5.38345.

Negroni, M. S., Marengo, A., Caruso, D., Tayar, A., Rubiolo, P., Giavarini, F., Dell'Agli, M. (2019). A Case Report of Accidental Intoxication following Ingestion of Foxglove Confused with Borage: High

Digoxinemia without Major Complications. *Case Rep. Cardiol.*, 2019, 9707428. doi:10.1155/2019/ 9707428.

Nikolaou, P., Papoutsis, I., Stefanidou, M., Dona, A., Maravelias, C., Spiliopoulou, C., & Athanaselis, S. (2012). Accidental poisoning after ingestion of "aphrodisiac" berries: diagnosis by analytical toxicology. *J. Emerg. Med.*, 42(6), 662-665. doi:10.1016/j.jemermed.2011.03.023.

Nyirimigabo, E., Xu, Y., Li, Y., Wang, Y., Agyemang, K., & Zhang, Y. (2015). A review on phytochemistry, pharmacology and toxicology studies of Aconitum. *J. Pharm. Pharmacol.* 67(1), 1-19. doi:10.1111/ jphp.12310.

Soler-Rodríguez, F., Martín, A., García-Cambero, J. P., Oropesa, A. L., & Pérez-López, M. (2006). Datura stramonium poisoning in horses: a risk factor for colic. *Vet. Rec.*, 158(4), 132-133. doi:10.1136/vr. 158.4.132.

Spiegl, F. W., DC: Taylor & Francis. ss. 21-22. ISBN. (1996). *Fritz Spiegl's Sick Notes: An Alphabetical Browsing-Book of Derivatives, Abbreviations, Mnemonics and Slang for Amusemen* New York: Parthenon.

Sunday, O. J., Babatunde, S. K., Ajiboye, A. E., Adedayo, R. M., Ajao, M. A., & Ajuwon, B. I. (2016). Evaluation of phytochemical properties and *in-vitro* antibacterial activity of the aqueous extracts of leaf, seed and root of Abrus precatorius Linn. against Salmonella and Shigella. *Asian Pacific Journal of Tropical Biomedicine*, 6(9), 755-759. doi:https://doi.org/10.1016/j.apjtb.2016.07.002.

Vetter, J. (2004). Poison hemlock (Conium maculatum L.). *Food Chem. Toxicol.*, 42(9), 1373-1382. doi:10. 1016/j.fct.2004.04.009.

Worbs, S., Kampa, B., Skiba, M., Hansbauer, E. M., Stern, D., Volland, H., Becher, F., Simon, S., Dorner, M. B., & Dorner, B. G. (2021). Differentiation, Quantification and Identification of Abrin and *Abrus precatorius* Agglutinin. *Toxins*, 13(4), 284. https://doi.org/10.3390/toxins13040284.

Worbs, S., Köhler, K., Pauly, D., Avondet, M. A., Schaer, M., Dorner, M. B., & Dorner, B. G. (2011). Ricinus communis intoxications in human and veterinary medicine-a summary of real cases. *Toxins (Basel)*, 3(10), 1332-1372. doi:10.3390/toxins3101332.

Chapter 23

Mushroom Poisonings

Zeynep Karakaya*, MD, Ahmet Kayali, MD and Serkan Bilgin, MD

Department of Emergency Medicine Katip Çelebi University Izmir, Izmir, Turkey

Abstract

Although about 135,000 mushroom species have been discovered so far, it is thought that there are about 2.2-3.8 million different types of mushrooms. It is known that 50-100 of these mushrooms are poisonous. The type of mushroom that causes the poisoning cannot be determined in mushroom poisonings. When classifying toxic fungi, first of all, the duration of effect after entry into the body and the systems they target are taken into account. Intoxication where symptoms begin in the acute period; Symptoms begin within the first 6 hours after ingestion of the toxic mushroom. These are mostly non-fatal poisonings. Gastrointestinal system irritants, hallucinogens, and neurotoxic, cholinergic, and disulfiram-like effects can be classified as allergic. Poisonings with late-onset of symptoms; Symptoms and signs begin to appear 6 hours after the ingestion of mushrooms. This group of poisonings is more serious and has a high probability of mortality. Therefore, they need to be evaluated more carefully. Amanita phalloides contains amatoxin and is responsible for 90% of deaths due to mushroom poisoning. Mushroom poisonings continue to be among the differential diagnoses that should always be kept in mind as an important cause of mortality and morbidity.

Keywords: mushroom, mushroom toxins, poisoning

Introduction

Humans have consumed mushrooms for many years. Although some mushroom species are poisonous, their consumption continues in this process. The incidence of poisoning varies according to the mushroom species found in the region, the region's culture, the consumption pattern, and the frequency of the mushrooms (Diaz, 2005). These poisonings can cause simple gastrointestinal symptoms and severe liver and kidney failure. They are still among the causes

---

* Corresponding Author's Email: zeynepkarakaya76@hotmail.com.

In: Environmental Emergencies and Injuries in Nature
Editors: Murat Yücel, Murat Güzel and İbrahim İkizceli
ISBN: 978-1-68507-833-1

of serious mortality and morbidity (Diaz, 2005). For this reason, studies on fungal species, their toxins, and treatments continue actively.

Epidemiology

The number of mushroom species discovered every day is increasing day by day. Although approximately 135,000 mushroom species have been discovered so far, it is thought that there are about 2.2-3.8 million different types of fungi (Hibbett et al., 2017; Hawksworth and Lucking, 2017). It is known that 50-100 of these mushrooms are poisonous (Goldfrank, 2019). Approximately 6,000 to 8,000 cases of mushroom poisoning are reported each year in the United States. As a result of these poisonings, 3-5 patients die in a year for the USA and 50 patients a year for Europe (Brandenburg and Ward, 2018).

The type of mushroom that causes the poisoning cannot be determined in mushroom poisonings. In mushroom poisoning, the way the mushroom is taken, the amount used, and other toxins taken together can change the degree of poisoning. For this reason, symptom-oriented treatment is mostly applied. For this purpose, while classifying toxic mushrooms, first of all, the duration of effect after entry into the body and the systems they target are taken into account (Diaz, 2005). The classification is divided into acute (before 6 hours) and late (after 6 hours) onset, based on the time of onset of symptoms, and then detailed according to the systems they target.

Poisonings in Which the Symptoms Begin in the Acute Period

Symptoms begin within the first 6 hours after ingestion of the toxic mushroom. These are mostly non-fatal poisonings. Gastrointestinal system irritants, hallucinogens, and neurotoxic, cholinergic, and disulfiram-like effects can be classified as allergic effects (Bren and Palmer, 2007).

Gastrointestinal System Irritants (*Chlorophyllum molybdites, Clitocybe nebularis, Omphalates illudens, Psilocybe cubensis, P. Mexicana*)

Symptoms usually begin within the first 2 hours after mushroom ingestion. Many types of fungi can cause gastrointestinal complaints. These are mostly non-fatal poisonings. Nausea, vomiting, cramps, and diarrhea are the most common symptoms (Bren and Palmer, 2007). Symptoms usually resolve within 12 to 24 hours. Although there are poisonings with a benign course, care should be taken because fungal species such as Amanita smithiana, which can cause severe toxicity, may also cause gastrointestinal symptoms (West et al., 2009).

There is no specific antidote in the treatment, and supportive treatment is sufficient. IV fluid therapy and the correction of electrolyte imbalance form the basis of treatment. Although antiemetics (ondansetron 0.15 mg/kg IV) are recommended because this does not change the amount of toxin absorbed, the use of antispasmodics are not recommended for similar reasons (Berger and Guss, 2005). Activated charcoal therapy (0.5-1.0 mg/kg PO) is recommended within the first hour after ingestion of mushroom poisoning. If the patient's oral intake is provided and symptoms such as nausea and vomiting have resolved, discharge of the patient may be considered (Berger and Guss, 2005).

Hallucinogenic Mushrooms (*Conocybe cyanopus, Gymnopilus aeruginosa, Panaeolous foenisecil*)

This group of mushrooms is known as magic mushrooms (Kalberler et al., 1962). Due to their hallucinogen effects, intoxications due to accidental intake are observed, but it is also common to deliberately take them. It is possible to encounter these small, brown, or golden mushrooms, often seen in warm climates, especially in the United States, Asia, and Australia (Stebelska, 2013).

Psilocybin found in these fungal species is converted to psilocin by alkaline phosphatase (Kalberler et al., 1962). These tryptamine group alkaloids are thought to be responsible for the hallucinogenic effects.

Clinically, patients present with symptoms and signs such as euphoria, impaired mood, mild tachycardia, hypertension, and dilated pupil, which starts 30-120 minutes after ingestion (Goldfrank, 2019).

There is no specific antidote for treatment. The symptomatic treatment approach is adopted. If necessary, benzodiazepines (midazolam 0.05 mg/kg, lorazepam 0.05-0.1 mg/kg) for sedation can be used. Rarely developing seizure attacks can also be treated with benzodiazepines. Symptoms usually last between 4 and 12 hours (Goldfrank, 2019).

Mushrooms Affecting the Central Nervous System (*Amanita muscaria, Amanita pantherina, Amanita gemmata*)

The agents responsible for the toxic effect in this group of mushrooms are muscimol and ibotenic acid (Stebelska, 2013). A. muscaria is the most well-known mushroom species of this group. It is recognized by its head with white dots on a red or orange background. Due to its neurological effects, its use has been consciously abused for years.

Muscimol has a depressant effect on the central nervous system through gamma-aminobutyric acid (GABA). On the other hand, ibotenic acid stimulates the central nervous system by affecting glutamic acid receptors (Taylor et al., 2019).

Clinical signs and symptoms begin to appear within 30 minutes to 3 hours after mushroom ingestion. Severe symptoms and signs that can progress to delirium and coma can often be seen, along with non-specific symptoms such as nausea, vomiting, and diarrhea (Moss and Hendrickson, 2019).

Benzodiazepines (midazolam 0.05 mg/kg, lorazepam 0.05-0.1 mg/kg) can be used in patients with agitation or seizures. The symptomatic treatment approach together with close monitoring will be sufficient for this patient group. The end of the effectiveness of toxins can vary between 4 and 24 hours (Moss and Hendrickson, 2019). Patients who do not have any additional pathology and whose complaints regress can be safely discharged during this period.

Mushrooms Containing Cholinergic Toxins (*Inocybe, Clitocybe*)

Muscarine toxin was the first fungal toxin identified (WASER, 1961). This toxin can be found in many fungal species (Goldfrank, 2019). Although Amanita muscoria has the term muscoria in its name, contrary to popular belief, it has a trace amount of this toxin. This amount is not enough to create cholinergic symptoms. Therefore, it does not produce cholinergic effects unless consumed in very excessive amounts.

Clinical findings occur when muscarine binds to postganglionic cholinergic receptors. Typical signs of cholinergic poisoning are seen clinically. *SLUGBAM:* Salivation, Lacrimation, Urination, Gastrointestinal findings (nausea, vomiting, diarrhea), Bradycardia, Bronchorea, Bronchospasm, Abdominal cramps, and Myosis are typical symptoms and signs (George and Hegde, 2013).

Symptoms and signs usually begin to appear within the first 30 minutes after ingestion of the toxin (Diaz 2005). It has a much better clinical course than the conditions that lead to other cholinergic poisonings, such as organophosphate poisonings. These toxins do not cross the blood-brain barrier and generally have a self-limiting effect (Pauli and Foot, 2005). A 12-hour follow-up is sufficient in these patients.

Atropine can be administered in patients with severe increased secretion or bradycardia (Diaz, 2005). Atropine can be administered at 0.5-1.0 mg IV in adults and 0.02 mg/kg IV in children. Inhaled β2-mimetics can be used for bronchospasm.

Mushrooms with Disulfiram-Like Effects (*Coprinus atramentarius*)

The clinically responsible agent is the coprin toxin. This toxin irreversibly inhibits the alcohol dehydrogenase enzyme 2 hours after entering the body (Haberl et al., 2017). If alcohol is consumed during this process, a disulfiram-like reaction occurs in the body.

Symptoms and signs of nausea, vomiting, headache, flushing, chest pain, shortness of breath, tachycardia, hypotension, and coma can be seen (Haberl et al., 2017).

Treatment is directed towards the symptoms. Gastrointestinal decompression or activated carbon therapy is of no benefit. In the case of hypotension, IV hydration can be administered. β-blockers can be used in severe sympathetic increase. Symptoms and signs may appear for up to 2 days and usually tend to be self-limiting (Michelot, 1992). Patients who do not have active complaints and tolerate oral intake can be safely discharged.

Poisonings with Late-Onset of Symptoms

Symptoms and signs begin to appear 6 hours after the ingestion of mushrooms. This group of poisonings is more serious and has a high probability of mortality. Therefore, they need to be evaluated more carefully.

Mushrooms Causing Acute Gastroenteritis and Late-Onset Kidney Failure
(*Amanita smithiana, A. boudieri, A. gracilior, and A. echinocephala*)

The most well-known mushroom of this group is Amanita smithiana. However, other Amanita species (A. boudieri, A. gracilior, and A. echinocephala) are similarly poisonous. While A. smithiana is mainly seen in America, other Amanita species are common in Europe and Asia (Kirchmair et al., 2012).

Although A. smithiana is mostly white in appearance, it can also be yellow, brown, or gray depending on the environment's weather conditions and the developmental stage. It has a non-specific head region. In particular, poisonings were observed in Japan due to the consumption of matsutake (Tricholoma magnivelare) mushrooms. While the cause of these poisonings was expected to be matsutake mushroom, it was understood that A. smithiana mushroom was investigated further (Guin, 1997).

In this group, the agent responsible for toxication is allenic norleukine (amino-hexadienoic acid). Although the exact mechanism of action has not been clarified, it is thought to cause necrosis and fibrosis in renal tubular epithelial cells (Kirchmair et al., 2012).

The onset of symptoms and signs after ingestion of the toxin ranges from 20 minutes to 12 hours. Gastrointestinal symptoms such as nausea, vomiting, diarrhea, and abdominal cramps usually begin after an asymptomatic period of 5-6 hours after ingestion of the fungus. Between the 3rd and 6th days, renal findings may begin to appear. Oliguria, anuria, high urea and creatinine can be seen. Renal damage is expected to be primarily reversible (Diaz, 2021).

In the patient's evaluation, first of all, the patient should be monitored, and biochemistry parameters including hemogram, liver function tests, kidney function tests, and electrolyte parameters should be studied (Tulloss and Lindgren, 1992). Antiemetics may be given for gastrointestinal symptoms. IV hydration of the patient should be provided by paying attention to the signs of overload. It should not be forgotten that the patient may be ovarian volemic as urine output will decrease (Leathem et al., 1997). Activated carbon can be given in the first hour. In the case of renal damage, Dialysis should be planned for the patient in the case of uremia, hyperkalemia, volume overload despite diuretic, and resistant metabolic acidosis (Warden and Benjamin, 1998). Although chromatographic methods can determine the causative agent, they cannot be applied in many clinics (Apperley et al., 2013). Since there is no specific antidote for the toxin, only symptomatic treatment can be used. Although its clinic is different, it can be confused with other Amanita species and other nephrotoxic toxins because it causes slight elevations in AST/ALT values. In this respect, care should be taken (West et al., 2009).

Mushrooms Causing Late-Onset Gastroenteritis and Liver Toxicity
(*Amanita phalloides (death mushroom), A. Virosa (destroyer angel),*
Amanita verna (dumb mushroom), Galerina autumnalis,
and Lepiota josserandii)

In this group, the clinically responsible toxin is amatoxin. Especially Amanita phalloides is the most common type of fungus in this group. It is stated that it is responsible for 90% of deaths due to mushroom poisoning (Ye and Liu, 2018). They often cause poisoning in Europe and Asia (Enjalbert, 2002).

Amatoxin inhibits mRNA transcription by inhibiting RNA polymerase in the liver, and hepatic necrosis develops due to the inhibition of protein synthesis (Horowitz and Moss, 2021).

Clinical findings begin to appear 6-12 hours after mushroom ingestion. Earlier onset gastrointestinal findings do not exclude amatoxin toxicity. In this group, clinical findings are examined in 3 phases (Giannini et al., 2007).

- Phase 1: This occurs between 6 and 24 hours. It is the stage in which gastrointestinal symptoms and signs are seen. Nausea, vomiting, abdominal cramps, and diarrhea may occur. Liver values are within normal limits.
- Phase 2: This occurs within 24-36 hours. In this stage, elevations in liver values are observed. Transaminases, bilirubin, and coagulation values begin to increase. This phase may last up to 3 days or may not be seen at all.
- Phase 3: This occurs between 48 and 96 hours. It is the phase in which fulminant hepatitis is seen, and liver damage becomes irreversible. AST/ALT values tend to decline after peaking at 72 hours. Hypoglycemia, coagulopathy, encephalopathy, renal failure, and multiorgan failure are seen due to hepatic failure. Generally, 30% of cases die within 1-2 weeks.

Since late-onset symptoms are expected in this group of poisonings, hemogram and biochemistry tests should be requested regarding hepatic toxicity at the first admission of the patients. Since the detection of amatoxin can be made at the 36th hour at the earliest, treatment should be initiated in the presence of clinical suspicion (Lopez and Hendrickson, 2014).

Patients should be monitored, and IV hydration should be performed to prevent fluid loss. It is stated that multiple applications of activated charcoal increase survival by reducing amatoxin absorption. Care should be taken in hypoglycemia, strict blood glucose monitoring should be performed, and replacement should be applied when necessary (Lopez and Hendrickson, 2014).

Silibinin dihemisuccinate is used in therapy because it inhibits the absorption and transport of amatoxin. After a 5 mg/kg IV loading dose, a maintenance dose of 20 mg/kg/day is recommended. Similarly, high doses of penicillin G (300,000-1,000,000 units/kg/day) and ceftazidime (4.5 g/2 hours) are also used to inhibit toxin absorption and transport to hepatocytes. However, they are recommended to be used in the absence of silibinin (Poucheret et al., 2010; Magdalan et al., 2010). N-Acetyl cysteine (NAC), vitamin C, and cimetidine are other agents that can be used as anti-oxidant therapy (Poucheret et al., 2010).

In addition to these treatments, many new treatment protocols are being tried. Recently, it has been stated that the medium cut-off membrane hemodialysis method also gives positive results (Huddam et al., 2021). Liver transplantation is applied as the last choice in patients who are not successful despite these treatments.

Mushrooms Causing Late-Onset Gastroenteritis, Seizures, and Liver Toxicity (*Gyromitra genus, Gyromitra esculenta (false morel)*)

This group includes gyromitra-type mushrooms, and they contain the gyromitra toxin. They are commonly found in the USA, Europe, and Asia. Amanitin-containing mushrooms are more common in winter, whereas this group of mushrooms is more common in summer. Gyromitra esculenta was named the false morel because it was confused with Morchella esculenta (morel) (Leathem and Dorran, 2007).

As a result of the hydrolysis of gyromitrin in the stomach, N-methyl-N-formylhydrazine and N-methylhydrazine are formed. N-Methylhydrazine binds to pyridoxine and inhibits enzymes that require pyridoxine as a cofactor. Therefore, the amount of γ-Aminobutyric acid (GABA) in the central nervous system decreases and causes seizure formation. N-Methyl-N-formylhydrazine is converted into a free radical in the liver and causes local liver necrosis by blocking the cytochrome P450 system, glutathione, and other liver enzyme systems. Although the seizure and liver toxicity mechanism has been elucidated, the cause of gastrointestinal symptoms has yet to be explained (Michelot and Toth, 1991).

Gastrointestinal symptoms, including nausea, vomiting, diarrhea, and abdominal cramps, begin 6-8 hours after ingestion of the mushroom. AST/ALT elevation due to liver damage, muscle cramps, headache, and seizure complaints are usually seen after the 2nd day. Death can occur within one week. The mortality rate is around 10-15% (Horowitz et al., 2021). There is no specific treatment available for hepatic injury. Pyridoxine (70 mg/kg) replacement can be applied to patients with seizures. Benzodiazepines can be used in seizure intervention (Horowitz et al., 2021).

Mushrooms Causing Late-Onset Kidney Failure (*Cortinarius orellanus, Mycena pura, and Omphalatus orarius*)

Orellanin, orellinin, cortinarin A, and cortinarin B are responsible for the toxic effect. It is believed that these toxins act by forming intestinal nephritis, edema, leukocyte infiltration, tubular necrosis, and fibrosis in the kidneys (Karlson-Stiber and Persson, 2003).

After the 6th hour, symptoms such as increased kidney values, decreased urine volume and flank pain occur following complaints such as nausea, vomiting, and fatigue.

There is no specific treatment protocol. If necessary, supportive treatment, dialysis, and kidney transplantation as a last choice can be applied (Danel et al., 2001).

Mushrooms Causing Rhabdomyolysis

The most well-known mushroom of these groups is Tricholoma equestre. Within 24-72 hours of intake, complaints such as vomiting and muscle cramps begin. Creatinine kinase (CK) is seen in potassium levels (Bedry et al., 2001).

Fungi such as Russula subnigrans can also cause onset rhabdomyolysis. These are available in Europe and Asia. Symptoms are seen within the first few hours of ingestion of the mushroom (Trakulsrichai et al., 2020).

There is no specific treatment for this group of fungi and treatment includes IV hydration, electrolyte disorders therapy and supportive therapy.

Shiitake Dermatitis

Itchy, erythematous, and linear-extending rashes are seen after consuming shiitake mushrooms. These can be seen within 1-2 days after ingestion of the mushroom. Treatment with topical antihistamines and corticosteroids is sufficient (Wang et al., 2013).

Conclusion

A new member of the mushroom population is being discovered every day, and the number of poisonous mushrooms is increasing in parallel with this. In cases of mushroom poisoning, the diagnosis cannot always be made, so the actual mortality and morbidity numbers cannot be accessed.

Since patients come to the clinic with non-specific symptoms and signs, and even if mushroom poisoning is suspected, the necessary tests (chromatography, ELISA, PCR) for fungus detection are not available for many clinics, so the treatment is mainly shaped according to the characteristics, the duration of the symptoms and signs, and the results of laboratory tests. For this purpose, besides the classical classification, new types of classifications and treatment protocols that can make diagnosis and treatment more effective and faster are also being studied. Mushroom poisoning continues to be among the differential diagnoses that should always be kept in mind for these reasons, as well as an important cause of mortality and morbidity.

References

Apperley, S., Kroeger, P., Kirchmair, M., Kiaii, M., Holmes, D. T., & Garber, I. (2013). Laboratory confirmation of Amanita smithiana mushroom poisoning. *Clinical toxicology* (Philadelphia, Pa.), 51(4), 249-251. https://doi.org/10.3109/15563650.2013.778995.

Bedry, R., Baudrimont, I., Deffieux, G., Creppy, E. E., Pomies, J. P., Ragnaud, J. M., Dupon, M., Neau, D., Gabinski, C., De Witte, S., Chapalain, J. C., Godeau, P., & Beylot, J. (2001). Wild-mushroom intoxication as a cause of rhabdomyolysis. *The New England journal of medicine*, 345(11), 798-802. https://doi.org/10.1056/NEJMoa010581.

Berger, K. J., & Guss, D. A. (2005). Mycotoxins revisited: Part I. *The Journal of emergency medicine*, 28(1), 53-62. https://doi.org/10.1016/j.jemermed.2004.08.013.

Brandenburg, W. E., & Ward, K. J. (2018). Mushroom poisoning epidemiology in the United States. *Mycologia*, 110(4), 637-641. https://doi.org/10.1080/00275514.2018.1479561.

Brent J., Palmer, R. B. Mushrooms. In: *Haddad and Winchester's Clinical Management of Poisoning and Drug Overdose,* 4th ed, Shannon M. W., Borron S. W., Burns M. J. (Eds), Saunders Elsevier, Philadelphia, PA 2007. p. 455.

Danel, V. C., Saviuc, P. F., & Garon, D. (2001). Main features of Cortinarius spp. poisoning: a literature review. *Toxicon: official journal of the International Society on Toxinology*, 39(7), 1053-1060. https://doi.org/10.1016/s0041-0101(00)00248-8.

Diaz, J. H. (2005). Evolving global epidemiology, syndromic classification, general management, and prevention of unknown mushroom poisonings. *Critical care medicine*, 33(2), 419-426. https://doi.org/10.1097/01.ccm.0000153530.32162.b7.

Diaz, J. H. (2005). Syndromic diagnosis and management of confirmed mushroom poisonings. *Critical care medicine*, 33(2), 427-436. https://doi.org/10.1097/01.ccm.0000153531.69448.49.

Diaz, J. H. (2021). Nephrotoxic Mushroom Poisoning: Global Epidemiology, Clinical Manifestations, and Management. *Wilderness & environmental medicine*, 32(4), 537-544. https://doi.org/10.1016/j.wem.2021.09.002.

Enjalbert, F., Rapior, S., Nouguier-Soulé, J., Guillon, S., Amouroux, N., & Cabot, C. (2002). Treatment of amatoxin poisoning: 20-year retrospective analysis. *Journal of toxicology. Clinical toxicology*, 40(6), 715-757. https://doi.org/10.1081/clt-120014646.

George, P., & Hegde, N. (2013). Muscarinic toxicity among family members after consumption of mushrooms. *Toxicology international*, 20(1), 113-115. https://doi.org/10.4103/0971-6580.111559.

Giannini, L., Vannacci, A., Missanelli, A., Mastroianni, R., Mannaioni, P. F., Moroni, F., & Masini, E. (2007). Amatoxin poisoning: a 15-year retrospective analysis and follow-up evaluation of 105 patients. *Clinical toxicology* (Philadelphia, Pa.), 45(5), 539-542. https://doi.org/10.1080/15563650701365834.

Goldfrank, L. R. Mushrooms. In: *Goldfrank's Toxicologic Emergencies*, 11th ed, Nelson L. S., Howland M., Lewin N. A., Smith S. W., Goldfrank L. R., Hoffman R. S. (Eds), McGraw-Hill Education, 2019. p. 1582.

Guin, J. Matsutake Mushroom: The White Gold Rush of the 1990s, *A Guide and Journal, Naturegraph Publishers*, 1997.

Haberl, B., Pfab, R., Berndt, S., Greifenhagen, C., & Zilker, T. (2011). Case series: Alcohol intolerance with Coprine-like syndrome after consumption of the mushroom Lepiota aspera (Pers.:Fr.) Quél., 1886 (Freckled Dapperling). *Clinical toxicology* (Philadelphia, Pa.), 49(2), 113-114. https://doi.org/10.3109/15563650.2011.554840.

Hawksworth, D. L., & Lücking, R. (2017). Fungal Diversity Revisited: 2.2 to 3.8 Million Species. *Microbiology spectrum*, 5(4), https://doi.org/10.1128/microbiolspec.FUNK-0052-2016.

Hibbett, D., Abarenkov, K., Kõljalg, U., Öpik, M., Chai, B., Cole, J., Wang, Q., Crous, P., Robert, V., Helgason, T., Herr, J. R., Kirk, P., Lueschow, S., O'Donnell, K., Nilsson, R. H., Oono, R., Schoch, C., Smyth, C., Walker, D. M., Porras-Alfaro, A., … Geiser, D. M. (2016). *Sequence-based classification and identification of Fungi. Mycologia*, 108(6), 1049-1068. https://doi.org/10.3852/16-130.

Horowitz, B. Z., Moss, M. J. Amatoxin Mushroom Toxicity. [Updated 2021 Aug 11]. In: *StatPearls* [Internet]. Treasure Island (FL): StatPearls Publishing; 2021 Jan-. Available from: https://www.ncbi.nlm.nih.gov/books/NBK431052/.

Horowitz, K. M., Kong, E. L., Horowitz, B. Z. Gyromitra Mushroom Toxicity. [Updated 2021 Jul 10]. In: *StatPearls* [Internet]. Treasure Island (FL): StatPearls Publishing; 2021 Jan-. Available from: https://www.ncbi.nlm.nih.gov/books/NBK470580/.

Huddam, B., Alp, A., Kırlı, İ., Yılmaz, M., Çağırtekin, A., Allı, H., Edebali, S. (2021) Medium Cut-Off Membrane Can Be a New Treatment Tool in Amanita phalloides Poisoning. *Wilderness Environ Med*. 2021 Jun;32(2):192-197. doi: https://10.1016/j.wem.2020.12.002. PMID: 33676852.

Kalberer, F., Kreis, W., & Rutschmann, J. (1962). The fate of psilocin in the rat. *Biochemical pharmacology*, 11, 261-269. https://doi.org/10.1016/0006-2952(62)90050-3.

Karlson-Stiber, C., & Persson, H. (2003). Cytotoxic fungi - an overview. *Toxicon: official journal of the International Society on Toxinology*, 42(4), 339-349. https://doi.org/10.1016/s0041-0101(03)00238-1.

Kirchmair, M., Carrilho, P., Pfab, R., Haberl, B., Felgueiras, J., Carvalho, F., Cardoso, J., Melo, I., Vinhas, J., & Neuhauser, S. (2012). Amanita poisonings resulting in acute, reversible renal failure: new cases, new toxic Amanita mushrooms. *Nephrology, dialysis, transplantation: official publication of the European Dialysis and Transplant Association - European Renal Association*, 27(4), 1380-1386. https://doi.org/10.1093/ndt/gfr511.

Leathem, A. M., & Dorran, T. J. (2007). Poisoning due to raw Gyromitra esculenta (false morels) west of the Rockies. *CJEM*, 9(2), 127-130. https://doi.org/10.1017/s1481803500014937.

Leathem, A. M., Purssell, R. A., Chan, V. R., & Kroeger, P. D. (1997). Renal failure caused by mushroom poisoning. *Journal of toxicology. Clinical toxicology*, 35(1), 67-75. https://doi.org/10.3109/15563659709001168.

Lopez, A. M., & Hendrickson, R. G. (2014). Toxin-induced hepatic injury. *Emergency medicine clinics of North America*, 32(1), 103-125. https://doi.org/10.1016/j.emc.2013.09.005.

Magdalan, J., Ostrowska, A., Piotrowska, A., Gomułkiewicz, A., Podhorska-Okołów, M., Patrzałek, D., Szelag, A., & Dziegiel, P. (2010). Benzylpenicillin, acetylcysteine and silibinin as antidotes in human hepatocytes intoxicated with alpha-amanitin. *Experimental and toxicologic pathology: official journal of the Gesellschaft fur Toxikologische Pathologie*, 62(4), 367-373. https://doi.org/10.1016/j.etp.2009.05.003.

Michelot, D. (1992). Poisoning by Coprinus atramentarius. *Natural toxins*, 1(2), 73-80. https://doi.org/10.1002/nt.2620010203.

Michelot, D., & Toth, B. (1991). Poisoning by Gyromitra esculenta - a review. *Journal of applied toxicology: JAT*, 11(4), 235-243. https://doi.org/10.1002/jat.2550110403.

Moss, M. J., & Hendrickson, R. G. (2019). Toxicity of muscimol and ibotenic acid containing mushrooms reported to a regional poison control center from 2002-2016. *Clinical toxicology* (Philadelphia, Pa.), 57(2), 99-103. https://doi.org/10.1080/15563650.2018.1497169.

Pauli, J. L., & Foot, C. L. (2005). Fatal muscarinic syndrome after eating wild mushrooms. *The Medical journal of Australia*, 182(6), 294-295. https://doi.org/10.5694/j.1326-5377.2005.tb06705.x.

Poucheret, P., Fons, F., Doré, J. C., Michelot, D., & Rapior, S. (2010). Amatoxin poisoning treatment decision-making: pharmaco-therapeutic clinical strategy assessment using multidimensional multivariate statistic analysis. *Toxicon: official journal of the International Society on Toxinology*, 55(7), 1338-1345. https://doi.org/10.1016/j.toxicon.2010.02.005.

Stebelska, K. (2013). Fungal hallucinogens psilocin, ibotenic acid, and muscimol: analytical methods and biologic activities. *Therapeutic drug monitoring*, 35(4), 420-442. https://doi.org/10.1097/FTD.0b013e31828741a5.

Taylor, J., Holzbauer, S., Wanduragala, D., Ivaskovic, A., Spinosa, R., Smith, K., Corcoran, J., & Jensen, A. (2019). Notes from the Field: Acute Intoxications from Consumption of Amanita muscaria Mushrooms - Minnesota, 2018. MMWR. *Morbidity and mortality weekly report*, 68(21), 483-484. https://doi.org/10.15585/mmwr.mm6821a4.

Trakulsrichai, S., Jeeratheepatanont, P., Sriapha, C., Tongpoo, A., & Wananukul, W. (2020). Myotoxic Mushroom Poisoning in Thailand: Clinical Characteristics and Outcomes. *International journal of general medicine*, 13, 1139-1146. https://doi.org/10.2147/IJGM.S271914.

Tulloss, R. E., Lindgren, J. E. (1992) Amanita smithiana - taxonomy, distribution, and poisonings. *Mycotaxon*; 45:373. http://www.cybertruffle.org.uk/cyberliber/index.htm (Accessed on October 20, 2009).

Wang, A. S., Barr, K. L., & Jagdeo, J. (2013). Shiitake mushroom-induced flagellate erythema: A striking case and review of the literature. *Dermatology online journal*, 19(4), 5.

Warden, C. R., & Benjamin, D. R. (1998). Acute renal failure associated with suspected Amanita smithiana mushroom ingestions: a case series. *Academic emergency medicine: official journal of the Society for Academic Emergency Medicine*, 5(8), 808-812. https://doi.org/10.1111/j.1553-2712.1998.tb02508.x.

Waser, P. G. (1961). Chemistry and pharmacology of muscarine, muscarone, and some related compounds. *Pharmacological reviews*, 13, 465-515.

West, P. L., Lindgren, J., & Horowitz, B. Z. (2009). Amanita smithiana mushroom ingestion: a case of delayed renal failure and literature review. *Journal of medical toxicology: official journal of the American College of Medical Toxicology*, 5(1), 32-38. https://doi.org/10.1007/BF03160979.

Ye, Y., & Liu, Z. (2018). Management of Amanita phalloides poisoning: A literature review and update. *Journal of critical care*, 46, 17-22. https://doi.org/10.1016/j.jcrc.2018.03.028.

Chapter 24

Mad Honey

Sinan Paslı[1], MD, Ali Aygün[2], MD
and Abdülkadir Gündüz[1,*], MD

[1]Karadeniz Technical University Faculty of Medicine, Department of Emergency Medicine, Trabzon, Turkey
[2]Ordu University Faculty of Medicine, Department of Emergency Medicine, Ordu, Turkey

Abstract

Due to the presence of a toxic substance called grayanotoxin in the extract of the flowers of the plants known as Rhododendron pontica and Rhododendron luteum, which grow in forest areas in the Black Sea Region of Turkey, honey collected from these plants can have a toxic effect. The toxic effects of grayanotoxin in the cell occur through the sodium channels, and it is also known that it exerts an inhibitory effect on the vagus nerve. Clinical findings related to mad honey poisoning are related to the action mechanism of grayanotoxin, which gives honey poisonous properties. The most common symptoms observed in patients after consuming mad honey are nausea, vomiting, drowsiness, dizziness and fainting. The most common findings in mad honey poisoning are related to the cardiovascular system. These findings are often accompanied by cardiac arrhythmias. When the patients admitted to the hospital are examined, the clinical findings seen in most of the patients are nausea, vomiting, hypotension and bradycardia. A few patients may experience fatigue, sweating, dizziness, drowsiness, and altered consciousness. Suspicion and a detailed anamnesis constitute the main points in the diagnosis of mad honey poisoning. Diagnosis of mad honey poisoning in current conditions; In patients who apply to the clinic with symptoms of hypotension and bradycardia, questioning the consumption of mad honey in the anamnesis is established by the presence of vital signs and clinical symptoms, when the complaints begin after eating mad honey. The treatment in mad honey poisoning is shaped according to the severity of the clinical situation. In mild cases, 2-6 hours of monitored follow-up and monitoring of vital signs are sufficient. Most patients generally improve with supportive treatment with saline and, if necessary, administration of 0.5-3mg of atropine.

In cases that do not respond to these treatments, the advanced cardiac life support guidelines for bradycardia should be applied. It should be noted that the diagnosis of mad honey poisoning can be made with a detailed history and suspicion. On discharge, it should be stated that in the case of a recurrence of symptoms, it is necessary to refer to the hospital

---

* Corresponding Author's Email: gunduzkadir@hotmail.com.

In: Environmental Emergencies and Injuries in Nature
Editors: Murat Yücel, Murat Güzel and İbrahim İkizceli
ISBN: 978-1-68507-833-1

again. In addition, there should be an instruction not to consume honey that is known or suspected to be mad honey.

Keywords: Mad honey, grayanotoxin, bradycardia

Introduction

Among the few known toxic effects of honey in the world, only Rhododendron species are grown in the northern region of Turkey, and the nectar accumulated in their flowers passes into honey. This honey, which is produced by bees feeding on the nectar of these plants and contains grayanotoxin, is called "mad honey" (Viccellio et al., 1993). Rhododendron honey (mad honey), produced mostly in Turkey, is a natural product formed by honeybees collecting the nectar and pollen of R. ponticum and R. luteum species of the Ericaceae family (Çeter and Güney, 2011).

Mad Honey in the Historical Process

During the Paleolithic and Mesolithic Ages, human beings made a living by hunting and gathering, and then they got rid of consumerism and passed into production. Beekeeping, as a trade element besides consumption, appeared in Egypt in 4000 BC. Considering the historical process, beekeeping is considered to be an important source of income, mostly in lands unsuitable for agriculture, and in rural and forested areas. According to the information from ancient sources, the poison found in mad honey is based on the "Rhododendron" (rhododendron) flower, which grows extensively in forests in some parts of the world (Oksuz et al., 2015; Plinius, 1980).

Mad honey poisoning was first mentioned in 401 BC as a condition that the Athenian historian and military commander Xenophon (430-355 BC) and his army were exposed to. In the book translated into Turkish as "Anabasis, the Return of the Tens", the mad honey poisoning and subsequent events that Xenophon and his soldiers who were fighting the Macrons in the city of Trabzon were exposed to, are described in detail: "The Greeks, reaching their climax, encamped in many villages with ample provisions. In this village, they encountered one thing that surprised them: There were many hives, and the soldiers who ate honey from the combs in these hives vomited, got diarrhea, and none of them could stand; those who ate little looked like people who were drunk, those who ate a lot looked like crazy madmen, even dying people. In this situation, many fell to the ground as if after a rout, and great despair began. No one was found dead the next day, and the drunkenness had ceased at about the time it had begun the day before.

On the third and fourth days, they stood up, exhausted, as if they had taken a laxative" (Oksuz et al., 2015; Gökçel, 2015). In the event described in this work, clinical findings caused by mad honey poisoning are also mentioned. In addition, the Makrons were the first to discover that mad honey could be used as a biological weapon, in addition to being a consumable item (Gökçel, 2015).

Worldwide: Although mad honey poisoning cases have been reported from Far East countries, North America and Europe, most of the cases reported so far are from Turkey, and the Black Sea region of Turkey is the region where poisoning cases are most common.

The toxic substance called grayanotoxin is found in honey produced by bees placed on the flowers of the plants known as "Rhododendron pontica" and Rhododendron luteum, which grow in forest areas in the Black Sea Region of Turkey. For this reason, this honey can have a toxic effect (Viccellio, 1993).

Grayanotoxins

Grayanotoxins (GTX) belong to the group of toxic diterpenes and are typed from GTX-I to form GTX-II and GTX-III. These natural toxins are found in substantial amounts in the leaves, flowers and nectar secretion of species such as Rhododendron and Kalmia. When honeybees collect the pollen and nectar secretion of these plants, they take these compounds to the honeycombs in the hive. These compounds do not detoxify when the nectar is transferred to the honeycomb. When this honey is consumed during the collection stage or in the next stage, the toxic effects of GTXs occur. So far, 60 different types of grayanotoxin have been identified, and those with primary toxic components are grayanotoxin I, III, and VI (Gunduz et al., 2008; Zhang et al., 2005).

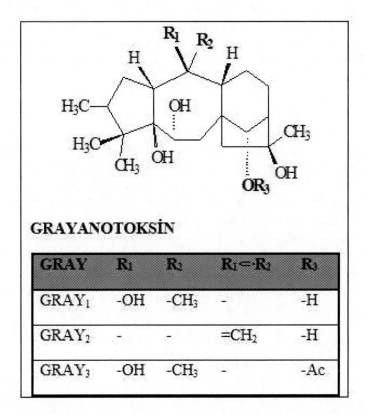

GRAY	R_1	R_2	$R_1=R_2$	R_3
GRAY$_1$	-OH	-CH$_3$	-	-H
GRAY$_2$	-	-	=CH$_2$	-H
GRAY$_3$	-OH	-CH$_3$	-	-Ac

Figure 1. Chemical structure of Grayanotoxin: General Chemical Structure of Grayanotoxin I, II and III (Gunduz et al., 2008).

The toxic effects of grayanotoxin in the cell occur via the sodium channels. According to the review by Maejima, grayanotoxin exerts its effect on voltage-dependent Na channels in 3 stages. First, grayanotoxin binds to these channels during the opening phase of voltage-dependent channels, then the channels are modified and finally the activation potential of the modified Na channels causes hyperpolarization. At the end of this process, voltage-dependent activation or inactivation occurs in the cell membrane (Maejima et al., 2003). Grayanotoxin is also known to exert an inhibitory effect on the vagus nerve. Onat et al. found that grayanotoxin causes bradycardia and respiratory depression in mice (Onat et al., 1991).

Clinical Findings of Mad Honey Poisoning

Clinical findings related to mad honey poisoning are related to the action mechanism of grayanotoxin (GTX). The most common findings in patients after consuming mad honey are nausea, vomiting, a feeling of lightheadedness, dizziness and fainting. When faced with this situation, which is known as "honey-sickness" among the people in regions where this honey is well known, people usually do not go to the hospital. People affected by the honey rest where they are, and natural treatment methods such as salted buttermilk and salt water are applied. After natural treatment or resting, patients recover spontaneously within a few hours (Gunduz et al., 2015).

Cardiovascular system findings are the most common findings in mad honey poisoning. These findings are often accompanied by cardiac arrhythmias. Cardiac arrhythmia is present in almost all of the cases reported to date. Although nonspecific arrhythmia, interatrial block, complete atrioventricular (AV) block, 2nd degree AV blocks and nodal rhythm have been reported, the most common arrhythmia is sinus bradycardia. Only one case with asystole has been reported in the literature (Gunduz et al., 2007, Osken et al., 2021).

When patients admitted to the hospital are examined, the clinical findings seen in most of the patients (90%) are nausea, vomiting, hypotension and bradycardia. Fatigue, sweating, dizziness, drowsiness and altered consciousness can also be seen in some of the patients (70%). Syncope is seen in approximately one-third of the patients. Decreased visual acuity and double vision are also clinical complaints reported in the literature. Although we encounter them at different rates, symptoms such as a feeling of something stuck in the throat, respiratory distress, increased salivation, headache, flushing, tremor, cyanosis, hypothermia, blurred vision, hallucinations, and peripheral numbness can also be seen due to mad honey poisoning (Aygun et al., 2016; Shrestha et al., 2018). There are also cases of mad honey poisoning with signs and symptoms consistent with acute coronary syndromes. The decrease and insufficiency in coronary blood flow secondary to hypotension and bradycardia are thought to cause an acute coronary event mechanism (Akıncı et al., 2008).

Diagnosis of Mad Honey Poisoning

Suspicion and a detailed anamnesis constitute the main points in the diagnosis of mad honey poisoning. Diagnosis of mad honey poisoning in current conditions; In patients who apply to the clinic with symptoms of hypotension and bradycardia, the questioning of mad honey consumption in the anamnesis is established by the presence of vital signs and clinical symptoms, as well as the onset of complaints after eating this honey. By using the LC-MS/MS method, the amount of GTX in the honey eaten by the patients and in body fluids such as blood and urine can be determined. However, in many clinics, this special laboratory test or method cannot be used to precisely measure or detect grayanotoxin levels in the body fluids of these patients and in the honey that they eat (Gunduz et al., 2014; Aygun et al., 2015).

Mad honey poisoning is not seen in everyone who consumes honey; the symptoms are dose-dependent and it is enough to consume 5-30 g of honey for poisoning. The mean age of the cases with poisoning is 49 years and the majority of cases are male (80.7%). Depending on the amount of honey consumed, onset of symptoms may be from a few minutes to more than two hours. It is stated that there is no correlation between clinical signs and symptoms and blood GTX levels after poisoning (Aygun et al., 2017). Symptoms can last from a few hours to a few days, depending on the severity of the poisoning. The clinical features mentioned in mad honey poisoning can be confused with many medical conditions and even many poisonings. For this reason, it is important to question the history of eating honey in patients presenting with these common symptoms, especially in regions where poisoning is endemic, in order to consider the possibility of mad honey poisoning. In the Black Sea region, where mad honey poisoning is endemic, it may be easy to think that the patient may have mad honey poisoning, but in European countries especially where people from the Black Sea region live outside the region, it can be quite difficult to understand that the cause of unexplained hypotension and bradycardia is mad honey poisoning (Gunduz et al., 2008; Gunduz et al., 2015; Gunduz et al., 2008).

Treatment of Mad Honey Poisoning

The treatment in mad honey poisoning is shaped according to the severity of the clinical situation. In mild cases, 2-6 hours of monitored follow-up and the monitoring of vital signs are sufficient. Most patients generally improve with supportive treatment with saline and, if necessary, administration of 0.5-3 mg of atropine. In cases that do not respond to these treatments, the advanced cardiac life support guide for bradycardia should be applied (Soar et al., 2021). A temporary pacemaker application may also be required for patients who do not improve despite this treatment. Significant signs and symptoms in untreated severe cases disappear within 24 hours at the latest. By the end of this period, all vital signs return to normal (Gunduz et al., 2008). Patients presenting with mild signs of intoxication can be safely discharged after being monitored for 2-6 hours.

Conclusion

It should not be forgotten that the diagnosis of mad honey poisoning can be made with a detailed anamnesis and suspicion. On discharge, it should be stated that in the case of a recurrence of symptoms, it is necessary to refer to the hospital again. In addition, there should be an instruction not to consume honey that is known or suspected to be mad honey.

References

Akıncı S, Arslan U, Karakurt K & Çengel A. (2008). An unusual presentation of mad honey poisoning: Acute myocardial infarction. *International Journal of Cardiology*, 129(2), e56-e58.

Aygun A, Gunduz A, Turedi S, Turkmen S, Karaca Y, Ayaz FA, ... & Kim S. (2015). Examination using LC-MS/MS determination of grayanotoxin levels in blood, urine, and honey consumed by patients presenting to the emergency department with mad honey intoxication and relations with clinical data: a preliminary study. *Annals of Saudi Medicine*, 35(2), 161-164.

Aygun A, Vuran HS, Aksut N, Karaca Y, Gunduz A & Turedi S. (2016). Mad honey poisoning–related hypothermia: A case series. *The Journal of Emergency Medicine*, 50(1), 51-54.

Aygun A, Sahin A, Karaca Y, Turkmen S, Turedi S, Ahn SY ... & Gunduz A. (2018). Grayanotoxin levels in blood, urine and honey and their association with clinical status in patients with mad honey intoxication. *Turkish Journal of Emergency Medicine*, 18(1), 29-33.

Çeter T, ve Güney K. 2011. Rhododendron and Mad Honey, *Uludağ Arıcılık Journal*, 11, 4, 124-129.

Gökçel T, Xenophon. (2011). *Anabasis*, Sosyal Yayınlar 2nd Edition, Sena Publishing. p. 143-4.

Gunduz A, Durmus I, Turedi S, Nuhoglu I & Ozturk S. (2007). Mad honey poisoning-related asystole. *Emergency Medicine Journal*, 24(8), 592-593.

Gunduz A, Tatlı O, Turedi S. (2008). Mad honey poisoning from the past to the present. *Turk J Emerg Med*, 8(1):46-49.

Gunduz A, Turedi S, Russell RM, Ayaz FA. (2008). Clinical review of grayanotoxin/mad honey poisoning past and present. *Clin Toxicology*, (Phila) 46:437-42.

Gunduz A, Eraydın I, Turkmen S, Kalkan OS, Turedi S, Eryığıt U, Ayar A. (2014). Analgesic effects of mad honey (grayanotoxin) in mice models of acute pain and painful diabetic neuropathy. *Hum Exp Toxicol*, 33(2):130-5.

Gunduz A., Tugrul O, Argın EC. (2015). *Clinical Diagnosis and Treatment of Mad Honey Intoxication*, Honey and Mad Honey. 1st Edition. Istanbul, Nobel Publishing. 147-53.

Maejima H, Kinoshita E, Seyama I, Yamaoka K. (2003). Distinct sites regulating grayanotoxin binding and unbinding to D4S6 of Na(v) 1.4 sodium channel as revealed by improved estimation of toxin sensitivity. *J Biol Chem*, 278:9464-71.

Oksuz H, Emir O. (2015). *Honey in the Historical Process*, Honey and Mad Honey, 1st Edition, Istanbul, Nobel Publishing. 2-7.

Onat FY, Yegen BC, Lawrence R. (1991). Mad honey poisoning in man and rat. *Rev Environ Health*, 9:3-92.

Ösken A, Aydın E, Özcan KS & Yaylacı S. (2021). Evaluation of Electrocardiographic Parameters and the Presence of Interatrial Block in Patients with Mad Honey Intoxication. *Cardiovascular Toxicology*, 1-9.

Plinius GS. (1980). *Natural History of Pliny*, (Translate J. Bostock and HT Riley), London: George Bell&Sons York Street.

Shrestha TM, Nepal G, Shing YK & Shrestha L. (2018). Cardiovascular, psychiatric, and neurological phenomena seen in mad honey disease: A clinical case report. *Clinical Case Reports*, 6(12), 2355.

Soar J, Böttiger BW, Carli P, Couper K, Deakin CD, Djärv T ... & Nolan JP. (2021). European Resuscitation Council guidelines 2021: Adult advanced life support. *Resuscitation*, 161, 115-151.

Viccellio P. (1993). *Systemic poisonous plant intoxication*. Handbook of Medical Toxicology. Washington: Library of Congress Cataloging, 718.

Zhang HP, Wang HB, Wang LQ, Bao GH & Qin GW. (2005). Note: A new 1, 5-seco grayanotoxin from Rhododendron decorum. *Journal of Asian Natural Products Research*, 7(1), 87-90.

Chapter 25

Organic Phosphate Poisoning

Aynur Şahin and Vildan Özer[*]
Department of Emergency Medicine, Karadeniz Technical University, Trabzon, Turkey

Abstract

Organophosphate compounds and carbamates have been a crucial public health problem across the world for many years. Nowadays, they pose a danger to human health because of both their utilization in agricultural areas and as weapons of mass destruction in organophosphate form. The World Health Organization is trying to actively fight against these chemicals and raise awareness in communities and governments. Still, millions of people are exposed to these chemicals every year, particularly due to agricultural use in Asia and terrorist attacks in the Middle East. Both acute-onset cholinergic and nicotinic effects and late-onset symptoms can be life-threatening for people who are exposed to these compounds. Atropine and oximes are well-known agents in antidotal therapy. However, more effective treatment protocols are trying to be established with many new-generation drugs and treatment approaches. This article aims to update our knowledge about organophosphate compounds and carbamates and discuss current/new-generation treatment approaches.

Keywords: atropine, acetylcholine, acetylcholinesterase, insecticides, organophosphate, oximes, toxidrome

Introduction

Initially, organophosphate (OP) compounds were chemicals developed as pesticides to protect animals, plants, houses, and communities from the direct and indirect effects of insects and the diseases they brought with them. However, they were rather used as chemical weapons in later periods (Eddleston, 2019a). OP compounds were first synthesized in 1854. According to estimations, more than 50,000 OP compounds have been synthesized since then (Soltaninejad & Shadnia, 2014). In history, they became most famous during the Second World War. Mass deaths were induced with chemical warfare agents containing OP, such as synthesized soman

---

[*] Corresponding Author's Email: dr.vilzan@hotmail.com.

In: Environmental Emergencies and Injuries in Nature
Editors: Murat Yücel, Murat Güzel and İbrahim İkizceli
ISBN: 978-1-68507-833-1

(GD), sarin (GB), tabun (GA), new-generation VX and others. These agents are called "nerve agents" since they specifically influence the autonomic nervous system (Soltaninejad & Shadnia, 2014). Nerve gases in OP form have been employed as weapons of mass destruction in many military conflicts and terrorist acts over the last fifteen years (Eddleston, 2019a).

According to the data of the World Health Organization (WHO), about 1 million accidental and 2 million intentional exposures to compounds containing OP occur annually, resulting in more than 300,000 deaths (Jeyaratnam, 1990). Exposure to these compounds may be accidental, intentional, or occupational, and the way of exposure for poisoning may even change by season and demographics in developed and developing countries (Baker et al., 1978; Jeyaratnam, 1990; van der Hoek et al., 1998; Eddleston, 2000; Clark, 2002). Especially in rural parts of Asia, they are often used for suicidal purposes, and almost 200,000 deaths have been reported (Eddleston, 2000). Occupational exposure is also commonly observed in developing countries because of the unprotected use of pesticides during agricultural spraying or unsafe areas where these compounds are stored (Koh & Jeyaratnam, 1996; Mishra et al., 2012). Mortality is substantially low in accidental exposures (Eddleston, 2019a). According to the WHO's pesticide classification, especially upon the prohibition of insecticides in the most toxic OP form, there was a 50% decrease in the poisoning rate in Sri Lanka, which shows that the regulations on the use of these chemicals were effective (Knipe et al., 2017a, 2017b; Gunnell et al., 2007).

Pharmacokinetics and Pharmacodynamics of Organophosphates

OP compounds are taken into the body via the mouth, skin, respiration, and eyes, rapidly absorbed and dispersed to all body tissues. However, they mostly accumulate in the liver, kidney, and adipose tissue. Poisoning can be acute or chronic. Depending on the agent, way of exposure, accompanying toxins, degree of exposure, and elimination and metabolic rate of the compound, signs and symptoms may be observed suddenly or after a few hours. Most OP compounds are lipophilic. Particularly the agents with a high virtual volume of distribution (disulfoton, fenthion, etc.) may be stored in the adipose tissue and lead to symptoms that act late and for a long time (Vohra, 2017). Oral exposure is frequently accidental in children and the elderly, whereas it is suicidal in young people and adults, especially in developing countries (Eddleston, 2019a; Mishra et al., 2012; London, 2009; London et al., 2012). In the case of oral ingestion, symptoms appear within minutes. After parenteral or intravenous administration, symptoms appear early, and the clinical picture is more mortal. Skin exposure to OP compounds is generally accidental or occupational. Absorption is extremely slow in this way. However, patients are brought to health institutions at a later time owing to the late awareness of patients about the exposure. For this reason, the exposure time is longer. In inhalation exposure, absorption rates are considerably high due to the high rate of solubility of OP compounds in oil. When respiratory or skin exposure takes place, taking the patient away from the environment and decontaminating the patient by removing his clothes are among the first field practices to decrease exposure to OP compounds (Eddleston, 2019a; Mishra et al., 2012).

Classification pf Organophosphate Compounds/Toxicity Mechanism

According to the WHO, OP compounds are divided into four groups (Eddleston, 2019a; World Health Organization, 2019) (Table 1). Group 1 consists of potent cholinesterase inhibitors. This is the group called phosphorylcholines, which were initially developed as warfare agents. These agents directly stimulate cholinergic receptors owing to their similarity to acetylcholine in structural terms. Group 2 consists of fluorophosphates, which are also volatile and quite toxic like Group 1 and are employed as chemical warfare agents. Cyanophosphates, such as tabun, which is a warfare agent, are the best known of the Group 3 compounds. Group 4 compounds have a wide range, and this group includes most of the insecticides used nowadays (Vohra, 2017; Eddleston, 2019a; World Health Organization, 2019).

Acetylcholine is a neurotransmitter in nicotinic, muscarinic, and CNS receptors and it enables transmission from the presynaptic zone to the postsynaptic zone along the nerve. Sometimes a gland, sometimes a muscle cell, and sometimes another nerve cell is the target cell. The transmission should be terminated after the targeted effect is achieved. The enzyme acetylcholinesterase breaks down acetylcholine by binding to acetylcholine and terminates the transmission by ending its activity. Thus, the target cell carries on its normal function. After exposure to OP compounds and carbamates, these compounds bind to both acetylcholinesterase (AChE) in red blood cells (RBCs) and butyrylcholinesterase, also known as pseudocholinesterase (PChE) or plasma cholinesterase, in the blood. As a result, they lead to the enzyme blockade, in other words, an inability to break down acetylcholine in the environment, along with an excessive increase in acetylcholine in the synaptic gap and excessive stimulation of the target cell (Casida & Quistad, 2004; Eddleston, 2019a, 2019b). The enzyme inhibition half-life is 0.7-0.8 hours *in vitro* in exposure to dimethoxy compounds, whereas it is 31-57 hours in diethoxy compounds (Eyer, 2003). However, the exposure dose is also significant because the reactivated enzyme will undergo inhibition again in high-dose exposures. The reactivation of the inhibited enzyme is accelerated by oximes. However, if oximes are administered late, an alkyl group on the OP-enzyme complex is lost, and "enzyme aging" takes place. The aging enzyme cannot be reactivated by oximes. The enzyme inhibition power of OP compounds also depends on conditions such as lipophilicity and the rate of enzyme inhibition of the compounds, other than their structures (Eyer, 2003; Eddleston, 2019a, 2019b).

Like OP compounds, carbamates also inhibit enzymes, but this happens reversibly and takes a shorter time. Since they cross the blood-brain barrier less than other OP compounds, their CNS effects are less evident. Physostigmine, pyridostigmine, and neostigmine are carbamates used to treat MG through the inhibition of the acetylcholinesterase enzyme. Moreover, there are carbamates that do not inhibit the enzyme (Eddleston, 2019a).

Clinical Picture

Onset times of symptoms differ according to the chemical structure, amount and way of exposure. As OP compounds in the oxon form are active even without being metabolized, their effects appear within minutes. However, OP compounds in the thion form exhibit their effects after they are transformed into the oxon form in the body. For example, the transformation of fenthion into its active form occurs within hours, while the transformation of parathion into its active form takes place within minutes, and symptoms appear quickly (Eyer, 2003). The rapid emergence of respiratory failure before reaching the hospital is considered to be the most important factor of mortality (Eddleston, 2019a).

Symptoms are classified considering the receptors influenced and the time of emergence.

Early Onset Symptoms

Clinical findings resulting from the excessive increase of the acetylcholine amount in the synaptic gap differ according to which receptor is affected in the autonomic nervous system. There are two types of receptors in the sympathetic and parasympathetic systems, which constitute the autonomic nervous system. For this reason, the typical cholinergic syndrome is divided into two subgroups as muscarinic and nicotinic. Cholinesterase inhibition may occur in a mixed clinical picture, which sometimes incorporates the symptoms of both sub-syndromes, as a result of the competing effects of ganglionic stimulation of both parasympathetic and sympathetic pathways (Vohra, 2017; Eddleston, 2019a).

Muscarinic Symptoms

Muscarinic receptors are the main receptors of the parasympathetic system, and the symptoms arising from their excessive activation are generally the most encountered symptoms in OP poisoning. As a consequence of the excessive activation of muscarinic receptors, bronchospasm, bradycardia, abdominal pain, vomiting, diarrhea, miosis, and excessive sweating develop. There are two mnemonics that make it easy to remember them in the clinical picture. DUMBBBELLS: diarrhea, urination, miosis, bradycardia, bronchorrhea, bronchospasm, emesis, lacrimation, lethargy, salivation, and SLUDGE+3B: salivation, lacrimation, urination, diaphoresis, gastrointestinal symptoms, emesis + bronchorrhea, bradycardia, bronchospasm (Vohra, 2017; Eddleston, 2019a).

Nicotinic Symptoms

The nicotinic effects mainly develop because of the excessive stimulation of the receptors at the neuromuscular junction resulting from the increased amount of acetylcholine. They are characterized especially by muscle weakness and tremors/fasciculations. Nicotinic receptors are located in the sympathetic nervous system. Therefore, tachycardia, hypertension, and mydriasis are observed. The mnemonic used to remember the symptoms refers to the days of the week: MTWTF (mydriasis, tachycardia, weakness, hypertension, fasciculations, seizures) (Vohra, 2017; Eddleston, 2019a).

CNS Symptoms

Central nervous system symptoms include agitation, lethargy, seizures, and coma (Vohra, 2017; Eddleston, 2019a).

Table 1. The classification of organic phosphorus compounds

Group 1	Leaving group	Examples of Each Group	Group 2	Leaving group	Examples of Each Group
Phosphorylcholines	Substituted quaternary nitrogen	Echothiophate iodide	Fluorophosphates	Fluoride	Dimefox Sarin Mipafox
Group 3	**Leaving group**	**Examples of Each Group**	**Group 4**	**Leaving group**	**Examples of Each Group**
Cyanophosphates, other halophosphates	CN-, SCN-, OCN-, halogen other than fluoride	Tabun	Multiple constituents	Dimethoxy	Azinphos-menthyl, bromophos, chlorothion, crotoxyphos, dicapthon, dichlorvos, dicrotophos, dimethoate, fenthion, malathion, mevinphos, parathion-methyl, phosphamidon, temephos, trichlorfon
				Diethoxy	Carbophenothion, chlorfenvinphos, chlorpyriphos, coumaphos, demeton, diazinon, dioxathion, disulfoton, ethion, methosfolan, parathion, phorate, phosfolan, TEPP
				Other dialkoxy	Isopropyl paraoxon, isopropyl parathion
				Diamino	Schradan
				Chlorinated and other substituted dialkoxy	Haloxon
				Trithioalkyl	Merphos
				Triphenyl and substituted triphenyl	Triorthocresyl phosphate (TOCP)
				Mixed substituent	Crufomate, cyanofenphos

(Eddleston, 2019a; World Health Organization, 2019)

Late-Onset Symptoms

Organic Phosphorous Compound-Induced Delayed Neuropathy (OPIDN)

OPIDN is a rare complication characterized by peripheral neuropathic symptoms that are observed upon the re-release of a lipophilic OP compound from the adipose tissue, where it is stored, into the system after 2-3 weeks. Inhibition of the neuropathic target esterase (NTE) enzyme in nerve tissues is considered in the pathogenesis. It occurs 14-28 days after exposure. Neuropathy is typically peripheral and symmetrical, and the clinical picture is accompanied by sensory weakness. However, sensory impairment is milder than motor impairment (Vohra, 2017; Eddleston, 2019a).

Neuromuscular Junction Dysfunction – Intermediate Syndrome

This is a clinical condition characterized by the paralysis of neck muscles (broken neck sign), respiratory muscles, and bulbar and proximal extremity muscles resulting from the impairment of muscle conduction in the presynaptic and postsynaptic zones after exposure to compounds containing OP. It appears 2-4 days after exposure. In the pathogenesis, many factors such as prolonged enzyme inhibition after severe toxicity, re-release of lipophilic compounds from adipose tissue, paralysis induced by prolonged nicotinic stimulation, desensitization or downregulation of postsynaptic acetylcholine receptors, and insufficient or delayed antidotal therapy have been brought forward. Early diagnosis is of extreme importance since it leads to respiratory failure by influencing the respiratory muscles. The clinical condition continues for 1-3 weeks, and no response to antidotal therapy is observed in general (Vohra, 2017; Eddleston, 2019a).

Miscellaneous Toxic Effects

Apart from the afore-stated clinical findings, pesticides have also been reported to cause rare symptoms such as Guillain-Barré syndrome, choreiform movement disorders, Parkinson's symptoms, glucose abnormalities, metabolic acidosis, acute coronary syndrome, hypotension, and pancreatitis. Furthermore, it should be kept in mind that clinical findings of acute lung injury, pulmonary edema and chemical pneumonia may also be encountered due to aspiration of hydrocarbon solvents since the said compounds are frequently combined with hydrocarbon compounds (Vohra, 2017; Eddleston, 2019a).

Diagnosis

Detailed anamnesis and recognition of cholinergic syndrome symptoms to identify the exposure agent are the most important elements in the diagnosis of exposure to OP compounds. In patients presenting with cholinergic toxidrome symptoms, the presence of cholinergic, nicotinic, and CNS symptoms should be examined in detail. In addition to the patient's vital signs, laboratory tests such as arterial blood gas, ECG, and biochemical tests including creatine kinase will be helpful for the diagnosis. In the differential diagnosis, drugs and toxins likely to cause cholinergic syndrome should be taken into account and tried to be excluded. Plasma pseudocholinesterase (PChE) and acetylcholinesterase (AChE) enzyme levels can be measured for diagnostic purposes. However, they are not used as diagnostic tools due to the lack of bedside measurement methods and because the results cannot be obtained immediately. The erythrocyte AChE level is more specific than the PChE level. More than a 50% decrease from the initial level indicates exposure to OP compounds, but the level may differ in patients taking oral contraceptives or malaria medication or infants compared to the normal population. Since these specific diagnostic tests are not accessible in clinical practice, the diagnosis should be established in line with the anamnesis and physical examination findings, and treatment should be initiated promptly (Vohra, 2017; Eddleston, 2019a, 2019b).

Treatment

Decontamination

The method of decontamination that will be applied to the patient differs according to the way of exposure to organophosphate compounds. After the clothes of the patient who contacted the OP compound are properly put in a nylon bag not to be worn again, the bag should be tied up firmly and buried in a pit with a minimum 30 cm depth (Eddleston, 2019a). Decontamination procedures, and resuscitation procedures and antidotal administrations in severe toxicities should not be delayed. When required, decontamination procedures should be carried out right after interventions such as resuscitation, maintaining the airway, and atropinization. No matter how the exposure occurred, clinicians and other involved health personnel should avoid contamination by wearing Level C protective clothes and neoprene/nitrile gloves during the application of this procedure in undecontaminated patients (Vohra, 2017; Eddleston, 2019a, 2019b). It should be remembered that contact with all body fluids, such as the patient's stomach and stool contents, will also be a source of contamination (Little & Murray, 2004). Despite all these risks, secondary contamination of hospital personnel is improbable as long as standard measures are taken (Roberts & Senarathna, 2004).

If the patient's exposure has been accidental or occurred intentionally by ingestion, but the patient has not vomited, the gastric contents of patients who are conscious and whose airway is maintained should be evacuated via gastric lavage within the first 2 hours following ingestion. Due to the presence of studies indicating that some OP compounds are absorbed by activated charcoal, activated charcoal at a dose of 1 gr/kg should be administered to the patient within the first two hours of ingestion. If the airway has not been maintained in admissions within the first 2 hours of ingestion, these procedures should be carried out after intubating the patient (Vohra, 2017; Eddleston, 2019a). Administration of activated charcoal at repeated doses is not recommended due to the lack of sufficient evidence for its benefits (Eddleston et al., 2008c). As in all patients, if there are contraindications to gastric lavage and activated charcoal administration, these interventions should definitely be avoided.

If the patient's exposure has occurred through the skin or mucous membranes, the exposure areas, including the hair and under the nails, should be washed with soap and rinsed with water after removing the patient's contaminated clothes. It should be remembered that exposed eyes should also be washed with a large amount of warm water (Vohra, 2017; Eddleston, 2019a). Washing/wiping should be done in a pinching manner to prevent spreading. In the case of exposure to an oil-based OP compound, it is recommended to wash the exposure area at least 3 times and shave the scalp when necessary (Eddleston, 2019a). In the military field, studies on skin decontamination with sponges containing cholinesterase enzyme are conducted, and the results of these studies are reported to be effective in skin decontamination of OP compounds (Gordon et al., 1999). If there is no soap and water in the exposure environment, dry decontamination can be performed with aluminum silicate or magnesium silicate gloves.

Principles of Emergency and Supportive Treatment (Abc)

Other than the afore-stated decontamination measures, if nerve gas exposure is suspected, people working in contaminated areas should also take respiratory protective measures and wear Type C CBRN-protective clothes. It is sufficient for healthcare personnel to wear Type D CBRN-protective clothes when a patient is brought to the emergency department after being decontaminated at the site. Airway respiration and circulation of each patient should be evaluated at the initial stage and stabilized. The patient should be evaluated for early advanced airway intervention if muscle fasciculations, muscle weakness, and bronchorrhea are observed. If the patient has seizures, benzodiazepines are the first agents to be used. In hypotensive episodes, inotropic agents such as dopamine or vasopressor agents such as noradrenaline should be preferred in addition to intravenous fluid therapy. In severe OP poisoning cases, magnesium should be used in the visible treatment of QT prolongation and torsades de pointes (TdP). In the acute phase of organophosphate poisoning, complications such as respiratory distress, aspiration pneumonia, seizures, and impairment in neurological functions may appear. In the acute period, patients should be monitored for these complications and the requirement for an increase or decrease in the atropine dose (Eddleston, 2019a, 2008a, 2008b, 2004a). In the evaluation of patients' response to treatment, monitoring of clinical signs and symptoms is more reliable than the measurement of the cholinesterase enzyme level. It is recommended to monitor patients for late-onset symptoms for 8-12 hours after becoming asymptomatic (Vohra, 2017).

Antidotal Therapy

Atropine

Atropine, which is an antimuscarinic agent in OP poisoning, is only used to reverse muscarinic symptoms since it does not affect nicotinic symptoms such as tremor/fasciculation in muscles and muscle weakness (Freeman & Epstein, 1995; Heath, 1992; Eddleston, 2019a). The antidotal use of atropine in OP poisoning in adolescents and adults is as follows: It is started as an intravenous bolus of 1-3 mg, and the previous dose is doubled every 5 minutes until the excessive cholinergic activity is brought under control and bronchial secretions dry up. In children, the starting dose is 0.05 mg/kg. In this intervention called atropinization, the important clinical situation is to bring the patient's cholinergic symptoms under control and reverse the symptoms resulting from the excessive cholinergic activity, especially to bring the life-threatening bronchorrhea under control. The tachycardia response likely to be observed during this high-dose atropine administration in the patient does not pose an absolute contraindication for atropinization (Eddleston, 2004a, 2004b).

In the prehospital period, 2 mg of atropine alone or a combination of 2 mg of atropine and 600 mg of pralidoxime/220 mg of obidoxime is administered in a disaster or military area. During exposure to OP compounds, particularly nerve gases, autoinjectors containing the combination of atropine and oxime can be administered IM to the anterolateral side of the thigh over clothes every 5-10 minutes, for 3 times in total, until the symptoms are improved. Physician evaluation is necessary to switch to IV administration in cases when symptoms are not improved (Henretig et al., 2002; Eddleston, 2019a, 2008a, 2008b).

Oximes

Oximes reverse the neuromuscular nicotinic effects by reactivating the acetylcholinesterase enzyme, which becomes inactive in OP poisoning. To be effective, oximes should be used before enzyme aging (irreversible phosphorylation of the cholinesterase enzyme) begins. The administration dose of pralidoxime, which is one of the oximes, is as follows: 30 mg/kg (maximum 2 g) in 100 cc sodium chloride after 15-30 minutes of infusion, continuous infusion of 8-10 mg/kg/hr (up to 650 mg/h) (Tang et al., 2013; Eddleston, 2019a). Continuation of oxime therapy is recommended until symptoms resolve and atropine is no longer needed for 12-24 hours (Eddleston, 2008a, 2004b). In toxicity associated with carbamate, one of the OP compounds, the need for using oximes in addition to atropine is quite rare (Burgess et al., 1994; Eddleston, 2019a).

New-Generation Treatments

Regarding OP poisoning, the therapeutic use of magnesium (Basher et al., 2013; Vijayakumar et al., 2017), clonidine (Perera et al., 2009), fresh frozen plasma (Guven et al., 2004; Pichamuthu et al., 2010), sodium bicarbonate (Roberts & Buckley, 2005) and lipid emulsions (Mir & Rasool, 2014; Zhou et al., 2010) to reduce the release of presynaptic acetylcholine has been investigated. However, these therapies are not recommended yet for the current treatment of OP poisoning as they are all at the experimental stage (Eddleston, 2019a).

Elimination

The EXTRIP (The Extracorporeal Treatments in Poisoning Work Group) group, which has published recommendations and guidelines on extracorporeal treatments to be applied in poisoned patients, has not recommended the interventions of hemodialysis, hemofiltration, or hemoperfusion in organophosphate poisoning to date (EXTRIP, 2021). In the literature, some publications have revealed that hemoperfusion is an effective method to eliminate organophosphate compounds from the blood; it improves cholinesterase activity; there is less need for atropine and lower mortality rates in patients undergoing hemoperfusion compared to the control group; the duration of coma is reduced and clinical outcomes such as earlier discharge are associated with hemoperfusion (Xiaoxia et al., 2000; Yang et al., 2011; Li & Xiao, 2009; Wang et al., 2004); these clinical outcomes are even better in patients who receive hemoperfusion at repeated doses compared to those who receive it once, therefore, repeated doses of hemoperfusion are recommended in the early period (Bo, 2014); hemoperfusion decreases the level of inflammatory mediators in organophosphate poisoning (Huo et al., 2012), and acute intermediate syndrome is observed less in patients undergoing hemoperfusion (Li et al., 2017). However, treatment options such as HD or HP are not recommended since organophosphate compounds usually have a large volume of distribution and data on treatment success are not sufficient (Eddleston, 2019a) (Vohra, 2017).

Follow-Up and Discharge

All suicidal exposures should be evaluated seriously. Particularly the cases presenting with symptoms of cholinergic syndrome should be followed up under intensive care conditions. Patients who have been administered an antidote but no longer need atropinization, who do not have any new signs of a cholinergic crisis or complications during their follow-up, and who are asymptomatic can be discharged after 48 hours of follow-up. Discharge after 12 hours of follow-up can be planned for patients who have been asymptomatic since the admission (Eddleston, 2019a).

Conclusion

An effective global action plan is needed to prevent the damage of organophosphate compounds to humans and nature. As in the Sri Lanka example, the rates of toxicity caused by OP compounds will be decreased by prohibiting the use of OP compounds with high toxicity rates and implementing more effective solutions for the storage and use of other OP agents.

References

Baker, E.L., Warren, M., Zack, M., Dobbin, R.D., Miles, J.W., Miller, S., Alderman, L., Teeters, W.R. (1978). Epidemic malathion poisoning in Pakistan malaria workers, *The Lancet*, 311(8054), 31-34.

Basher, A., Rahman, S.H., Ghose, A., Arif, S.M., Faiz, M.A., Dawson, A.H. (2013). Phase II study of magnesium sulfate in acute organophosphate pesticide poisoning. *Clin Toxicol.*, 51(1), 35-40.

Bo, L. (2014). Therapeutic efficacies of different hemoperfusion frequencies in patients with organophosphate poisoning. *Eur Rev Med Pharmacol Sci*, 18(22), 3521-3523.

Burgess, J.L., Bernstein, J.N., & Hurlbut, K. (1994). Aldicarb poisoning—a case report with prolonged cholinesterase inhibition and improvement after pralidoxime therapy. *Arch Intern Med.*, 154(2), 221-224.

Clark, R.F. (2002). Insecticides: organic phosphorus compounds and carbamates. *Goldfrank's Toxicological Emergencies* (7), 1346–1360.

Casida, J.E., Quistad, G.B. (2004). Organophosphate toxicology: safety aspects of nonacetylcholinesterase secondary targets. *Chem Res Toxicol.*, 17, 983-998.

Eddleston, M. (2019a). Insecticides: Organic Phosphorus Compounds And Carbamates. Goldfrank's Toxicological Emergencies (9), 1486-1502.

Eddleston, M. (2019b). Novel clinical toxicology and pharmacology of organophosphorus insecticide self-poisoning. *Annual review of pharmacology and toxicology*, 59, 341-360.

Eddleston, M., Dawson, A.H. & Buckley, N.A. (2008a). Management of acute organophosphorous pesticide poisoning. *Lancet.*, 371, 597-607.

Eddleston, M., Buckley, N.A., Eyer, P., Dawson, A.H. (2008b). Medical management of acute organophosphorus pesticide poisoning. *The Lancet*, 371(9612), 597-607.

Eddleston, M., Juszczak, E., Buckley, N.A., Senarathna, L., Mohamed, F., Dissanayake, W., Hittarage, A., Azher, S., Jeganathan, K., Jayamanne, S., Sheriff, R., Warrell, D.A. (2008c). Multiple-dose activated charcoal in acute self-poisoning: a randomised controlled trial. *The Lancet*, 371(9612), 579-587.

Eddleston, M., Dawson, A., Karalliedde, L., Dissanayake, W., Hittarage, A., Azher, S., Buckley, N.A. (2004a). Early management after self-poisoning with an organophosphorus or carbamate pesticide—a treatment protocol for junior doctors. *Crit Care.*, 8(6), 1-7.

Eddleston, M., Buckley, N.A., Checketts, H., Senarathna, L., Mohamed, F., Sheriff, R., Dawson, A. (2004b). Speed of initial atropinisation in significant organophosphorus pesticide poisoning—a systematic comparison of recommended regimens. *J Toxicol Clin Toxicol.*, 42(6), 865-875.

Eddleston, M. (2000). Patterns and problems of deliberate self-poisoning in the developing world. *Qjm*, 93(11), 715-731.

Eyer, P. (2003). The role of oximes in the management of organophosphorus pesticide poisoning. *Toxicol Rev.*, 22(3), 165-190.

EXTRIP (2021, December 27). https://www.extrip-workgroup.org/recommendations

Freeman, G., & Epstein, M.A. (1955). Therapeutic factors in survival after lethal cholinesterase inhibition by phosphorus insecticides. *N Engl J Med.*, 253(7), 266-271.

Gordon, R.K., Feaster, S.R., Russell, A.J., Lejeune, K.E., Maxwell, D.M., Lenz, D.E., Ross, M., Doctor, B.P. (1999). Organophosphate skin decontamination using immobilized enzymes. *Chem Biol Interact*, 119, 463-470.

Gunnell, D., Fernando, R., Hewagama, M., Priyangika, W.D.D., Konradsen, F., Eddleston, M. (2007). The impact of pesticide regulations on suicide in Sri Lanka. *Int. J. Epidemiol*, 36(6), 1235–1242.

Guven, M., Sungur, M., Eser, B., Sarı, I., & Altuntas, F. (2004). The effects of fresh frozen plasma on cholinesterase levels and outcomes in patients with organophosphate poisoning. *J Toxicol Clin Toxicol.*, 42(5), 617-623.

Heath, A.J.W. (1992). Atropine in the management of anticholinesterase poisoning. In: Ballantyne B, Marrs T, eds. *Clinical and Experimental Toxicology of Organophosphates and Carbamates.*, 543-554.

Henretig, F.M., Mechem, C., & Jew, R. (2002). Potential use of autoinjector-packaged antidotes for treatment of pediatric nerve agent toxicity. *Ann Emerg Med.*, 40(4), 405-408.

Huo, J., Fan, C.B., Li, Q., & Tong, H. (2012). Sequential hemoperfusion and continuous veno-venous hemofiltration in treatment of severe organophosphorus pesticide poisoning. *Journal of Hainan Medical University.*

Jeyaratnam, J. (1990). Pesticide poisoning: a major global health problem. *World Health Statist. Quart.*, 43(3), 139-144.

Knipe, D.M., Gunnell, D., Eddleston, M. (2017a). Preventing deaths from pesticide self-poisoning—learning from Sri Lanka's success. *Lancet Global Health*, 5(7), 651–652.

Knipe, D.W., Chang, S.S., Dawson, A., Eddleston, M., Konradsen, F., Metcalfe, C., Gunnell, D. (2017b). Suicide prevention through means restriction: impact of the 2008–2011 pesticide restrictions on suicide in Sri Lanka. *PLoS one*, 12(4), e0176750.

Koh, D., & Jeyaratnam, J. (1996). Pesticides hazards in developing countries. *Sci. Total Environ.*, 188(1), 78-85.

Li, H., & Xiao, Y.H. (2009). Observation of effects of hemoperfusion associated with hemodialysis on severe organophosphorous poisoning. *Modern Medicine & Health*, 2009, 13.

Li, Z., Wang, G., Zhen, G., Zhang, Y., Liu, J., & Liu, S. (2017). Application of hemoperfusion in severe acute organophosphorus pesticide poisoning. *Turkish journal of medical sciences*, 47(4), 1277-1281.

Little, M., Murray, L. (2004). Consensus statement: risk of nosocomial organophosphate poisoning in emergency departments. *Emerg Med Australas.*, 16(5-6), 456-458.

London, L. (2009). Neurobehavioural methods, effects and prevention: workers' human rights are why the field matters for developing countries. *Neurotoxicology*, 30(6), 1135-1143.

London, L., Beseler, C., Bouchard, M.F., Bellinger, D.C., Colosio, C., Grandjean, P., Harari, R., Kootbodien, T., Kromhout, H., Little, F., Meijster, T., Moretto, A., Rohlman, D.S., Stallones, L. (2012).

Neurobehavioral and neurodevelopmental effects of pesticide exposures. *Neurotoxicology*, 33(4), 887-896.

Mir, S.A., & Rasool, R. (2014). Reversal of cardiovascular toxicity in severe organophosphate poisoning with 20% intralipid emulsion therapy: case report and review of literature. *Asia Pac J Med Toxicol.*, 3(4), 169-172.

Mishra, A., Shukla, S. K., Yadav, M. K., Gupta, A. K. (2012). Epidemiological study of medicolegal organophosphorus poisoning in central region of Nepal. *J Forensic Res*, 3(9), 1-5.

Perera, P.M., Jayamanna, S.F., Hettiarachchi, R., Abeysinghe, C., Karunatilake, H., Dawson, A.H., Buckley, N.A. (2009). A phase II clinical trial to assess the safety of clonidine in acute organophosphorus pesticide poisoning. *Trials.*, 10(1), 1-9.

Pichamuthu, K., Jerobin, J., Nair, A., John, G., Kamalesh, J., Thomas, K., Jose, A., Fleming, J.J., Zachariah, A., David, S.S., Daniel, D., Peter, J.V. (2010). Bioscavenger therapy for organophosphate poisoning—an open-labeled pilot randomized trial comparing fresh frozen plasma or albumin with saline in acute organophosphate poisoning in humans. *Clin Toxicol.*, 48(8), 813-819.

Roberts, D., Senarathna, L. (2004). Secondary contamination in organophosphate poisoning. *Qjm.*, 97(10), 697-698.

Roberts, D., & Buckley, N.A. (2005). Alkalinisation for organophosphorus pesticide poisoning. *Cochrane Database Syst Rev.*, (1).

Soltaninejad, K., Shadnia, S. (2014). History of the use and epidemiology of organophosphorus poisoning. *In Basic and Clinical Toxicology of Organophosphorus Compounds*, 25-43.

Van Der Hoek, W., Konradsen, F., Athukorala, K., Wanigadewa, T. (1998). Pesticide poisoning: a major health problem in Sri Lanka. *Soc. Sci. Med.*, 46(4-5), 495-504.

Vijayakumar, H.N., Kannan, S., Tejasvi, C., Duggappa, D.R., Gowda, K.M.V., Nethra, S.S. (2017). Study of effect of magnesium sulphate in management of acute organophosphorous pesticide poisoning. *Anesth Essays Res.*, 11(1), 192-196.

Vohra R. (2017). Organophosphorus and carbamate insecticides. Poisoning and Drug Overdose (7), 353-360.

Tang, X., Wang, R., Xie, H., Hu, J., Zhao, W. (2013). Repeated pulse intramuscular injection of pralidoxime chloride in severe acute organophosphorus pesticide poisoning. *Am J Emerg Med.*, 31(6), 946-949.

Wang, J.S., Liu, H.Y., & Gao, J.H. (2004). Application of therapeutic plasma exchange to severe active organic phosphorus intoxication. *Chinese Journal of Critical Care Medicine*, 24(6), 394-395.

World Health Organization. (2019). The WHO recommended Clasification of Pesiticides by Hazard and Guidelines to Clasification.

Xiaoxia, Y.U., Lixin, W., & Zenglu, L.U. (2000). Efficacy study of hemoperfusion in treating intermediate syndrome following acute organophosphorus pesticide poisoning. *Chinese Journal of Nephrology*, 03.

Yang, L.S., Li, W.F., & Ma, X. (2011). Study of the cholinesterase energy recovery on Hemoperfusion application in acute organophosphorus pesticide poisoning. *Ningxia Medical Journal*, 6.

Zhou, Y., Zhan, C., Li, Y., Zhong, Q., Pan, H., & Yang, G. (2010). Intravenous lipid emulsions combine extracorporeal blood purification: a novel therapeutic strategy for severe organophosphate poisoning. *Med Hypotheses.*, 74(2), 309-311.

Chapter 26

Lead Poisoning

Mehmet Tevfik Demir[*], MD and Metehan Yılman, MD

Department of Emergency Medicine, Samsun Training and Research Hospital,
Samsun, Turkey

Abstract

Lead poisoning is the most common cause of chronic metal poisoning. It constitutes an important environmental health problem, especially in developing countries. In the early phase of lead poisoning, symptoms such as fatigue, irritability, headache, abdominal pain, and constipation are observed non-specifically. In severe poisoning, many symptoms are observed, affecting many systems and requiring hospitalization. In children, acute lead encephalopathy is characterized by abnormal behavior, growth retardation, ataxia, vomiting, seizures, and sometimes cerebral edema, resulting in increased intracranial pressure, coma, and death. Adults with high blood lead concentrations also have similar neurological signs such as encephalopathy, confusion, headaches, seizures, and blindness. Measurement of the blood lead level is the best indicator in diagnosing lead poisoning. The medical treatment of patients with high blood lead levels consists of decontamination, supportive care, and chelation therapy.

Keywords: lead exposure, poisoning, environmental emergencies, chelation therapy

Introduction

Lead poisoning is the most common cause of chronic metal poisoning. It constitutes a significant environmental health problem, especially in developing countries. While most lead exposures in adults are due to workplace conditions as required by their profession, in children, they mainly occur due to putting the objects in their hands into their mouths and swallowing them.

Batteries and battery manufacturing are one of the leading uses of lead. Another important area of use is the insulation of communication cables. Besides these, lead is often used in glass

---

[*] Corresponding Author's Email: mehmetevfik@yahoo.com.

In: Environmental Emergencies and Injuries in Nature
Editors: Murat Yücel, Murat Güzel and İbrahim İkizceli
ISBN: 978-1-68507-833-1

and ceramic works, in the water insulation of high voltage lines, the manufacture of weapons, and the packaging industry (Tintinalli, 2019).

Lead is found in inorganic or organic forms. Absorption of inorganic lead is mainly via the respiratory or gastrointestinal tract, whereas dermal absorption is generally not expected. Organic lead exposure occurs through the skin, and respiratory and gastrointestinal routes (Wani et al., 2015).

The entry of inorganic lead into the body is mostly via inhalation and less frequently via the gastrointestinal tract. Inorganic lead is not transformed in the body; however, when organic lead is taken into the body, it is converted into water-soluble lead trialkyls in the liver. The nervous system, cardiovascular system, kidneys, and hematopoietic system are primarily affected. Lead poisoning usually occurs with chronic absorption of more than 0.4-0.5 mg/dl (Stone et al., 2006).

Pathophysiology

The pathophysiology of lead poisoning is quite complex and affects almost every organ system. It primarily affects the neurological, cardiovascular, renal, and hematopoietic systems. Lead has a strong affinity for the sulfhydryl, amine, phosphate, and carboxyl groups in the body and acts by binding to various proteins (Mitra et al., 2017). Due to its similarity to +2, cations such as calcium and zinc act on many cellular mechanisms regulated and mediated by these cations. 90% of the lead in the body is stored in the bones. It can also easily pass through the placenta (Wani et al., 2015). The half-life of lead in bone is approximately 30 years.

By inhibiting glutamate reuptake and glutamate synthesis in the astroglia, lead stops glutamate production, the main excitatory neuro mediator of the central nervous system (Hardej D, Trombetta LD, 2004). The toxic effects of lead in the central nervous system damage astrocytes, with secondary damage to the microvascular structure, disruption of the blood-brain barrier, cerebral edema, and increased intracranial pressure; a reduction in cyclic adenosine monophosphate and protein phosphorylation contributes to memory and learning loss. Changes in calcium homeostasis lead to the spontaneous and uncontrolled release of neurotransmitters (Tintinalli 2019). As a result of central toxicity, cognitive and behavioral changes, seizure, increased intracranial pressure, encephalopathy, cerebral edema, and coma can be seen. The main target of lead in the peripheral nervous system is the motor axons. Here it causes segmental demyelination and axonal degeneration (Wani et al., 2015).

Lead causes anemia by affecting the functions of enzymes involved in maintaining the integrity of the erythrocyte cell membrane and various enzymes involved in heme synthesis, leading to decreased erythrocyte production and increased erythrocyte destruction, respectively (Mitra et al., 2017).

While reversible renal tubular dysfunction from the renal effects of lead is generally seen in children with acute lead poisoning, chronic interstitial nephropathy characterized by vascular sclerosis, tubular cell atrophy, interstitial fibrosis, and glomerular sclerosis is irreversible. Maternal lead easily crosses the placenta and affects the fetus. Prenatal low-dose lead exposure may result in low birth weight and premature birth (WHO, Lead, cadmium, and mercury, 1996).

Exposure to lead is associated with atherosclerotic vascular disease and hypertension (Dingwall-Fordyce et al., 1963).

Lead negatively affects osteoblast and osteoclast functions in bone. Increased calcium deposition in the epiphyseal plaque with chronic lead exposure can be seen as "lead lines" on the radiographs of long bones (Tintinalli, 2019).

Clinical Findings

In the early phase of lead poisoning, symptoms such as fatigue, irritability, headache, abdominal pain, and constipation are observed non-specifically. In severe poisoning, a wide variety of symptoms affecting many systems are observed.

While encephalopathy, seizure, altered consciousness, papilledema, optic neuritis, and ataxia are observed in the central nervous system, acute toxicity, chronic toxicity, headache, restlessness, depression, fatigue, mood and behavioral changes, memory deficit, and sleep disturbances are seen. In peripheral nervous system toxicity, paresthesia, motor function deficit (drop-in wrist), and deep tendon reflex loss are seen. Exposure to organic lead compounds causes more dramatic acute encephalopathy than exposure to inorganic lead. Delirium and hallucinations are the observed symptoms (Stone et al., 2006).

Among the gastrointestinal findings: metallic taste, blue-gray gingiva, constipation, diarrhea, and toxic hepatitis are present with abdominal pain, mostly seen in acute poisonings.

In renal involvement: interstitial nephritis, renal failure, hypertension, and gout are seen in chronic toxicity, while Fanconi syndrome is seen in acute toxicity.

Hematological, hypoproliferative and/or hemolytic anemia and rarely nonspecific basophilic punctuation are seen.

In the reproductive system: decreased libido, impotence, sterility, abortions, premature birth, and decreased or abnormal sperm production are seen.

Children are more susceptible to the effects of lead than adults. In children, acute lead encephalopathy characteristically manifests as abnormal behavior, growth retardation, ataxia, vomiting, seizures, and sometimes cerebral edema with consequent increased intracranial pressure, coma, and death. This condition is usually seen in children with a high blood lead concentration (over 70-100 mcg/dl). It has been proven that IQ decreases inversely with the lead level in the blood. For every 10 mcg/dl increase in blood lead level, IQ decreases by about 6 points (Stone et al., 2006).

Adults with high blood lead concentrations also have similar neurological signs such as encephalopathy, confusion, headaches, seizures, and blindness (Mitra et al., 2017; Lidsky et al., 2003; de Souza et al., 2013; Needleman, 2004).

Diagnosis

The most important criterion for diagnosing lead poisoning is the patient's exposure history. The scarcity of diagnostic findings and the frequency of nonspecific symptoms lead to misdiagnosis (Keogh, 1992). Occupational and environmental lead exposure in the story, lead-related interests in questioning about hobbies, bullet cores remaining in the body after gunshot injury, and exposure in children's developmental and nutritional history (pica) guide the diagnosis. Lead poisoning should be kept in mind in children presenting with encephalopathy. The diagnosis of inorganic lead poisoning in adults requires the detection of excessive lead absorption, a demonstration of the effects of lead on the target organ, and the exclusion of other causes of diseases.

Lead poisoning may occur years later, depending on the bullet core remaining in the body after a firearm injury. Hyperthyroidism, pregnancy, fever, re-injury, and immobilization of the affected limbs increase lead release from these objects remaining in the body after years of sleep mode (Tintinalli, 2019).

The blood lead level measurement is the single best indicator for diagnosing lead poisoning. Within hours after acute exposure, blood lead levels rise rapidly and remain elevated for several weeks (Landrigan, 1994). Although the ideal blood lead level is zero, < 10 mcg/dl in children and < 25 mcg/dl in adults are acceptable levels in healthy individuals. Values above 70 mcg/dl are quite serious and require hospitalization (Stone et al., 2006). The blood lead level can be determined from fingertip capillary blood but should be confirmed by obtaining a venous blood sample in the case of abnormal results. Unlike inorganic lead poisoning, the urine lead level is relatively higher than the blood lead level.

Table 1. Agents used in chelation therapy

Chelation agent	Indicator	Dosage/ Route	Contraindications
Dimercaprol (BAL)	Blood Pb level ≥ 70µg/dl (If blood Pb level > 100µg/dl, additionally edetate calcium disodium)	3-5 gün boyunca her 4 saatte bir 4-5 mg/kg (IM) For every 4 hours 4-5 mg/kg (IM route) for 3 to 5 days	Glucose 6 phosphate dehydrogenase enzyme deficiency Peanut allergy Iron deficiency anemia treatment at the same period
Edetate calcium disodium (CaNa₂EDTA)	Blood Pb Level ≥ 45µg/dl or presence of Pb encephalopathy	1000 mg/m2 /day or 50 mg/kg (maximum 1g/day) IV route (inside normal saline or 5% dextrose solution) for 5 days period and IM therapy for 8-12 hour periods about 2 to 4 days. Therapy (IM and IV) will be repeated after a period without medication.	Renal failure Dehydratation
D-Penicillamine	Blood Pb Level 45-69 µg/dl	Adults: 250 mg for each 6 hours Children over 6 months: 10-15 mg/kg (ORAL) for 4-12 weeks period	Penicillin Iron deficiency anemia therapy at the same period Renal failure
DMSA (Dimercapto succinic acit, succimer)	Blood Pb level 45-69 µg/dl	10mg/kg every 8 hours for five days period or 350mg/m2; and then every 12 hours in14 days period. It can be repeated after two weeks period without medication. With a minimum rest period without medication, 30mg/kg/day minimum of five days. The therapy (Oral) is not preferred for children under 12 months	High ALT, AST enzyme levels Glucose 6 phosphate dehydrogenase enzyme deficiency

Although the blood lead level is helpful in the follow-up of diagnosis and treatment, and as it may take a long time for the results to come from the laboratory, diagnostic studies, especially in the emergency department, should focus on radiographic examinations to investigate anemia and detect lead exposure. An increased reticulocyte count and normocytic/microcytic anemia are present in lead poisoning. The serum-free heme level increased due to impaired heme biosynthesis and an increased erythrocyte destruction rate. Basophilic punctuation is seen as a nonspecific finding.

In acute and subacute poisoning, radiopaque materials can be seen in the gastrointestinal tract on abdominal radiographs. Long bone radiographs taken in children show horizontal, metaphyseal lead lines, which indicate failure in bone remodeling rather than lead deposition, especially in the knee (Tintinalli, 2019).

Treatment

The first step of treatment in lead poisoning is determining the patient's cause of exposure and eliminating this cause. Medical treatment of high blood lead levels consists of decontamination, supportive care, and chelation therapy (Table 1).

Although its incidence is low, seizures developing in patients with encephalopathy with high mortality and morbidity are treated with benzodiazepines and phenobarbital. When necessary, seizures are controlled with general anesthesia.

If a patient with encephalopathy has a history of lead exposure, chelation therapy can be started without waiting for the patient's blood lead level results. Chelation therapy should be applied to children with a blood lead level above 45 mcg/dl, and adults with 70-100 mcg/dl or more, and any patient with lead encephalopathy. This procedure should be done under the direction of a toxicologist (Kosnett et al., 2007).

Agents such as dimercaprol (formerly known as British anti-Lewisite (BAL)), calcium disodium ethylenediaminetetraacetic acid (CaNa$_2$EDTA), and succimer (dimercaptosuccinic acid or DMSA) used in chelation therapy can be used alone or in combination depending on the clinical situation and blood lead level. Another chelating agent is D-penicillamine. The side effects of these drugs are shown in Table 2.

Table 2. Side effects of chelation agent

Dimercaprol (BAL)	Edatate calcium disodium (CaNa$_2$EDTA)	D-Penicillamine	DMSA (Dimercapto succinic acit, succimer)
Hypertension Fever, pain, abscess formation in the injection area Nausea, vomiting, diarrhea, abdominal pain Headache, lacrimation, rhinorrhea Hemolysis in patients with glucose 6 phosphate dehydrogenase enzyme deficiency	Renal failure Arrhythmias, Hypotension Tetany, hypocalcemia, Bone marrow depression, prolonged bleeding time Respiratory depression Dermatitis	Thrombocytopenia, leukocytopenia, aplastic anemia Anorexia, nausia and vomiting Pemphigus, lupus erythematosus, polymyositis/dermatomyositis, membranous glomerulopathy, and autoimmune cases like hypersensitivity pneumonia	Gastrointestinal distress Skin reaction Mild neutropenia, thrombocytosis, eosinophilia Increase in liver enzymes Paraesthesia

Prognosis

While the mortality rate was 65% in cases of encephalopathy due to lead poisoning before chelation therapy; after the combination of BAL+CaNa$_2$EDTA, this rate decreased below 5% (Ennis et al., 1950; Coffin et al., 1966). Persistent neurological sequelae such as mental retardation, hemiparesis, and epileptic seizures remain in many patients who survive even after successful chelation therapy of acute lead encephalopathy (Coffin et al., 1966) (Wani et al., 2015). While abdominal colic generally regresses within days after chelation therapy, other acute findings resolve within 1-16 weeks (Wani et al., 2015).

Conclusion

Lead poisoning, the most common chronic metal poisoning, causes a broad spectrum of symptoms with multisystem involvement in adults and children. This condition may require hospitalization. Complete treatment can be provided using a detailed history, appropriate diagnostic methods, and early treatment methods.

References

Keith Stone C., Roger L. (2006). Humphries. *Lange Current emergency Diagnosis and Treatment*. 5th edition. p:988-989.

Coffin, R., Phillips, J. L., Staples, W. I., & Spector, S. (1966). Treatment of lead encephalopathy in children. *The Journal of pediatrics*, 69(2), 198–206. https://doi.org/10.1016/s0022-3476(66)80320-7.

de Souza, A., Narvencar, K. P., Desai, P. K., D'Costa, Z., & Nilajkar, G. (2013). Adult lead encephalopathy. *Neurological research*, 35(1), 54–58. https://doi.org/10.1179/1743132812Y.0000000115.

Dingwall-Fordyce, I., & Lane, R. E. (1963). A FOLLOW-UP STUDY OF LEAD WORKERS. *British journal of industrial medicine*, 20(4), 313–315. https://doi.org/10.1136/oem.20.4.313.

Ennis, J. M., & Harrison, H. E. (1950). Treatment of lead encephalopathy with PAL (2.3-dimercaptopropanol). *Pediatrics*, 5(5), 853–868.

Hardej D, Trombetta L. D. (2004) *Metals*. Alındı: Clinical Toxicology Barile FA (Ed), Chapter 24, CRCpres LLC, London, p. 308-310.

Judith E. Tintinalli (2019). *Tintinalli's Emergency Medicine: A Comprehensive Study Guide*, Seventh Edition Section: 15. p: 1308-1311.

Keogh J. P. Lead. In: Sullivan J. B. Jr, Krieger G. R., eds. *Hazardous materials toxicology: clinical principles of environmental health*. Baltimore: Williams & Wilkins, 1992:834–44.

Kosnett, M. J., Wedeen, R. P., Rothenberg, S. J., Hipkins, K. L., Materna, B. L., Schwartz, B. S., Hu, H., & Woolf, A. (2007). Recommendations for medical management of adult lead exposure. *Environmental health perspectives*, 115(3), 463–471. https://doi.org/10.1289/ehp.9784.

Landrigan P. J. (1994). Lead. In: Rosenstock L, Cullen M. R., eds. *Textbook of clinical occupational and environmental medicine*. Philadelphia: Saunders, 1994:745–54.

Lidsky, T. I., & Schneider, J. S. (2003). Lead neurotoxicity in children: basic mechanisms and clinical correlates. *Brain : a journal of neurology*, 126(Pt 1), 5–19. https://doi.org/10.1093/brain/awg014.

Mitra, P., Sharma, S., Purohit, P., & Sharma, P. (2017). Clinical and molecular aspects of lead toxicity: An update. Critical reviews in clinical laboratory sciences, 54(7-8), 506–528. https://doi.org/10.1080/10408363.2017.1408562.

Needleman H. (2004). Lead poisoning. *Annual review of medicine*, 55, 209–222. https://doi.org/10.1146/annurev.med.55.091902.103653.

Wani, A. L., Ara, A., & Usmani, J. A. (2015). Lead toxicity: a review. *Interdisciplinary toxicology*, 8(2), 55–64. https://doi.org/10.1515/intox-2015-0009.

WHO. *Lead, cadmium and mercury*. Trace elements in human nutrition and health. Geneva, 1996; 195-203) (Case studies in environmental medicine: lead toxicity. U.S Department of Human Service, Public Health Service, Agency of Toxic Substance and Disease Registry. 0.

Chapter 27

Mercury Poisoning

Muhammet A. Oruç, MD and İrfan Bayhan*, MD

[1]Department of Family Medicine, Faculty of Medicine, Ahi Evran University, Kırsehir, Turkey
[2]Department of Chief Physician, Bafra State Hospital, Samsun, Turkey

Abstract

Mercury, with the element symbol Hg, is a heavy metal that is in liquid form at room temperature. Metallic (elemental) mercury is found in nature as inorganic salts and organic compounds, and any form of mercury can be toxic. It is widely used in modern technology, especially as a catalyst in the production of plastics, in various measuring and control devices, in the electricity and cement industries, in mining, in the production of cellulose, in the paint and paper industries, and as a filling material in dental treatments. Potential health risks may occur in individuals exposed to mercury in various ways. The effect of mercury and its compounds is related to the dose, the age of the affected person, the duration of exposure, the route of exposure, and the health and nutritional level of the affected person. Diagnosis of affected individuals is established by evaluating the history, symptoms, findings, and laboratory results. The first thing to do in treatment is to remove the patient from the source. While supportive treatment is sufficient in some cases, chelation therapy should be considered in the presence of findings such as high urine and blood mercury levels, respiratory distress, or acrodynia.

Keywords: mercury, intoxication, chemical, disease

Introduction

Derived from the Latin word "hydragyros" meaning liquid silver, mercury, with the element symbol Hg, is a heavy metal that is liquid at room temperature. It is in the 2B group in the periodic table, its atomic number is 80, its atomic weight is 200.59 g/mol, its freezing point is -38.84°C, its boiling point is 356.95°C, and its density is 13.546 g/cm3. It is not soluble in water, and it is 13.55 times heavier than water, and seven times denser than air (Clarkson et al., 2003).

---

* Corresponding Author's Email: drirfanbayhan@gmail.com.

In: Environmental Emergencies and Injuries in Nature
Editors: Murat Yücel, Murat Güzel and İbrahim İkizceli
ISBN: 978-1-68507-833-1

Besides being naturally found in the earth's crust, industrial processes, especially coal-fired power plants and coal-fired activities (such as heating), processes such as waste incineration and metal mining, and scrap metal processing are human-induced activities that cause mercury to be present in the environment (Finster et al., 2015).

Once released into the atmosphere, mercury is a substance that can survive in the environment for 3,000 years in a cycle called the "global mercury cycle."

The amount of mercury in the air (weighted by time) should not exceed 0.05 milligrams per cubic meter. In terms of occupational exposure, the 15-minute weighted value should not exceed 0.03 mg per cubic meter, and the eight-hour weighted value should not exceed 0.01 mg. The normal balancing pressure of mercury in air is well above this value. The presence of volatile mercury in the environment therefore causes undesirable inhalation of mercury.

Mercury is a metal widely used in nature. Cas No: 7439-97-6.

Mercury and its components are used as a catalyst in the production of synthetic industrial materials such as acetaldehyde and vinichlorite, as an electrode in the production of sodium hydroxide and chlorine from sodium chloride, in the production of thermometers and electrical tools, in industrial control devices, as a fungicide in the production of pesticides, and also in the paint and paper industries (Akcan and Dursun, 2008).

When evaluated in terms of exposure routes, mercury can be exposed through the following routes: orally through food (fish and sea products), by inhalation of mercury vapors in the effluent of mercury-containing fossil fuels (such as coal-fired power plants) and incinerators, by types of mercury from dentistry and medical treatments, by workplace-related respiratory and skin contact, and by its use in cultural, ethnic and traditional materials, and rituals.

Mercury, metallic (elemental) mercury, is found in nature in the form of inorganic salts and organic compounds, and any form of mercury can have toxic effects (Counter and Buchanan, 2004).

Metallic mercury can be formed as a result of industrial plants and coal burning, can be found in various materials used in daily life, and dental fillings, while inorganic mercury is more related to occupational exposures, and organic or methyl mercury are the forms mainly found in food.

Mercury is a substance that can cause adverse health effects when even exposed at low amounts. Listed by the World Health Organization (WHO) as one of the ten chemicals that pose a major public health concern, mercury causes deformation in many tissues and organs, and is considered as the third most toxic element in terms of human health.

According to the International Agency for Research on Cancer-IARC classification, metallic mercury and inorganic mercury compounds are classified as Group 3, and methyl mercury as Group 2B.

Mercury, which has become an increasingly serious problem in terms of public health, has also been the focus of an international convention (Minamata Convention). An international agreement on this issue was prepared in 2013, ratified by 98 countries and came into force in 2017. This convention provides for management and reduction measures, limits the production, import and export of mercury-containing products and materials, and provides for the effective disposal of mercury-containing wastes, and countries are expected to develop strategies to reduce mercury-related emissions.

Types of Mercury and Clinical Features

Elemental Mercury

Elemental mercury is a shiny, silvery, odorless and easily volatile substance. Elemental mercury is an element that has not formed compounds with other elements. It is the only metal that is liquid at room temperature. It evaporates at standard room temperature and pressure, and as the room temperature increases, the vapor pressure of mercury increases (for every 10 degrees Celsius increase, the vapor pressure of mercury doubles). Mercury vapor is odorless and very toxic. It can enter the body through the mouth, skin and respiratory tract. The most toxic form of contact is the inhalation of mercury vapor through the respiratory tract. 80% of the inhaled mercury vapor is absorbed from the lungs and enters the bloodstream and accumulates especially in the central nervous system where it demonstrates its toxic effects. It rarely causes toxic effects when taken orally. This is because less than 0.01% of the amount taken from the gastrointestinal tract can be absorbed. When it comes into contact with the skin, it is absorbed much less. Excretion from the body is mostly through the kidneys. The half-life ranges from 30-60 days, however, the half-life of mercury accumulated in the brain can be many years (Langford and Ferner 1994).

High levels of elemental mercury can cause symptoms in the nervous system, respiratory system, and cardiovascular system, and on the skin. The primary causes of mortality after high levels of mercury exposure are lung damage, pulmonary edema, erosion of the bronchial epithelium, severe acidosis, and coma, and death may occur. Cough, fever, tremor, weakness, dyspnea, gingivitis, hallucinations, neurological findings, erythema and peeling of the hands and feet are among the symptoms that can be observed (Fisher et al., 2005).

The bright, gray appearance of elemental mercury is very attractive to children (Nakayama et al., 1984). Children playing with liquid mercury, which they bring home from the school laboratory because of its attractive and mystical appearance, may be exposed to the toxic effect of mercury vapor during their game or by being in the same room, especially in poorly ventilated areas (Tominack et al., 2002). Contact with elemental mercury in children and young people is mostly with mercury brought into the home environment from outside (industrial areas or school) (Cherry at al., 2002). When mercury diffuses into the environment, it spreads onto carpets, furniture, floors, walls and other items and begins to evaporate over time. Since mercury vapors are heavier than air, they settle on the ground and accumulate more in poorly ventilated areas. If there is a ventilation system, vapors can spread into other rooms and areas through this system. In general, if the spilled/scattered mercury is 35 ml and above, it is considered as a high amount of mercury scattering (Vaizoğlu and Çamur, 2012).

Organic Mercury

Organic mercury compounds are compounds such as methyl, ethyl, and phenyl mercury. The absorption and release values, physical and chemical properties, and distribution and accumulation patterns in tissues are different in all three forms.

Methyl mercury is the most common organic mercury compound, which is formed by microorganisms most commonly found in nature and transformed in natural processes. Methyl mercury is obtained as a result of methylation of inorganic mercury and biological transformations. Methyl mercury has the ability to pass through cell membranes and accumulate in living tissues. It is a neurotoxin that has the ability to be stored in lipid. Its solubility in lipid is not high, but it binds to proteins with strong sulfhydryl bonds, accumulates in biological tissues and causes toxic effects (Clarkson, 1994).

Methyl mercury is teratogenic. It can cross the placenta and affect breast milk (Akcan and Dursun, 2008).

Organic mercury compounds are rapidly absorbed from the gastrointestinal tract and distributed rapidly throughout the body. Particularly, they accumulate in the cerebral cortex, the brain, membranes of peripheral sensory nerves, and the kidneys. Therefore, they cause sensory deficiencies. In the past, organic mercury compounds were used in disinfection substances. Today, substances with fewer toxic effects are used instead of organic mercury compounds (Önal, 1995).

In addition to mild symptoms, severe paresthesia, dysarthria, ataxia, visual field narrowing, hearing loss, blindness, microcephaly, spasticity, paralysis, and coma may develop in organic mercury poisonings (Akcan and Dursun, 2008).

Inorganic Mercury

When mercury is combined with chlorine, sulfur and oxygen, inorganic mercury compounds are formed. Inorganic mercury compounds are called mercury salts. Inorganic mercury is found in nature in two forms of salts, mercuric (divalent) and mercureuse (monovalent). The most well-known of these salts is mercuric mercury, which is more toxic because of its higher solubility in water. It is also highly corrosive and can cause fatal gastrointestinal erosion (Erkekoğlu and Kadıoğlu, 2013).

Inorganic mercury compounds can attach to epithelial cells, blood cells, and plasma proteins, and accumulate in organs, glands and the central nervous system. Since inorganic mercury salts have low lipid solubility, they cannot easily cross the placenta and blood-brain barrier; however, they can cause neurological damage. The acute lethal oral dose of mercury chloride is approximately 1-4 grams (Park and Zheng, 2012).

Dental amalgam usually contains inorganic mercury at the ratio of 50%. Along with mercury, copper, tin, zinc and silver are also found in amalgams. It is stated that this composition of amalgams causes mercury exposure, which "increases more easily with chewing, eating, tooth brushing, and hot drink consumption" (Tatlı and Avşar, 2016).

It has been observed that mercury in the cerebrospinal fluid (CSF) of multiple sclerosis (MS) patients is 7.5 times higher than in healthy patients. MS patients with and without amalgam fillings were compared, the group whose fillings were removed had less depression, less aggression, and less psychotic behavior. After the removal of amalgam fillings in MS patients, the pathological oligoclonal band disappeared in the CSF (Martı Akgün and Akgün, 2012).

Acute Mercury Exposure

As a result of the exposure of individuals to inorganic mercury at a concentration of 3.1 mg/m3 for 10 minutes, 2.1 mg/m3 for 30 minutes, 1.7 mg/m3 for 60 minutes, 0.67 mg/m3 for 4 hours, and 0.33 mg/m3 for 8 hours, serious and long-lasting toxic effects may occur. Lower levels cause a feeling of discomfort in the individual, and in sensitive individuals, certain side effects begin to appear. On the other hand, exposure to air containing higher concentrations of inorganic mercury can have life-threatening effects and cause death. Severe and prolonged toxic effects may occur as a result of individuals' exposure to inorganic mercury at the concentrations and durations of 16 mg/m3 for 10 minutes, 11 mg/m3 for 30 minutes, 8.9 mg/m3 for 60 minutes, 2.2 mg/m3 for 4 hours, and 2.2 mg/m3 for 8 hours (Erkekoğlu and Kadıoğlu, 2013).

Initially, fever, headache and muscle pain, a burning sensation in the mouth and throat, gingivostomatitis, a metal taste in the mouth, nausea, vomiting, diarrhea, and abdominal cramps are observed. Metallic mercury vapor is easily absorbed from the lungs and reaches the brain. Central nervous system symptoms such as tremor, extreme irritability, forgetfulness, weakness and visual disturbances develop. It should be kept in mind that acute respiratory distress syndrome (ARDS) may develop within the first 4 hours. This can cause fatal chemical pneumonia and non-cardiogenic pulmonary edema, and rarely acute kidney and liver damage may develop.

Chronic Mercury Exposure

Permanent damage to the nervous system and kidneys may occur in chronic poisoning. Especially industrial workers are among the risk group. Common findings include irritability, delirium, neurasthenia, and erethism as neurological disorders. Neurasthenia is fatigue, depression, headache and concentration disorder. Erethism is easy embarrassment characterized by extreme shyness. Gingivostomatitis can produce a metallic taste and mucosal ulcers. Less frequently, muscle paralysis is seen. These findings should be meticulously checked by occupational physicians. Low levels of oliguria, anuria, uremia, proteinuria, and bicarbonate can be observed as a result of proximal tubule damage in kidneys, and nephrotic syndrome may develop.

Mercury Decontamination

Actions to be taken:

The area must be evacuated. Make sure the area is well ventilated. Beads should touch each other to try to reduce the surface area. A syringe or injector should be used to remove the mercury. The mercury should be taken into a tightly sealed container filled with water. If spilled on a carpet, blankets, upholstery or other soft material, these should be discarded. Whenever possible, mercury in the ambient air should be measured.

In the mercury removal process, in order to remove mercury from the skin, the clothes on the patient should be removed, the contaminated area should be washed with plenty of soapy water, and corneal washing should also be performed.

Don'ts:

Mercury should not be in contact with bare hands. A vacuum cleaner should not be used. It should not be poured into sinks, toilets and waste water drains. Any application that may cause the mercury to disperse or blister should be avoided. The place where mercury is spilled should not be stepped on or walked over. Such materials should not be attempted to be recovered.

In the case of oral poisoning, patients should not induce vomiting as there is no absorption of metallic mercury.

Diagnosis

Diagnosis is established by evaluating the history, symptoms, findings and laboratory results.

As a specific method, urine and blood mercury levels should be measured (Refik Saydam Hygiene Center Presidency Poison Research Directorate Labs reference values: 0.6-59 microgram/L in whole blood, 0.1-20 microgram/L in urine). The most specific indicator in measuring the amount of Hg in the body, especially due to the binding property of mercury to hemoglobin, is the erythrocyte Hg concentration. The blood Hg level reflects the amount of both methyl mercury and inorganic Hg. It is recommended to evaluate the values in the blood and urine (24-hour) levels together in determining a person's Hg contact.

The concentration of organic mercury in erythrocytes is about 20 times higher than in plasma, while the concentration of inorganic mercury in plasma is about 2 times higher than the organic mercury (Erkekoğlu and Kadıoğlu, 2013)

The mercury vapor content in the air can be measured by "silver amplification autoradiography," and the mercury content in the tissues can be measured by "atomic absorption spectrometry" (AAS). In addition, "instrumental neutron activation analysis" (INAA), and for more sensitive measurements, "radiochemical neutron activation analysis" (RNAA) can also be used (Küçükeşmen, 2007).

The half-life in the blood is short, as mercury is rapidly distributed into body compartments. The half-life in the body averages two months. Almost all of the absorbed mercury is excreted in the urine. Therefore, the amount of mercury in the 24-hour urine is preferred for diagnosis in urinalysis.

The urine and blood mercury levels are below 5 micrograms/L in individuals who have not been exposed to mercury before. In those exposed to mercury in the workplace, the level should be below 15 micrograms/L in blood and 35 micrograms per gram creatinine in urine on weekly measurements.

Treatment

The first thing to do in treatment is to remove the patient from the source.

While supportive treatment is sufficient in some cases, chelation therapy should be considered in the presence of findings such as high urine and blood mercury levels, respiratory distress, or acrodynia.

Fluid loss due to the ingestion of mercury salt should be reversed.

If there is bronchospasm, beta2 agonist bronchodilators (salbutamol) are administered by spray in adults (4-8 sprays every 20 minutes in the first 4 hours, then 2-4 sprays every 4 hours) or by nebulizer (2.5-5 mg repeated as needed), and in children by nebulizer (0.10-0.15 mg/kg, maximum 2.5 mg, repeated as needed).

While supportive treatment is sufficient in some cases, chelation therapy should be considered in the presence of findings such as high urine and blood mercury levels, respiratory distress, or acrodynia.

Among the antidotes that can be used in chelation therapy, BAL (dimercaprol), DMSA (dimercaprol succinic acid), and DMPS (2.3-Dimercapropropan-1-sulfonate) can be used.

If mercury salt has been taken by mouth: British anti-Lewisite (BAL, dimercaprol) is given 3-5 mg/kg intramuscularly every 4 hours for a duration of 2 days in adults and children, every 12 hours for 7-10 days until the patient's symptoms subside. If the patient can take it orally: Dimercaptosuccinic acid (DMSA, Succicaptal® 200 mg), at the dose of 10 mg/kg or 350 mg/m^2, is given every 8 hours for 5 days and every 12 hours for the following 14 days.

If organic mercury compounds have been taken orally: DMSA is given with the protocol mentioned above. BAL is not used because it causes redistribution of mercury to the central nervous system and increases its toxic effect on the nervous system.

If metallic mercury has been inhaled: Dimercaptosuccinic acid (DMSA, Succicaptal® 200 mg), at the dose of 10 mg/kg or 350 mg/m^2, is given every 8 hours for 5 days, and every 12 hours for the following 14 days, or penicillamine (Metalcaptase® 300 film-coated tablet, 300 mg) is given by mouth at the dose of 1000-1500 mg per day (maximum 2 g) in adults, 25-100 mg/kg/day in children (maximum 1 g) in 2 or 4 divided doses up to 5 days, and if longer treatment is required, 40 mg/kg/day is given without exceeding this dose.

Oral intake of metallic mercury: The absorption of metallic mercury is very slow and will delay fecal excretion. Unless there is a slowdown in digestive tract motility, this does not cause acute poisoning.

Conclusion

Heavy metals, which are not necessary for the human body, are taken into the body primarily by food, water or the respiratory tract, causing a "metal load." These metals, which are accumulated in the body of living organisms due to metal load, cause many chronic and degenerative diseases.

In Minamata disease, as a result of the release of methyl mercury into the industrial wastewater from the chemical factory of Chisso Corporation, which continued from 1932 to 1968, this toxic chemical biologically mixed into the waters and infected the fish in the Shiranui Sea and the surrounding environment. Local people who ate Minamata sheep or surrounding fish have had mercury poisoning. In a study conducted in Turkey, the level of mercury was found to be 0.013 ± 0.002 ppm in anchovy caught in the Black Sea (Mud et al.,). The American Food and Drug Administration (FDA) recommends that women of childbearing age and children completely avoid swordfish, shark meat, and mackerel, and that they consume crab and tuna in a limited regime. The United States Centers for Disease Control and Prevention also make recommendations for breastfeeding mothers to prevent exposure to mercury, especially in regard to foods with high mercury levels. It is estimated that mercury, which is specifically exposed due to mercury accumulation in fish, causes cognitive effects at a rate of 1.5-17 per thousand in children in some communities that are economically dependent on fishing due to their consumption of mercury-containing fish. It is estimated that 75.000 newborns in the USA each year suffer from learning difficulties due to exposure to mercury in the womb. The European Commission recommended limiting the consumption of fish with high mercury levels, despite the fact that consumption of fish is actually beneficial for health by consuming 1-4 servings per week, considering the effect of fish/seafood consumption during pregnancy on the functional results of the nervous system development of children and on cardiovascular diseases in adults.

The preferability of amalgam as a restorative material is being reduced due to concerns about environmental pollution, aesthetics, and harmful health effects. Patients and dentists no longer prefer amalgam as a restorative material for filling carious tooth cavities due to the incompatibility of the metallic color of amalgam compared to the natural tooth color (Rathore et al, 2012). In a study conducted with dentists who worked for an average of 5 years (n=98, age range 24-49; average 32), it was determined that they showed decreased performance in neurobehavioral tests and their aggression scores were higher than those of controls. The airborne mercury levels measured in this study were 0.0007-0.042 mg/m3 (mean: 0.014 mg/m3) and blood levels were found to be 0.6-57 µg/L (mean: 9.8 µg/L) (Küçükeşmen, 2007).

As the ages of children decrease, the toxic effects of mercury vapor on the central nervous system increase, and it can cause death as a result of respiratory failure, especially in infants (Counter and Buchanan 2004). Mercury poisoning in children is quite common in Turkey. The majority of these cases (88.5%) are with metallic mercury in school children (Oto Geçim et al., 2006). Although the amount of mercury (1 ml) in instruments such as thermometers and barometers is considered to be low, it has been observed that exposure to mercury can be quite high due to the presence of various additional factors (such as the use of a vacuum cleaner to remove mercury) in accidents that may occur in the school environment (Akyıldız et al., 2012). Apart from the use of instruments such as thermometers and barometers leaving their places to alternative methods, it is important to make environmental regulations regarding heavy metals.

Thimerosal is a preservative that contains mercury and is added to vaccines to prevent them from spoiling. The harmful side effects of thimerosal have been proven. The American Academy of Pediatrics (AAP) recommends thimerosal to not be used as a preservative in vaccines. The World Health Organization (WHO) stated that thimerosal can be used in vaccines.

In the literature, Bhattacharya et al., reported a case of chemical pneumonitis and pneumothorax in a 5-month-old female patient due to exposure to mercury vapor. This case was treated with respiratory support in the intensive care unit without the need for chelation therapy (4). Smith et al., reported an atypical case of mercury intoxication, stating that a 15-year-old male patient had a wound on his arm as a result of its contact with a broken thermometer (5). Wossmann et al., suspected mercury poisoning in an 11-year-old girl who was presented with hypertension and tachycardia, due to the fact that urinary catecholamine excretion was high, but a mass compatible with pheochromocytoma could not be detected by imaging methods, accompanied by complaints such as insomnia and weight loss. It was emphasized that mercury intoxication should be kept in mind in the differential diagnosis of patients with complaints such as hypertension, tachycardia, weight loss and insomnia, even if there is no history of contact with mercury in patients or high levels of mercury in the urine and blood (6). Echeverria et al., had findings that supported genetic determinants associated with neurobehavior and mood dimensions (polymorphism in the serotonin transporter gene), which are known to be affected by metallic mercury, increase susceptibility to mercury poisoning (Echeverria et al., 2010). A T2-weighted brain MRI showed hyperintense lesions in the paracentral gyrus, posterior frontal region, parietal region, and posterior cingulate gyrus white matter, left globus pallidus, and putamen in a 10-year-old patient with symptoms of acrodynia, seizure, and blurred vision as a result of metallic mercury poisoning (Abbaslou and Zaman 2006). The clinical and radiological manifestations of this subject completely resolved after 9 months of chelation therapy.

As a result, mercury is used extensively in industry and reaches living organisms through industrial wastes. The only way to help the body in this struggle against heavy metals is to remove heavy metals from the body and eliminate the possibility of re-exposure. In a world where the use of heavy metals is increasing, care should be taken to live with caution before exposure. Mercury poisoning, due to the fact that it has widespread organ distribution in patients and causes permanent brain damage in the case of a delayed diagnosis, should be absolutely considered in the differential diagnosis, without losing time in regard to initiating the treatment.

References

Abbaslou P. and Zaman T. (2006). A child with elemental mercury poisoning and unusual brain MRI findings. *Clin Toxicol* 44,85-8.

Akcan A. B. and Dursun O. (2008). Mercury poisonings. *Current Pediatrics*, 6,72-75.

Akyildiz BN, Kondolot M. and Kurtoğlu S. (2012). Case series of mercury toxicity among children in a hot, closed environment. *Pediatr Emerg Care*, 28,254-8.

Bhattacharya B., Banerjee S. and Singhi S. (1997). Acute mercury vapour poisoning in an infant. *Ann Trop Paediatr*, 17, 57-60.

Önal. B. (1995). Amalgam toxicology, *Journal of İzmir Chamber of Dentists*, 6,28-34.

Bigham M. and Copes R. (2005), *Balancing the Risk of Adverse Effects with the Risk of Vaccine-Preventable Disease, Drug Safety*, 28, 89-101.

Cherry D., Lowry L. and Velez L. (2002). Elemental mercury poisoning in a family of seven. *Fam Community Health*, 24,1–8.

Clarkson TW., Magos L. and Myers GJ. (2003). The toxicology of mercury-Current exposures and clinical manifestations. *N Engl J Med*, 349, 1731-7.

Clarkson TW. (1994). The toxicology of mercury and its compounds. In Mercury Pollution: Integration and Synthesis. CRC Press, 631-41.

Cope WG., Leidy RB. and Hodgson E. (2004). Classes of Toxicants: Use Classes. Hodgson E. (Eds.) *A Textbook Of Modern Toxicology* 3rd ed.,(p.52) New Jersey: John Wiley & Sons.

Counter SA. and Buchanan LA. (2004) Mercury exposure in children: *Review. Toxicol and Appl Pharmacol*, 198,209-30.

Çamur D., Güler Ç., Vaizoğlu SA. and Özdilek B. (2016). Determining mercury levels in anchovy and in individuals with different fish consumption habits, together with their neurological effects. *Toxicol Ind Health*, 32, 1215-23.

Echeverria D., Woods JS. and Heyer NJ. (2010). The association between serotonin transporter gene promotor polymorphism (5-HTTLPR) and elemental mercury exposure on mood and behavior in humans. *J Toxicol Environ Health*, 73,1003-20.

Ellenhorn MJ. (1997). Metals and Related Compounds. In Ellenhorn MJ., Schonwald S., Ordog G. and Wasserberger J. (Eds.) *Ellenhorn's Medical Toxicology* 2nd. Edition, (p. 1532-1613), Baltimore: Williams and Wilkins Publishing.

Erkekoğlu P. and Kadıoğlu E. (2013). Mercury poisoning and treatment. *Toxicology Bulletin*, 37, 6-9.

Mercury in Europe's environment (2018). European Environment Agency (EEA), A priority for European and global action, Retrieved from https://www.eea.europa.eu/publications/mercury-in-europe-s-environment.

Fischbach FT. (1992). A manual of laboratory & diagnostic testing. 4th ed. (p. 214-6) Philadelphia: J. B. Lippincott Company.

Finster ME., Raymond MR., Scofield MA. and Smith KP. (2015). Mercury-impacted scrap metal: Source and nature of the mercury. *J Environ Manage*, 161,303-308.

Harada M. (1995). Methyl mercury poisoning in Japan caused by environmental pollution. *Crit Rev Toxicol*, 25,1-24.

Mercury Poisoning and Precautions to be Taken (2021). T. R. *Ministry of Health Environmental Health Department*, Retrieved from https://hsgm.saglik.gov.tr/tr/cevresagligi-ced/ced-birimi/c%C4%B1va-zehirlenmesi-ve-al%C4%B1nmas%C4%B1-gereken-%C3%B6nlemler.

Fisher F. J. and Amler S. N. (2005). Mercury exposure: Evaluation and intervention The inapropriate use of chelating agents in the diagnosis and the treatment of putative mercury poisining. *NueroToxicology*, 26,691-699.

Kahvecioğlu Ö., Kartal G., Güven A. and Timur S. (2004). Environmental effects of metals. III. *Journal of Metallurgy*, 138, 64-71.

Küçükeşmen Ç. (2007). Effects of Dental Amalgam on Human Organism. S. D. U. *Faculty of Medicine Journal*, 14, 52-61.

Langford NJ. and Ferner RE. (1994) Toxicity of mercury. *J Hum Hypertens*, 13, 651-6.

Lewis R. (2003). Occupational Exposures Metals. In LaDou J. (Eds.) *Current Occupational and Environmental Medicine* 3rd edition (p. 429-459.) USA; McGraw-Hill Medical.

List of classifications (2021). *Agents Classifed by the IARC Monographs*, 1,129.

Martı Akgün Ö. and Akgün H. (2012 *Effects of Amalgam Fillings on Human Tissues*., 16, 83-6.

Mercury Emissions: The Global Context (2021), *U.S. Environmental Protection Agency*, Retrieved from https://www.epa.gov/international-cooperation/mercury-emissions-global-context.

Mercury in food (2021). *European Commission Food Safety*, Retrieved from https://ec.europa.eu/food/safety/chemical-safety/contaminants/catalogue/mercury_en.

Mercury and health (2021). *World Health Organization (WHO) fact sheet*, Retrieved from http://www.who.int/ipcs/assessment/public_health/mercury/en/ Accessed.

Mercury (2021). *WHO International Programme on Chemical Safety*, Retrieved from http://www.who.int/ipcs/assessment/public_health/mercury/en/ Accessed.

Mercury (2021). Centers for Disease Control and Prevention (CDC). *Breast feeding mothers should minimize exposure to mercury in their diets, at home, and at work*, Retrieved from https://www.cdc.gov/breastfeeding/breastfeeding-special-circumstances/environmental-exposures/mercury.

Nakayama H., Shono M. and Hada S. (1984). Mercury exanthem. *J Am Acad Dermatol*, 13, 848-52.

Ng DK., Chan CH. And Soo MT. (2007). Low-level chronic mercury exposure in children and adolescents: metaanalysis. *Pediatr Int.*, 49,80-7.

Nielsen JB. and Andersen O. (1991). Effect of four thiol-containing chelators on disposition of orally administered mercuric chloride. *Hum Exp Toxicol*, 10, 423-430.

Oto Geçim N., Cesaretli Y. and Gönül N. (2006) Evaluation of childhood heavy metal poisoning cases reported to the national poison center. *Turkey Clinics J Pediatr Sci*, 2, 84-6.

Park J. and Zheng W. (2012). Human exposure and health effects of inorganic and elemental mercury. *J Prev Med Public Health*, 45, 344–52.

Rathore M., Singh A. and Vandana A. P. (2012). The Dental Amalgam Toxicity Fear: A Myth Or Actuality. *Toxicol Int*, 19, 81–88.

Rowens B., Guerrero-Betancourt D., Gottlieb CA., Boyes RJ. and Eichenhorn MS. (1991). Respiratory Failure and Death Following Acute Inhalation of Mercury Vapor. *Chest*, 99,185- 190.

Strategic Advisory Group of Experts. Vaccines and biologicals: Recommendations from the Strategic Advisory Group of Experts (2002, September, 13). *Wkly Epidemiol Rec*, 77, 305-11.

Smith SR., Jaffe DM. and Skinner MA. (1997). Case report of metallic mercury injury. *Pediatr Emerg Care,* 13, 114-6.

Şen AE. (2012). *Amalgam Toxicology and Its Effects on Human Health. Ege University Faculty of Dentistry, Department of Dental Diseases and Treatment.*

Tatlı EC and Avşar AFY. (2016). *Dental Amalgam-Mercury Toxicity Ankara Med J,* 4, 383-386.

Diagnosis and Treatment Guidelines for Poisoning for Primary Care (2007). *T. R. Ministry of Health RSHMB,* p.227-32.

Tominack R., Weber J. and Blume C. (2002) Elemental mercury as an attractive nuisance: Multiple exposures from a pilfered school supply with severe consequences. *Pediatr Emerg Care,* 18, 97-100.

Toxicological Profile for Mercury. (1999). U.S. Department of Health and Human Services Agency for Toxic Substances and Disease Registry (p.6), Retrieved from https://www.atsdr.cdc.gov/toxprofiles/tp46.pdf.

Vaizoğlu SA. and Çamur D. (2012). Mercury. In Güler Ç (Eds.). *Environmental health* (with Environment and Ecology Links). (p. 1045-1059). Ankara: Yazıt publishing.

Wossmann W., Kohl M., Gruning G. and Bucsky P. (1999). Mercury intoxication presenting with hypertension and tachycardia. *Arch Dis Child,* 80,556-7.

Chapter 28

Carbon Monoxide Poisoning

Seda Ozkan and Afsin Ipekci[*]

Department of Emergency Medicine, Cerrahpaşa School of Medicine, İstanbul University-Cerrahpaşa, İstanbul, Turkey

Abstract

Carbon monoxide is a colorless, odorless, tasteless, non-irritant, and environmental toxicant gas produced by the incomplete combustion of hydrocarbons and is an invisible hazard to humans. Carbon monoxide poisoning is one of the important causes of emergency room admissions and is the leading cause of poisoning-related deaths. Carbon monoxide toxicity is the combination of tissue hypoxia-ischemia resulting from carboxyhemoglobin formation and cellular damage caused by carbon monoxide. The early symptoms of carbon monoxide poisoning are usually non-specific and can be easily confused. The clinical manifestations of carbon monoxide range from headache and malaise to altered consciousness, hypotension, dysrhythmia, myocardial ischemia, and coma. Measuring the blood carboxyhemoglobin level is the most useful test in the definitive diagnosis of carbon monoxide poisoning. The mainstay of treatment is the administration of 100% normobaric oxygen with a non-rebreathing mask. Hyperbaric oxygen therapy is a treatment option for patients with significant CO exposures. Early diagnosis and treatment prevent much of the mortality and morbidity associated with CO poisoning.

Keywords: carbon monoxide, carboxyhemoglobin, environmental exposure, hyperbaric oxygen

Introduction

Carbon monoxide (CO) is a colorless, odorless, tasteless, non-irritant, and environmental toxicant gas produced by the incomplete combustion of hydrocarbons and is an invisible hazard to humans. CO has a molecular weight of 28.01 daltons and a gas density of 0.968 (air = 1.0). Control measures are required for carbon monoxide, a ubiquitous pollutant in our environment

---

[*] Corresponding Author's Email: afsin.ipekci@iuc.edu.tr.

In: Environmental Emergencies and Injuries in Nature
Editors: Murat Yücel, Murat Güzel and İbrahim İkizceli
ISBN: 978-1-68507-833-1
© 2022 Nova Science Publishers, Inc.

to protect public health. Ten per cent of the carbon in the universe is stored as CO (Raub et al., 2000; Tomaszewski, 2011).

There are two main sources of CO, endogenous and exogenous. CO is an endogenously produced neurotransmitter and is referred to as a gasotransmitter together with nitric oxide and hydrogen sulfide. Although there are many minor sources of endogenous CO, the most important source is the enzymatic catabolization of heme by heme oxygenase. Therefore, 0-5% carboxyhemoglobin (COHb) can be found in the human body at a non-toxic level (Vreman et al., 2001; Hopper et al., 2021).

The sources of exogenous CO are very diverse. Forest fires and volcanic eruptions, which cause rare toxicity to humans, are natural sources of CO. Hepatic metabolism of methyl chloride in dye removers by cytochrome CYP2E1 is another source of CO. Fuels used in industry, wood- or coal-burning stoves, gas ovens and stoves, exhaust gases of motor vehicles, propane-operated tools, indoor grills, house fires, and volatile anesthetic agents are other important sources of CO. Cigarette and hookah smoke are also an exogenous CO source and COHb levels can be measured up to 10% in smokers (Chenoweth et al., 2021; Yucel & Guzel, 2020).

Humanity has had a complex relationship with CO since the stone age. Although it is stated in historical documents about CO that Erasistratus said "coal fumes affect normal respiration" around 275 BC and that Aristotle said "coal fumes cause severe headache and death" around 350 BC, its toxic effects were first explained by Claude Bernard in 1865 (Hopper et al., 2021; Yucel & Guzel, 2020). Carbon monoxide poisoning is one of the important causes of emergency room admissions and the leading cause of poisoning-related deaths (Weaver, 2009). CO caused 137 poisoning cases per million and 4.6 deaths per million worldwide in 2017. Although the incidence of CO poisonings does not change over time, the rate of mortality due to CO poisonings has decreased over the years. The risk of mortality due to CO poisoning declined by 36% between the years 1992 and 2017, from 7.2 cases to 4.6 cases per million population (Mattiuzzi & Lippi, 2020).

CO exposure varies according to societies, climatic conditions, development levels of countries, and occupational groups. While industrial accidents, exhaust gases, and suicide attempts are important causes in developed countries, household poisonings due to using heating equipment such as stoves and boilers are at the forefront in cold countries, especially in winter, depending on the climatic conditions. There is also a higher risk of poisoning in some professional occupations, such as firefighters, police, and industrial workers (Yavuz, 2019).

Pathophysiology

CO enters the body, especially through the respiration tract after the inhalation of fumes and gases, and diffuses through the alveolar-capillary membrane similar to oxygen, causing toxicity. CO toxicity is the combination of tissue hypoxia-ischemia resulting from COHb formation and cellular damage caused by CO (Fan et al., 2012).

Hemoglobin has a 200-250 times greater affinity to CO than oxygen. Fetal hemoglobin has an even higher affinity and causes severe fetal toxicity. The most devastating effect of CO poisoning is that COHb, which is formed by the binding of CO to hemoglobin, deprives the tissues of oxygen. Although the partial pressure of oxygen in the blood is sufficient, the COHb complex cannot carry as much oxygen as hemoglobin, resulting in tissue hypoxia (Maloney, 2011).

In addition, 10-15% of the CO passing from the lungs to the blood binds to cellular heme-containing proteins such as cytochrome P450 enzymes, myoglobin, guanylyl cyclase, nitric oxide (NO) synthase, and cytochrome C oxidase, activating many pathways independent of hypoxia pathways, leading to cell necrosis and apoptosis. These effects cause various signs and symptoms other than hypoxia in patients with CO poisoning (Rose et al., 2017).

The task of the cytochrome C oxidase, mitochondrial enzyme, is the reduction of oxygen to water in the electron transport chain. The inhibition of mitochondrial cytochrome C oxidase by CO causes mitochondrial dysfunction and cellular respiratory dysfunction. As a result, oxygen radicals and reactive oxygen species (ROS) are formed and oxidative stress-induced cellular damage occurs (Rose et al., 2017).

NO is a naturally occurring vasodilator that can cause systemic hypotension, and also a signaling molecule. CO binds to the NO point on the heme proteins in cells and causes an increase in the amount of NO in the cells and the circulation. Increased NO is thought to be responsible for cerebral vasodilation, hypotension, and loss of consciousness. Increasing NO can cause the activation of xanthine oxidase, the formation of oxidative radicals, and oxidative damage by targeting the adhesion molecule B2-integrin which affects the adhesion of neutrophils to the endothelium. NO can also induce lipid peroxidation in the brain, which is thought to be responsible for delayed neurological sequelae (DNS), formation of peroxynitrite causing tissue hypoxia, platelet-neutrophil aggregation, neutrophil degranulation, the release of proteases and free oxygen radicals causing oxidative stress, and cell apoptosis (Bleecker, 2015; Chenoweth et al., 2021).

Myoglobin is a cytoplasmic hemoprotein that is released in cardiac myocytes and oxidative skeletal muscle fibers. Myoglobin stores oxygen in the muscles and releases oxygen in cases of hypoxia or anoxia. The affinity of CO for myoglobin is 60 times greater than that of oxygen. CO can bind to the myoglobin of the heart and skeletal muscle, reducing oxygen availability in the heart, leading to arrhythmias and cardiac dysfunction, however, it can directly cause skeletal muscle toxicity and rhabdomyolysis (Megas et al., 2021).

Clinical Manifestations

A wide range of non-specific clinical manifestations are seen in CO poisoning. Clinical effects and findings of CO can be seen as acute, delayed, and chronic.

Acute Effects

The early symptoms of CO poisoning are usually non-specific and can be easily confused with other diseases like viral infections. Headache was reported as the first symptom in volunteers exposed to 200 ppm COHb (15-20%). Nausea has also been reported in those exposed to 500 ppm COHb for a shorter period (Stewart et al., 1973). CO has a greater effect on the brain and heart because their oxygen requirements are greater. Early neurological symptoms are weakness, dizziness, and headache. As the CO level rises, patients may experience altered consciousness, confusion, syncope, seizures, acute stroke-like symptoms, and coma. Early cardiac symptoms are often due to hypoxia. Stable angina and exercise intolerance have been reported in 2% to 4% of subjects exposed to low-grade CO (Allred et al., 1989). In more severe exposures, hypotension, dysrhythmia, myocardial ischemia, infarction, and cardiac arrest may occur. Ventricular dysrhythmias are the most important cause of early death due to CO exposure. The skin and mucous membranes are other target organs in CO poisoning. Blisters and cherry-red mucous membranes can be seen in high COHb levels, often an important autopsy finding. CO poisoning can also cause rhabdomyolysis, acute renal failure, and non-cardiogenic pulmonary edema. Clinical manifestations of CO poisoning related to ambient concentration in parts per million (ppm) are listed in Table .1 (Stoller, 2007; Fan et al., 2012; Maloney, 2011; Peers & Steele, 2012).

Table 1. Clinical manifestations related to ambient concentration of COHb in ppm

Concentration (ppm)	Symptoms	Time of exposure
35 ppm	Headache and dizziness	6 to 8 hours
100 ppm	Slight headache	2 to 3 hours
200 ppm	Slight headache and loss of judgment	2 to 3 hours
400 ppm	Frontal headache	within 1 to 2 hours
800 ppm	Dizziness, nausea, and convulsions; insensible	45 minutes to 2 hours
1600 ppm	Headache, tachycardia, dizziness, and nausea; Death	within 20 minutes less than 2 hours
3200 ppm	Headache, dizziness, and nausea; Death	in 5 to 10 minutes within 30 minutes
6400 ppm	Headache and dizziness; Convulsions, respiratory arrest, and death	in 1 to 2 minutes less than 20 minutes
12800 ppm	Unconsciousness; Death	after 2 to 3 breaths less than 3 minutes.

Adopted from Fan et al., (2012).

Infants and children may be more susceptible to CO poisoning than adults because of their rapid respiratory rate, higher metabolic rate, and oxygen uptake. Pediatric patients can have non-specific symptoms as in adults. Moreover, CO can cross the placenta and bind much more tightly to fetal than adult hemoglobin. Pregnant patients with only mild-moderate symptoms have had devastating fetal outcomes. The fetal mortality rate exceeds 50% in cases of severe poisoning (Engel et al., 1969; Fan et al., 2012).

Delayed Effects

The effects of CO intoxication are not limited to acute exposure. Animal studies have shown that CO poisoning causes transient degradation of myelin basic protein (MBP), axonal damage in the hippocampus, and lipid peroxidation resulting in delayed CO-mediated neuropathology. DNS-related symptoms include dementia, amnesia, psychosis, chorea, memory loss, confusion, ataxia, seizures, emotional lability, disorientation, hallucinations, Parkinsonism, mutism, cortical blindness, psychosis, and gait motor disorders. The incidence of DNS caused by CO poisoning ranges from 2.75% to 40%. Most patients who develop DNS have altered consciousness in acute phase poisoning. Risk factors for the development of DNS are age (> 36 years), longer exposure to CO, higher COHb (> 10% or 25%), and damage to the globus pallidus or white matter. DNS development occurs 2 to 40 days (mean 22.4 days) after the recovery period. Cerebral demyelination of white matter fibers may be seen in DNS. Increased hypoperfusion of bilateral white matter and some parts of the cerebral cortex may be seen in cranial imaging. In addition, necrosis was detected in the white matter, globus pallidus, cerebellum, and hippocampus in autopsies performed weeks after exposure (Sert et al., 2021; Weaver, 2009; Lo et al., 2007).

Chronic Effects

The extent of sequelae after acute CO exposure is unpredictable and may be permanent. Approximately 6 years after poisoning, cognitive problems and abnormal neurological evaluations were seen in 19% and 37% of patients, respectively. Chronic effects are also seen in patients with prolonged exposures to low CO concentration. People with chronic CO poisoning may experience different symptoms such as chronic fatigue, headache, and dizziness, cognitive impairment, personality disorders such as dementia and psychosis, sleep disorders, peripheral neuropathy and paresthesias, recurrent infections, polycythemia, abdominal pain, and diarrhea (Fan et al., 2012; Maloney, 2011).

Diagnosis

Detailed history and clinical suspicion, especially in patients with vague symptoms or unconsciousness are the most important parts of the early diagnosis of CO poisoning. However, measuring the blood COHb level is the most useful test in the definitive diagnosis of CO poisoning.

A co-oximeter should be used to measure COHb levels because it can measure oxyhemoglobin (O_2Hb), deoxygenated hemoglobin, methemoglobin, and COHb as a percentage of total hemoglobin in the blood sample by differentiating wavelength absorbance values. Arterial or venous blood sampling is no different in the case of COHb levels in poisoned patients, so both blood samples can be used. Routine blood gas analyzers without co-oximeters cannot recognize the abnormal hemoglobins and pulse oximetry is also not reliable in predicting O_2Hb saturation in patients exposed to CO. Pulse co-oximeters and newer pulse oximeters can measure COHb levels noninvasively. They can be used in the field for screening, and in the emergency department setting for potential CO-exposed patients with nonspecific symptoms because of their noninvasive mechanism. Both the CO concentration and the exposure time correlate with the severity of clinical symptoms. On the other hand, oxygen therapy reduces COHb levels over time. Even so, whenever CO intoxication is suspected, COHb levels should be measured. Symptoms related to CO exposure differentiate according to the COHb levels. Low levels of COHb (15-20%) cause mild symptoms, while levels above 60% to 70% are usually quickly fatal. Clinical manifestations related to levels of COHb are listed in Table 2 (Plante et al., 2007; Tauger et al., 2010; Fan et al., 2012).

Table 2. Clinical symptoms related to COHb levels

COHb (%)	Symptoms
0-10	Asymptomatic
10-20	Weakness, headache
20-30	Severe headaches, nausea, vertigo
30-40	Nausea, vomiting, blurred vision, muscle weakness
40-50	Loss of consciousness, tachypnea, tachycardia
50-60	Coma, convulsions
> 60	Cardiovascular collapse, respiratory distress

Adopted from Fan et al., (2012).

Additional laboratory tests may be informative about the severity of poisoning cases. Arterial or venous blood gas analysis is useful to show the presence or degree of acidosis and to measure serum lactate levels. The time of exposure, the severity of clinical symptoms, or adverse neurological sequelae are associated with the level of acidosis. Elevated lactate levels may serve as a reliable index of the severity of poisoning. Troponin and creatine phosphokinase may be elevated depending on the degree of myonecrosis and rhabdomyolysis. Serum S100B protein may predict the development of DNS after acute CO poisoning (Zhang et al., 2021; Park et al., 2020; Kim et al., 2018; Maloney, 2011).

Cardiac monitoring and 12 lead electrocardiography (ECG) are essential to demonstrate dysrhythmias and ischemia. There is no specific ECG finding for CO poisoning. ECG findings range from normal ECG to Qt prolongation and ST-elevation myocardial ischemia. Echocardiography can define cardiac injury (Yilmaz, 2021; Park et al., 2020). Chest radiograph may identify non-cardiogenic pulmonary edema. Also, fetal monitoring is essential to identify fetal compromise in pregnant patients.

Neuroimaging methods such as magnetic resonance imaging (MRI), computed tomography (CT), single-photon emission CT (SPECT), and positron emission tomography (PET) can be used and be informative in CO poisoning, even if lesions seen in these methods are not specific for CO poisoning. There are single or bilateral, round, low-density areas in the globus, especially in the globus pallidus, putamen, and caudate nuclei. MRI is superior in detecting basal ganglia lesions. Diffusion-weighted MRI can detect changes in the subcortical white matter within hours in serious CO poisoning. SPECT can identify perfusion defects in CO poisoning. PET can be used to evaluate regional blood flow and oxygen metabolism in the brain in CO poisoning (Hopkins et al., 2006; Moon et al., 2018; Liu et al., 2020).

Several neuropsychiatric tests have been designed specifically to screen for cognitive dysfunction in CO poisoning and this technique can also be used to predict the development of neurologic sequelae.

Management

The first step of treatment starts with removal from the site of exposure. Administration of supplemental oxygen and general supportive care such as airway management, blood pressure support, and stabilization of cardiovascular status are other steps of the treatment.

The mainstay of treatment is an administration of normobaric oxygen (NBO2) by either a non-rebreathing mask or endotracheal tube because oxygen immediately enhances the dissociation of COHb. The half-life of COHb is 240 to 320 minutes in a person breathing restroom air (21% oxygen), compared to 40 to 80 minutes with 100% NBO2. Pregnant patients and patients with mild symptoms or who do not meet the criteria for HBO treatment should receive 100% NBO2 delivered by a tight-fitting facemask until their symptoms resolve completely or the COHb level falls below 5% (Yucel & Guzel, 2020).

High flow nasal cannula (HFNC) systems deliver oxygen at high flow rates (up to 60 L/min) and increase the concentration of inspiratory oxygen (FiO2) from 0.21 (room air) to 1.0 (pure oxygen). Recently, studies have been conducted on the use and effectiveness of HFNC in the treatment of patients with CO poisoning, especially in the emergency department setting. These studies reported that HFNC therapy has similar effectiveness at reducing the half-life of COHb as conventional NBO2 therapy; however, HFNC therapy reduces COHb levels more effectively than conventional NBO2 therapy (Young-Min et al., 2020; Tomruk et al., 2019; Yesiloglu et al., 2020). Even so, recently, animal studies have been conducted with photo-extracorporeal membrane oxygenation (ECMO) and hyperbaric photo-ECMO to reduce the half-life of CO and positive results have been obtained, but these are limited to experimental studies (Fischbach et al., 2021; Zazzeron et al., 2017).

Cardiac monitoring and intravenous (IV) access are necessary for the stabilization of cardiovascular status and blood pressure. Hypotension can be treated with IV fluids and inotropes. Advance cardiac life support protocols can be used to treat life-threatening dysrhythmias. Treatment with bicarbonate in patients with metabolic acidosis is controversial. Correction of acidemia with bicarbonate therapy may cause the O2Hb dissociation curve to shift to the left, resulting in further cellular damage (Tomaszewski, 2011).

Table 3. Suggested indications for HBO therapy

COHb levels > 25%
Pregnant with COHb levels > 20%
Metabolic acidosis (pH < 7.1)
Exposed to CO ≥ 24 hours
Age ≥ 36 years
Fetal distress in pregnancy
End-organ ischemia (ECG changes, chest pain)
Presence of neurological symptoms such as syncope, altered mental status or confusion, seizure, focal neurological deficits, and coma

Adopted from Tomaszewski (2011).

The hyperbaric oxygen (HBO) chamber applied for medical purposes was described in 1622 and the first application was used in CO intoxication in the 19th century (Megas et al., 2021). Administration of 100% oxygen at 2.5 atmospheres of pressure decreases the half-life of COHb to approximately 20 minutes, compared to 40 to 80 minutes with 100% NBO2. HBO increases and accelerates the dissociation of CO from hemoglobin, and allows the lung to excrete excessive CO. HBO therapy is a treatment option for patients with significant CO exposures. HBO may also have a role in preventing adverse neurologic sequelae in CO poisoning. Therapeutic one session of HBO at 2.5 to 3.0 atmospheres of absolute pressure for

60-90 minutes is recommended initially, with further sessions considered if symptoms persist. Suggested indications for HBO therapy in CO-exposed patients are given in Table 3 (Sen & Sen, 2021; Maloney, 2011).

CO-exposed patients with impaired consciousness or neurological or cardiovascular dysfunction may require hospitalization because these patients should be monitored for the development of comorbidities such as cardiac ischemia, burns, or hypotension.

Conclusion

Carbon monoxide poisoning is one of the important causes of emergency room admissions and the leading cause of poisoning-related deaths. CO poisoning may have lifelong effects in humans with its delayed and chronic effects. Early diagnosis and treatment with 100% oxygen prevent much of the mortality and morbidity associated with CO poisoning. Using a CO-detecting device at home and the workplace may prevent many unintentional poisonings.

References

Allred, E. N., Bleecker, E. R., Chaitman, B. R., Dahms, T. E., Gottlieb, S. O., Hackney, J. D., Pagano, M., Selvester, R. H., Walden, S. M., & Warren, J. (1989). Short-term effects of carbon monoxide exposure on the exercise performance of subjects with coronary artery disease. *The New England journal of medicine, 321*(21), 1426–1432.

Bleecker M. L. (2015). Carbon monoxide intoxication. *Handbook of clinical neurology, 131,* 191–203.

Chenoweth, J. A., Albertson, T. E., & Greer, M. R. (2021). Carbon Monoxide Poisoning. *Critical care clinics, 37*(3), 657–672.

Engel, R.R., Rodkey, F. L., O'neal, J. D., Collison, H.A. (1969); Relative Affinity of Human Fetal Hemoglobin for Carbon Monoxide and Oxygen. *Blood,* 33 (1), 37–45.

Fan, H. C., Juan, C. J., Chen, S. J. (2012) Carbon monoxide: sources, uses and hazards. D. DiLoreto, I. *Corcoran* (Ed.), (pp. 31-47); UK, Novthe a Science Publishers.

Fischbach, A., Traeger, L., Farinelli, W. A., Ezaka, M., Wanderley, H. V., Wiegand, S. B., Franco, W., Bagchi, A., Bloch, D. B., Anderson, R. R., & Zapol, W. M. (2021). Hyperbaric phototherapy augments blood carbon monoxide removal. *Lasers in surgery and medicine,* 10.1002/lsm.23486.

Hopkins, R. O., Fearing, M. A., Weaver, L. K., & Foley, J. F. (2006). Basal ganglia lesions following carbon monoxide poisoning. *Brain injury, 20*(3), 273–281.

Hopper, C. P., Zambrana, P. N., Goebel, U., & Wollborn, J. (2021). A brief history of carbon monoxide and its therapeutic origins. *Nitric oxide : biology and chemistry, 111-112,* 45–63.

Kim, H., Choi, S., Park, E., Yoon, E., Min, Y., & Lampotang, S. (2018). Serum markers and development of delayed neuropsychological sequelae after acute carbon monoxide poisoning: anion gap, lactate, osmolarity, S100B protein, and interleukin-6. *Clinical and experimental emergency medicine, 5*(3), 185–191.

Liu, J., Si, Z., Liu, J., Lin, Y., Yuan, J., Xu, S., He, Y., Zhang, T., & Wang, A. (2020). Clinical and Imaging Prognosis in Patients with Delayed Encephalopathy after Acute Carbon Monoxide Poisoning. *Behavioural neurology, 2020,* 1719360.

Lo, C. P., Chen, S. Y., Lee, K. W., Chen, W. L., Chen, C. Y., Hsueh, C. J., & Huang, G. S. (2007). Brain injury after acute carbon monoxide poisoning: early and late complications. *AJR. American journal of roentgenology, 189*(4), W205–W211.

Malone, G. (2011). Carbon Monoxide. J. E. Tintinalli, J. S. Stapczynski, O. J. Ma, D. M. Cline, R. K. Cydulka, G. D. Mecker (Eds.), Tintinalli's Emergency Medicine. *A Comprehensive Study Guide* (pp. 1410-1413), New York; USA; McGraw Hill.

Mattiuzzi, C., Lippi. G. (2020). Worldwide epidemiology of carbon monoxide poisoning. *Human and Experimental Toxicology,* 39(4), 387–392.

Megas, I. F., Beier, J. P., & Grieb, G. (2021). The History of Carbon Monoxide Intoxication. *Medicina (Kaunas, Lithuania), 57*(5), 400.

Moon, J. M., Chun, B. J., Baek, B. H., & Hong, Y. J. (2018). Initial diffusion-weighted MRI and long-term neurologic outcomes in charcoal-burning carbon monoxide poisoning. *Clinical toxicology (Philadelphia, Pa.), 56*(3), 161–169.

Park, J. H., Heo, R., Kang, H., Oh, J., Lim, T. H., & Ko, B. S. (2020). Diagnostic performance and optimal cut-off values of cardiac biomarkers for predicting cardiac injury in carbon monoxide poisoning. *Clinical and experimental emergency medicine, 7*(3), 183–189.

Peers, C., & Steele, D. S. (2012). Carbon monoxide: a visignalingling molecule and potent toxin in the myocardium. *Journal of molecular and cellular cardiology, 52*(2), 359–365.

Plante, T., Harris, D., Savitt, J., Akhlaghi, F., Monti, J., & Jay, G. D. (2007). Carboxyhemoglobin is monitored by bedside continuous CO-oximetry. *The Journal of trauma, 63*(5), 1187–1190.

Raub, J. A., Mathieu-Nolf, M., Hampson, N. B., & Thom, S. R. (2000). Carbon monoxide poisoning--a public health perspective. *Toxicology, 145*(1), 1–14.

Rose, J. J., Wang, L., Xu, Q., McTiernan, C. F., Shiva, S., Tejero, J., & Gladwin, M. T. (2017). Carbon Monoxide Poisoning: Pathogenesis, Management, and Future Directions of Therapy. *American journal of respiratory and critical care medicine, 195*(5), 596–606.

Sen, S., & Sen, S. (2021). Therapeutic effects of hyperbaric oxygen: integrated review. *Medical gas research, 11*(1), 30–33.

Sert, E. T., Kokulu, K., & Mutlu, H. (2021). Clinical predictors of delayed neurological sequelae in charcoal-burning carbon monoxide poisoning. *The American journal of emergency medicine, 48*, 12–17.

Stewart, R. D., Peterson, J. E., Fisher, T. N., Hosko, M. J., Baretta, E. D., Dodd, H. C., & Herrmann, A. A. (1973). Experimental human exposure to high concentrations of carbon monoxide. *Archives of environmental health, 26*(1), 1–7.

Stoller K. P. (2007). Hyperbaric oxygen and carbon monoxide poisoning: a critical review. *Neurological research, 29*(2), 146–155.

Tomaszewski, C. (2011) Carbon monoxide. L. S. Nelson, N. A. Lewin, M. A. Howland, R. S. Hoffman, L. R. Goldfrank, N. E. Flomenbaum (Ed.), *Goldfrank's Toxicologic Emergencies* (pp. 1658-1670). New York; USA; McGraw Hill.

Tomruk, O., Karaman, K., Erdur, B., Armagan, H. H., Beceren, N. G., Oskay, A., & Bircan, H. A. (2019). A New Promising Treatment Strategy for Carbon Monoxide Poisoning: High Flow Nasal Cannula Oxygen Therapy. *Medical science monitor : international medical journal of experimental and clinical research, 25*, 605–609.

Touger, M., Birnbaum, A., Wang, J., Chou, K., Pearson, D., & Bijur, P. (2010). Performance of the RAD-57 pulse CO-oximeter compared with standard laboratory carboxyhemoglobin measurement. *Annals of emergency medicine, 56*(4), 382–388.

Vreman, H.J., Wong, R.J., Stevenson, D.K. (2001). Sources, sinks, and measurements of carbon monoxide. R. Wang (Ed.), *Carbon Monoxide and Cardiovascular Functions* (pp. 273–307). CRC press.

Weaver L. K. (2009). Clinical practice. Carbon monoxide poisoning. *The New England journal of medicine, 360*(12), 1217–1225.

Yavuz, E. (2019). Carbon Monoxide Poisoning. *Eurasian J. Tox.*, 1 (1), 1-6.

Yesiloglu, O., Gulen, M., Satar, S., Acehan, S., & Akoglu, H. (2021). Response to Comment on Treatment of carbon monoxide poisoning: high-flow nasal cannula versus non-rebreather face mask. *Clinical toxicology (Philadelphia, Pa.), 59*(8), 769.

Yilmaz G. (2021). ECG Intervals on Acute Carbon Monoxide Poisoning. *Journal of the College of Physicians and Surgeons--Pakistan : JCPSP, 30*(6), 668–672.

Yucel, M., Guzel, M. (2020) Carbon monoxide. S. Satar, O. Guneysel, Y. Yurumez, S. Turedi, A. Akici (Ed.), *Clinical Toxicology Diagnosis and Treatment* (pp. 809-815). Antalya; Turkey; Cukurova Nobel Tip Publishing.

Zazzeron, L., Liu, C., Franco, W., Nakagawa, A., Farinelli, W. A., Bloch, D. B., Anderson, R. R., & Zapol, W. M. (2017). Pulmonary Phototherapy to Treat Carbon Monoxide Poisoning in Rats. *Shock (Augusta, Ga.)*, *47*(6), 735–742.

Zhang, L., Zhao, J., Hao, Q., Xu, X., Han, H., & Li, J. (2021). Serum NSE and S100B protein levels for evaluating the impaired consciousness in patients with acute carbon monoxide poisoning. *Medicine*, *100*(25), e26458.

Chapter 29

Chemical, Biological, Radioactive and Nuclear (CBRN) Emergencies

Volkan Ülker*, MD, PhD and Fatih Güneysu, MD

Clinics of Emergency Medicine, Sakarya University Research and Education Hospital, Sakarya, Turkey

Abstract

Chemical, biological, radiological and nuclear (CBRN) events can be seen due to warfare situations and accidental exposure in industry. First of all, according to prevention measures, workers and health authorities have to know the initial signs and symptoms, decontamination procedures, use of antidotes especially for time-sensitive agents, the medical transfer route of affected casualties, and the agent-specific medical therapy and blocking patterns of secondary contaminations. There are many effects of CBRN agents like acute and chronic phases. There are new researches to guide CBRN exposure within the improvement of technology. Globally, new trained, allocated and specified personnel are needed for each agent to manage and treat CBRN agent casualties.

Keywords: antidotes, decontamination, global health, emergencies, mass casualty incidents

Introduction

CBRN events in the environment can result in injury, illness, morbidity and mortality through the whole society. After exposure to CBRN threats, many victims can apply to emergency departments (EDs) which are the main areas of decontamination and management of CBRN material effects through the human body. And also, EDs are at the front line of the CBRN response with health care workers (HCW) as first responders. EDs have obligatory duties and responsibilities to prepare, decontaminate, plan and respond to CBRN threats immediately. ED workers should receive special training for the management of CBRN victims and maintain regular drills.

---

* Corresponding Author's Email: volkanulker07@yahoo.com.

In: Environmental Emergencies and Injuries in Nature
Editors: Murat Yücel, Murat Güzel and İbrahim İkizceli
ISBN: 978-1-68507-833-1

Chemical Hazardous Material Exposure

Through the development of civilization, chemical threats have been part of society. Many chemicals have been developed through the years, and most of these commercial chemicals have been stored and transported through and between human lives. Because of this connection, there is a resulting risk for environmental and health effects. Also, some chemicals have been developed to harm or kill humans over the last decades.

Chemicals were used as weapons in ancient years. According to archaeological discoveries, the Assyrians poisoned the wells of their enemies in the 6th century BC and in 1000 BC Persians used bitumen and sulfur against the Romans to asphyxiate them when attempting to take the fortress by tunneling into it. Also in 670 AD, Byzantine Greeks developed an effective weapon called Greek fire that contained naphtha, sulfur, saltpeter and pitch. By the 18th century, the harmful effects of of cyanide and chlorine were discovered. During World War I (WWI) large-scale production and use of harmful chemicals like chlorine, phosgene, diphosgene and chloropicrin became common. These chemicals made the soldiers choke and gasp and also caused lethal pulmonary edema. Within these chemicals, the Germans introduced sulfur mustard to defeat their enemies. The ease of chemical weapon manufacture concluded in new research, weaponizations and deposition of chemical materials. In Germany, in the 1940s, the organophosphate nerve agents were developed as insecticides. The first two nerve agents, tabun and sarin, were weaponized and stockpiled during World War II (WWII). After that another nerve agent called soman was developed but none of them used in WWII. The first battlefield use of these nerve agents was by Iraq against Iranian forces, The war of Iran-Iraq was between 1984 and 1987. The sarin agent was also used in the Tokyo subway attack of 1995. Despite the prohibition of the use of chemical warfare methods with the Geneva protocol signed on June 17, 1925, similar hazardous material attempts continue to be experienced, unfortunately. Despite the reduced death ratio that has been seen from chemical substances, much more public distress is created due to the psychological effects on the victims. Because of this effect, public authorities are concerned about the possible terrorist use of toxic industrial chemicals.

On the other hand, the use of chemicals throughout the world via globalization and the rapid development of the chemical industry led to accidents that may cause environmental disasters. In the light of the World Health Organization (WHO) data, while more than fifteen million chemical substances are available, approximately seventy thousand chemicals are used continuously.

A chemical accident that may lead to an environmental disaster is defined as the sudden and serious functional disruption in the society due to the scattering or spreading of toxic chemicals. The worst example of chemicals that cause an environmental disaster in recent years can be cited as the Bhopal disaster (India), in which nearly eight thousand people died in 3 days in 1984 and nearly three hundred thousand people were affected. The gas cloud containing fifteen tons of methylisocyanate leaking from the pesticide factory led to the death of people in the region and to injuries that still continue today. In 1976, due to the release of 2, 3, 7, 8 tetrachlorodibenz-p-dioxin (TCDD) because of the disruption of the cooling process in the pesticide and herbicide factory located in Seveso town, 20 km from the city of Milan in Italy, burns and physiological effects were detected in the local people and 80 thousand animal deaths and agricultural areas were impacted. Cyanide leaked in the dam accident that occurred as a result of a technological accident in the Baia Mare region of Romania in 2000 caused much environmental damage. Within these accidents and environmental disasters authorities and governments were directed to lead the classification, packaging and labeling of dangerous preparations and the events to be applied in any chemical incident were accepted on the international platform with some planned directives.

Chemical-induced events that can lead to environmental disasters need special planning and preparation. There is a plan for the treatment of chemically injured casualties and to reduce the harm caused directly to HCW. Although industrial workers are most injured, local people, law enforcement officers, civil defense workers, firefighters and HCW are faced with agent and transfer related exposures.

Chemical Substances, Clinical Considerations and Treatment Modalities

Chemical agents are suspected when there is an odd smell or abnormal color in the air and many patient admissions through EDs with similar acute symptoms. Chemical agents can be used in a terrorist attack to make a mass casualty incident and also in an industrial manner. There are many species of chemical agents like cyanides and nerve agents that have specific antidotes called time-sensitive materials. Pulmonary intoxicants, blister agents, choking agents, incapacitants, riot control agents and toxic industrial chemicals (ammonia, carbon monoxide, chlorine, ethylene oxide, sulfur dioxide, etc.) are other classifications of hazardous chemical materials.

Chemical hazardous agents can be used as warfare agents by missiles, explosive rockets, shells, spray devices, bombs, and mines and also through intentional and commercial accidents. Water containers have a risk for contamination. A substance scattered from an airplane or by missiles is an indication of chemical war assessment. Spray delivered from an air vehicle may not be seen and vapors can be occulted by meteorological situations.

Hazardous chemical materials can affect the body via many routes like being inhaled, as vapors, gases, and aerosols by the airway. Another route for absorption is through the top layer of airways of the nose, throat, mouth, and/or the alveoli parts of the thorax. Liquid particles and solid substances may be absorbed by the eyes, skin, and top layer of each organ. Hazardous chemical agents can pollute food and beverages, and are routed through the gastrointestinal system. Abrasions are more susceptible than intact skin to absorb the hazardous material. Additional situations that affect absorption can be warm and moist environments.

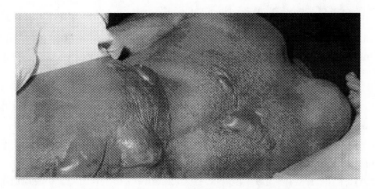

Figure 1. The skin effect of a vesicant chemical agent (Republic of Turkey Ministry of National Education, Emergency Health Services, Emergency Assistance in CBRN Hazards, 2011).

Diagnosis of injury from chemical agents can vary according to different properties of the agent. Some agents have odors, but many are essentially odorless. Observations of signs and symptoms of applied victims are important for diagnosis including a brief history, evaluation of the eye region (pupils, conjunctiva and lids), assessment of the respiratory pattern, the quality of membranes and skin and level of consciousness. Also, the identification of chemical hazardous materials can be made by special detector papers and tapes. There are some agent-specific papers (M8 and M9 chemical agent detector tape) and improved chemical agent monitors and detector kits (M256 chemical agent detector kit). They have false positive reactions and limitations to detect vapors of agents.

After exposure to a chemical agent, the treatment of victims consists of triage, basic initial assistive treatment using antidotes, decontamination, emergency advanced medical treatment, evacuation of victims and continuing protection of new casualties.

In order to prevent and reduce the chemical exposure after accidents and warfare, the steps of management of the victims are activated. The intervention begins with the preparation of medical intervention, emergency aid and rescue teams at the scene, and the isolation and security of the scene with scanning. The chemical properties of the substance are determined, and the crime scene is divided into three parts as hot, warm, and cold.

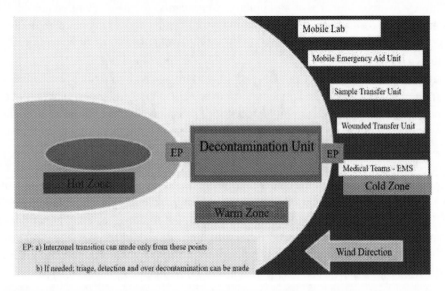

Figure 2. Management of the Scene of a CBRN accident.

The hot area is the polluted area where the incident occurred. Only firefighters and specially trained personnel (STP) can enter the polluted area with personal protective equipment (PPE). HCW who will administer emergency medical treatment wait in the safe zone. The works carried out in the hot area are planned and implemented by STP and military teams. A chemical substance is detected by them while wearing the highest level of PPE (Type A PPE); through electronic detectors, kits and sampling methods. The security of the area is evaluated and there is a wait until the scene is safe. After ordering the safe area; triage is done. Affected casualties are evacuated from the area as soon as possible. First aid is not applied in the hot zone. After the rescue and forensic studies, environmental purification is carried out. The warm area is the area between the hot and cold areas, which is actually clean and polluted by those coming from the hot area. At least 300 meters from the hot area, there should be a flat area of land suitable for the wind direction, with safety measures provided, and easy access for vehicles. There should be a water source in the area, and it should be close to other facilities. Purification and decontamination systems are installed in the warm area. The strength and direction of the wind are assessed attentionally. Warm area studies are performed by decontamination personnel with at least type C PPE. Airway, respiratory and circulatory support are provided. Bleeding is controlled. Triage is done. Treatment of the wounded and rescuers is carried out. The cold zone is the clean zone that has never been affected by the event. The cold zone is where the ambulances and HCW wearing personal protective suits (at least D level) are located. Triage is done. Medical care is administered. The antidote is applied. The injured/victims are transported to the hospital.

Table 1. Personal protective equipment

Personal Protective Equipment levels for hazardous materials and emergency response				
Protected region	Level D	Level C	Level B	Level A
Skin (Dermal layer)	Underwear: normal street clothes Outerwear: all-enveloping workwear or other protective clothes	Underwear: Streetwear or workwear providing environmental heat resistant insulation Outerwear: Chemical resistant clothing with hood		Underwear: Fully capsular chemical protective clothing outerwear: Authorized disposable protective clothing
Skin Especially hand region	Disposable gloves	Disposable gloves, chemical resistant inner and outer gloves		Chemical resistant outer glove on capsular suit
Respiratory airways		Air-purifying respirator (APR)	Respiratory equipment in capsular clothing (SCBA)	
Eyes		APR	SCBA	
Foot protection	Boots and shoes suitable for completing the task		Chemical resistant steel toe boots	Chemical resistant steel toe boots on capsular suit
	Known factor		Unknown factor	
	Skin contamination,		Skin contamination,	
	Inhalation,		Inhalation exposure,	
	No risk of harmful substance contact		Evident of eye exposure	

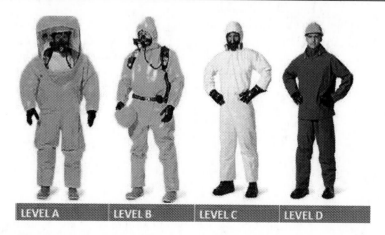

Figure 3. Types of Personal Protective Equipment.*
*(https://www.cbrnpro.net/news-bedford/2019/9/3/i-dont-think-you-are-doing-that-right-equipment-selection-and-use-in-cbrn-operations-part-1, Accessed November 19, 2021).

All around the world; CBRN preparations begin at the hospital when the news reaches the rescue first responder teams and the team gathers and goes to the scene. Incident management strategies are activated in accordance with the compliance of the hospital staff. The team, structural elements and infrastructure must be ready for an intervention. The establishment of the decontamination system, the detection phase, the arrival of the patients from the warm area after safety is ensured, starting the rescue process and the first patient's admission time may vary depending on the size of the event. During this time, some injured will die, everyone who thinks they are affected comes to the hospital without being ordered, and hospitals become inoperable. Hospitals can be contaminated by chemical vapors emitted from patients. Therefore, patients need to undergo a secondary decontamination. This decontamination should not be done for the injured or dead among the HCW and the intervention is not interrupted. Medical support should be planned by stakeholder institutions and organizations due to the application of sudden and unplanned patients. It is necessary to prepare antidotes and drugs in advance. In order to avoid such undesirable situations, each hospital should prepare a hospital disaster plan (HDP) in accordance with the characteristics of the local region. The hospital is then prepared for the CBRN event, e.g., preparation for communication, personnel and backup personnel planning, training of personnel, protective materials, sufficient antidotes and drugs, sufficient medical devices, equipment, a purification system, and where the purification will be carried out. Under the guidance of the incident management team (IMT), the personnel involved in the HDP should have practiced many times before and be experienced in recognizing certain toxidromes. Antidote storage is an essential component in chemical accidents and attacks. It should be determined in the HDP that the hospital should stock an antidote in accordance with the demographic, geopolitical and economic characteristics of the region where the hospital is located. Known as the time-sensitive antidote, diazepam, atropine, cyanide antidote kits, and pralidoxime are vital for the management of multiple injuries in chemical accidents and assaults. Antidotes should be readily available against industrial accident and chemical attack weapons

Table 2. Antidotes of specific chemical agents

Antidotes	Chemical Hazardous material
Calcium	Fluoride or hydrofluoric acid
Hydroxycobalamin	Cyanide
Atropine	Nerve agents, organophosphate, carbamate
Amyl nitrite	Cyanide, sulfides, nitriles
Methylene blue	Compounds that form methemoglobin
Oxygen	Simple-systemic asphyxiants, carbon monoxide, cyanide, azides, hydrogen sulfide, methemoglobin forming compounds
Oximes	Organophosphate, nerve agents
Pyridoxine	Hydrazones

Chemical exposure resulting from chemical accidents and assaults should be suspected early on and detected by experienced and well-equipped personnel, and the first decontamination process should be carried out by establishing hot, warm and cold areas in the field, and by ensuring interinstitutional coordination. There are general properties for any possible mass casualty incident by chemical materials. Decontamination and purification are the most important issues. Decontamination of patients faced with chemical material is essential to save their lives and also more significant in order to prevent secondary contamination of the rest of the victims, HCW and treatment modalities. With communication between stakeholders, the transfer of victims exposed to chemical substances to the relevant hospital, the functional division of labor by the hospital with HDP activation and the preparation of all drugs and antidotes, and appropriate intervention in the patients who underwent secondary decontamination will significantly reduce the number of deaths. The physical removal of contaminated clothes and equipment is more effective than all other known catalytic or chemical methods of decontamination. Soap and water, applied as soon as possible and in adequate amounts, are an efficient decontaminant for a chemical material on the surface of the skin.

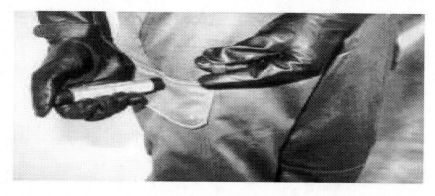

Figure 4. Automatic usage of antidotes (atropine) in chemical warfare incidents.*
* (Agency for Toxic Substances and Disease Registry – ATSDR. Medical Management Guidelines for Phosgene. http://www.atsdr.cdc.gov/mmg/mmg.asp?id=1201&tid=182 (Accessed November 19, 2021).

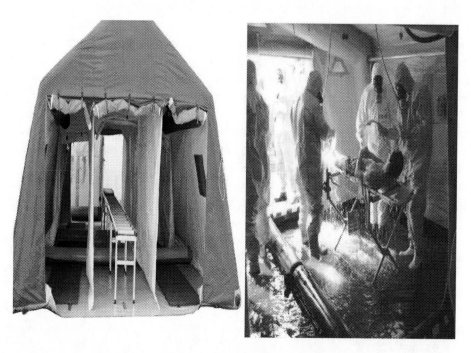

Figure 5. Decontamination Unit and Application of Decontamination with PPE.*
*(https://twitter.com/uprojectfield/status/1367071789470392320, Accessed November 19, 2021).

Also, within detection and first aid administration, triage is ordered at the scene and secondarily at the entrance to hospital EDs. Triage is a dynamic and continuing process and recorded in each level. First responders and HCW protect themselves with the use of PPE. HCW aim to save many casualties. In the triage of those affected by chemical agents, physiological effects and changes in vital signs are classified. There are 4 types of classification in triage victims; life-threatening (red color), urgent (yellow color), minor (green color) and dead (black color). Red ones need immediate treatment (casualties have strict respiratory distress, loss of consciousness, convulsions, apnea), yellow ones need urgent treatment (destroyed respiratory tract, skin and eye irritation), green ones need delayed treatment (minor skin irritation and fully oriented) and black ones need no treatment (cardiopulmonary arrest, high level burns). In chemical accidents; evacuating the victim from the hot zone and detailed decontamination may be lifesaving; as may instant application of the agent-specified antidotes that are suitable for time-sensitive chemicals (e.g., organophosphates, cyanide). On the other hand, in any chemical incident, clinical symptoms can be caused by prevalent, pre-diagnostic chronic diseases (e.g., ischemic cardiovascular diseases, diabetes, asthma, epilepsy), which may be seen by the situation.

P1	LIFE THREATENING	Breathe only after airway cleared or RR less than 9 or more than 30bpm or CRT more than 2 secs	IMMEDIATE TREATMENT
P2	URGENT	Unable to walk *and* RR 10bpm-29bpm *and* CRT 2 secs or less	URGENT TREATMENT
P3	MINOR	Walking	DELAYED TREATMENT
P4	DEAD	Not breathing even after airway cleared	NO TREATMENT

Figure 6. Triage categorization of CBRN casualties.

After the whole event, the preparation, intervention and rehabilitation phases, it is important that the institution is decontaminated and returned to its normal functionality in the recovery phase. During the entire intervention, patients, hospital staff, visitors, and the media should be informed within specified intervals of what is planned in the HDP. Notes taken during the response to the incident should be shared for archiving, reports should be written after the incident, and plans organized, making financial evaluations and creating a resource for the research of the international community. During the continuation of the entire event, the corpses of the dead due to chemical exposure should be kept separate from non-chemical deaths to avoid cross-contamination. Behavioral support is essential for healthcare professionals and victims, from the onset of the event to its end, and also beyond.

In chemical incidents, understanding the chemical hazard labels is significant for the management of casualties. There are some codes, numbers and groups that are known globally. Emergency Action Code (EAC) guides provide information to the health authorities about urgent situations (if there is fine or coarse spray, foam/a dry agent to fight any fire; the suitable PPE needed for the agent, safe spilth orientation) to make safe first action at the scene. The United Nations Substance Identification Number (SIN) is a globally agreed four-digit code that identifies the chemical material. The diamond-shaped symbol shows to which of the 9 UN Hazard Groups the material belongs. And also, a Chemical Abstract Service number (which has the form XXX-XX-X) is a unique identification number of chemical material given to a chemical by the CAS.

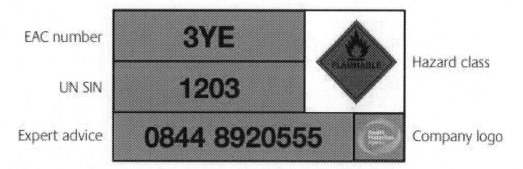

Figure 7. Classification of chemical substances according to international data.*
*(www.inchem.org, Accessed November 19, 2021).

Table 3. United Nations hazard groups

The nine selected *United Nations Hazard Groups* are:	
Class 1:	Explosive e.g., ammunition, fireworks, hydrazine (1.1: mass explosion, 1.4: not significant)
Class 2:	Gases (2.1: flammable, 2.2: non-toxic, 2.3: toxic)
Class 3:	Flammable liquids (e.g., diesel, methanol, xylene, alcohol)
Class 4:	Flammable solids e.g., sodium, barium (4.1: flammable solid, 4.2: spontaneous combustion risk)
Class 5:	Oxidizers (5.1) or organic peroxides (5.2)
Class 6:	Toxic (6.1 – includes nerve agents, sarin, mustard, pesticides, lewisite) or infectious (6.2) substances
Class 7:	Radioactive substances (sources in the nuclear industry, radiotherapy, the military)
Class 8:	Corrosive substances (e.g., chlorine, sodium hydroxide, fluorine, nitric acid)
Class 9:	Miscellaneous dangerous substances (e.g., mace, pepper spray, asbestos)

(https://www.ukfrs.com/guidance/search/un-system, Accessed November 19, 2021).

In this chapter, we focus on the acute effects of poisoning of chemical agents. There could be a more general emphasis is needed on the long-term effects, but this is still controversial. Examples of these long-term effects include: pulmonary fibrosis seen after recovery from poisoning with oxides of nitrogen; delayed neovascularization and blindness seen in Iranian war veterans poisoned with sulfur mustard; possible carcinogenesis seen after sulfur mustard poisoning, especially in the lung; and questions of chronic neurologic dysfunction in survivors of nerve agent poisoning.

At present, the disaster medicine community lacks a standardized medical review process, unfortunately. With improvements of technology, there are still some obstacles. For instance, we must have more drills, full-scale exercises and tactical operations to reduce the effects of a chemical incident. We have to have organized, standardized and usable plans for an immediate response for the needs of victims with our local and governmental stakeholders.

Table 4. Chemical agent properties and health effects

Chemical	Agent	Symbol	Odor	Mechanism	Eyes			Nose and Throat
					Pupils	Conjunctiva	Other parts	
NERVE	Tabun Sarin Soman VX Cyclosarin	GA GB GD VX GF	Faint sweetness, paint-like or fruity	Anticholinesterase materials	Miosis	Redness	Dimness or vision, Headache, Lacrimation Pain	Increased salivation and rhinorrhea
BLISTER	Mustard Sulfur mustard Nitrogen Mustard	H HD HN	Horseradish or garlic, irritating Fishy like, irritating	Alkylating agent, damages DNA Vesicants, bone marrow depressant,		Edema redness, irritation, pain	Pain, photophobia, edema of lids lacrimation, corneal ulceration, and scarring	Swelling, irritation, occasional edema of larynx, discharge
	Lewisite And other arsenical vesicants	L	Fruity to geranium like, irritating	Vesicants, Arsenical poisons		Prompt redness, edema, irritation	Immediate burning sensation, iritis, corneal injury	Deep irritation
	Mustard/Lewisite mixture	HL	Garlic like odor	Like lewisite and mustard	LIKE HN, HD, AND L			
LUNG DAMAGING (CHOKING)	Phosgene Oxime Chloropicrin	CX PS	Unpleasant and irritating	Powerful vesicant		Violently irritating, redness, edema	Lacrimation, corneal injury with blindness	Very irritating to mucous membranes
	Phosgene Diphosgene	CG DP	New-mown hay Green corn, or grass	Lung damaging agent		Irritation	Lacrimation (after respiratory symptoms)	Irritation
RIOT CONTROL	Vomiting agents (Adamsite, Diphenylchloroarsine, diphenylcyanoarsine)	DM DA DC	Burning fireworks, very irritating	Irritant, induces vomiting		Irritation	Lacrimation	Tightness, sneezing, pain, rhinorrhea / Tightness
	Irritant agents (chloroacetophenone, bromobenzylcyanide,	CN CA	Irritating	Local irritant		Redness, irritation	Pain, blepharospasm, lacrimation, photophobia	Irritation, burning / Tightness, burning
	O-chlorobenzylidene malononitrile, dibenz (b,f)-1,4-oxazepine)	CS CR	Pungent, pepper-like, very irritating	Local irritant		Intense irritation	Lacrimation blepharospasm, photophobia, pain	Burning, irritation, tightness / Tightness, burning

Chemical	Agent	Symbol	Odor	Mechanism	Eyes			Nose and Throat
					Pupils	Conjunctiva	Other parts	
CYANOGEN (BLOOD)	Hydrogen Cyanide	AC	Bitter almonds, faint odor	Interferes with oxygen utilization at the cellular level				
	Cyanogen Chloride	CK	Irritating	Lung irritant		Irritant	Lacrimation	Irritant
INCAPACITATING	Incapacitating agents	BZ	None	Anticholinergic	Mydriasis		Loss of vision	Dry eye
		LSD	None	Psychotomimetic	Mydriasis			
TOXIC INDUSTRIAL CHEMICALS	Ammonia	NH3	Urine or sweat	Activation of the NMDA receptor		Chemical burns	Irritation	Irritation and chemical burns
	Carbon-monoxide	CO	None	Prevents the blood system carrying oxygen				
	Hydrogen sulfide, and oxides of nitrogen	NOx	Rotten eggs	Inhibits cytochrome c oxidase, Binds to hemoglobin				
SMOKES	Hexachloroethane, zinc oxide containing mixtures,	HC	None	Production of reactive oxygen species		Irritation	Lacrimation	Irritation, burning, Tightness, stridor
	Fog oil, diesel fuel	SGF2	None	Burns, irritation				
	Titanium tetrachloride	FM	Strong penetrating odor	Thermal burns				
	Red phosphorus	RP	None	Reduced the heat release due to radical trapping				
	White phosphorus	WP	Garlic like odor	Burns in air and causes severe burns				

Table 5. Chemical agent properties and health effects

Chemical	Respiratory Tract	Skin	Gastrointestinal Tract	Cardiovascular System	Genitourinary System	Central Nervous System	Other
NERVE	Restlessness in chest, bronchoconstriction, increased bronchial secretion, dyspnea, cough, wheezing	Pallor, sweating, then cyanosis	Nausea, vomiting, salivation, epigastric tightness abdominal cramps, heartburn, diarrhea, tenesmus, involuntary defecation, anorexia,	Transient tachycardia and/or hypertension followed by bradycardia, arrhythmias, and hypotension	Urinary incontinence frequent micturition	Cheyne-Stokes respiration, convulsions, apprehension, headache, giddiness, insomnia, poor memory, confusion, weakness, ataxia, coma with areflexia	Fasciculations, cramps, easy fatigue, weakness paralysis (including respiratory muscles)
BLISTER	Tightness, irritation, hoarseness, cough, fever, dyspnea, rales, pulmonary edema in severe cases, pleural effusions, pneumonia	Redness and burning blisters surrounded by redness and itching. Necrosis, delayed hyper-hypo pigmentation, risk of secondary infection	Pain, hepatic failure, nausea, vomiting, diarrhea	Shock after severe exposure, hemoconcentration, hemolytic anemia	Renal failure	Depression, anxiety	Bone marrow depression, malaise, systemic arsenic poisoning (Lewisite)
LUNG DAMAGING (CHOKING)	Rapid irritation, coughing, choking, laryngospasm, later pulmonary edema, frothy sputum, rales, pneumonia, fever	Severe irritation and intense pain. Affected area turns white and swollen and blistering. Necrosis, long recovery. Possible cyanosis can be seen following cardiogenic edema	Nausea	Shock, hypertension, altered mental status, and tachycardia		Anxiety, depression	
RIOT CONTROL	Tightness, uncontrollable coughing, difficulty breathing, pain	Stinging (especially around the eyes and mouth), occasional dermatitis, may blister	Salivation, nausea and vomiting			Altered mental status, severe headache	May cause to remove protective mask in agitation

Chemical	Respiratory Tract	Skin	Gastrointestinal Tract	Cardiovascular System	Genitourinary System	Central Nervous System	Other
CYANOGEN (BLOOD)	Deep respiratory pattern followed by dyspnea, cough, gasping, choking, then cessation of respiration	Initially pink buffer than may change to purple	Nausea and vomiting	Hypertension		Initial agitation, then depression, giddiness, ataxia, headache, irritational behavior, convulsions or coma	
INCAPACITATING		Dry, flushed, sweaty palms, cold extremities	Constipation	Elevated blood pressure tachycardia	Urinary retention, urgency	Disorientation headache, drowsiness, hallucinations, maniacal behavior. Ataxia and/or lack of coordination, tremor	Pyrexia
TOXIC INDUSTRIAL CHEMICALS	Tightness and irritation in chest, Chemical burns in airways	Chemical burns on skin	Irritation Nausea	Secondary effects due to displacement of oxygen, Hypertension		Initial excitation, then depression, ataxia, irritational behavior, coma or convulsions and death	Respiratory failure, cardiovascular collapse and death
SMOKES	Dyspnea, coughing, stridor.	Chemical burns on skin	Irritation Nausea Gastritis	Shock after sever exposure, hypertension, and tachycardia		Excitation followed by loss of consciousness and stupor, coma	Bronchial constriction and respiratory collapse

Table 6. Chemical agent decontamination styles and treatment modalities

Chemical	Agent	Symbol	Decontamination	Treatment
NERVE	Tabun Sarin Soman VX Cyclosarin	GA GB GD VX GF	Remove contaminated clothes. For skin use nerve agent specific M291 kit. For individual equipment use M295 Packet	Pretreatment with pyridostigmine for Soman Postexposure medication: 1) Enzyme reactivation: oximes (2-PAM C1) 2) Cholinergic blockade: atropine 3) Antiepileptic: diazepam 4) Suction for respiratory secretions 5) Assisted ventilation, ocular atropine ointment
BLISTER	Mustard Nitrogen Mustard Lewisite And other arsenical vesicants Mustard /Lewisite mixture	H HD HN L HL	For obvious contamination of eyes, initially irrigate with many cups of water, sodium bicarbonate or saline eye wash. Remove clothes. For skin use specific kit. Use M295 Packet	Eyes: antibiotics, atropine drops and systemic analgesia (morphine may be needed to control pain) Skin: local antibiotics for infection Respiratory inflammations: iv antibiotic fluids BAL in oil IM systemic chelation. BAL ointment for eye and skin
LUNG DAMAGING (CHOKING)	Phosgene Oxime Chloropicrin Phosgene Diphosgene	CX PS CG DP	Wash with copious amounts of isotonic sodium bicarbonate or water Removal of victim to uncontaminated/fresh air	Apply dressings of sodium bicarbonate systemic analgesics. Debridate as any other necrotic skin lesions Enforced rest, warmth, and observation Steroids iv and by inhalation may be lifesaving. Oxygen, rest, antibiotics
RIOT CONTROL	Vomiting agents (adamsite, diphenylchloroarsine, diphenylcyanoarsine) Irritant agents (chloroacetophenone, bromobenzylcyanide, O-chlorobenzylidene malononitrile, dibenz-1,4-oxazepine)	DM DA DC CN CA CS CR	Wash eyes with amounts of water. Bleach should not be used because it produces irritation by-products from these materials, Decontaminate clothing by airing for a few hours	Wear mask in spite of symptoms; spontaneous improvement Antiemetics for prolonged symptoms. Acetaminophen or aspirin for headaches and general discomfort Analgesic for eyes and nose drops Symptoms disappear rapidly in fresh air

Chemical	Agent	Symbol	Decontamination	Treatment
CYANOGEN (BLOOD)	Hydrogen Cyanide	AC	Unnecessary.	A. Drugs binding cyanide: - Methemoglobin formers; nitrites or DMAP
	Cyanogen Chloride	CK	Remove clothes and decontaminate underlying surface with soap/water solutions	- Cleaners; dicobalt edetate and hydroxycobolamin B. Provision of S-Groups, thiosulfate C. Assisted respiratory support D. Oxygen, correct metabolic acidosis
INCAPACI-TATING	Incapacitating agents	BZ	Wash with soap and/or water	Cool the surroundings restraint, physostigmine
		LSD		Restraint, reassurance, emergent, diazepam
TOXIC INDUSTRIAL CHEMICALS	Ammonia	NH3	Generally, water or soap/water solutions.	Urgent aid: termination of contact and immediate wash/clean
	Carbon monoxide	CO		Removal from exposure area/decontamination of liquid agents.
	Hydrogen sulfide, and oxides of nitrogen	NOx		Monitor and guide for shock. Supportive/symptom-oriented treatment. Agents with respiratory effects may require supplemental oxygen, suctioning, assisted ventilation and advanced airway management
SMOKES	Hexachloroethane, grained aluminum, and zinc oxide containing mixtures,	HC	Eyes: saline/water. Skin: copious amounts of water or soap/water solution	Oxygen supply, if needed. Bronchial constriction due to HC smoke can be treated with epinephrine hydrochloride, as needed
	Fog oil, diesel fuel	SGF2		
	Titanium tetrachloride	FM		
	Red phosphorus	RP		
	White phosphorus	WP		

Biological Substances, Clinical Considerations and Treatment Modalities

Microorganisms and the toxins they produce are called biological weapons if used for biological warfare or terrorism. If these microorganisms are used to purposefully kill or create an outbreak among humans, animals, or plants, it is called bioterrorism. These agents can be found in the world but cannot be produced in a laboratory, despite the antibiotic resistance or infectivity that can be acquired. Unlike bioterrorism, bio crime intends to murder or make sick only a small group of people to take revenge or gain money by extortion. Nevertheless, bio crime is not intended for religious, political, or philosophical purposes. On the other hand, bioterrorism aims to create an atmosphere of terror, economic loss, social disruption, and panic based on political and religious beliefs.

There were 37 bioterrorist attacks worldwide from 1981 to 2018. The Centers for Disease Control and Prevention (CDC) list anthrax, botulism, plague, smallpox, tularemia, and viral hemorrhagic fevers as dangerous agents for national security, in category A, the highest-risk group. These dangerous agents listed by the CDC will be discussed in this section.

Anthrax

Bacillus anthracis is an agent found in soil that is capable of forming spores, and transmitted to humans via the skin, and respiratory and gastrointestinal tract through contact with contaminated animals and animal products. This microorganism can increase its virulence by producing toxins. Anthrax spores can easily pass through the skin pores. An anthrax vaccine has been discovered, but sequential vaccination is demanded as an effective dose. It is diagnosed by gram staining.

Anthrax contaminates in three main ways: skin, gastrointestinal tract, and inhalation.

1. *Inhalational anthrax*: This is caused by the accumulation of Bacillus anthracis spores in the lung alveoli and is usually fatal. After accumulation, macrophages, neutrophils, and dendritic cells absorb these spores. Then the spores begin to multiply and produce toxins in the regional lymph nodes. As a result of this process, there is septic shock. Symptoms usually occur a few days after infection, making diagnosis challenging.
2. *Dermal anthrax:* This appears when spores of Bacillus anthracis contact the subcutaneous tissue through the skin pores. They reproduce in this area and deliver spores and toxins. Expected edema and cutaneous ulceration are noticed on the skin. Injection of anthrax, which has emerged recently, is primarily seen in intravenous drug users in Northern Europe. Although its clinical course is similar to cutaneous anthrax, it causes infection in deeper tissues, especially myositis.
3. *Gastrointestinal anthrax:* This occurs when spores penetrate the gastrointestinal tract and replicate there due to eating meat contaminated with Bacillus anthracis. The disease progresses with mucosal ulceration and bleeding.

The CDC has designed straightforward guidance for anthrax exposure and clinical assessment. The disease diagnosis can be made by gram staining and cultures of samples taken from blood and body fluids or by analyzing the stool polymerase chain reaction (PCR). Routine diagnostic methods such as complete blood count (CBC) and radiological examination can also be valuable in patients.

It should be comprehended that cases of inhalation anthrax may be a bioterrorist event. Moreover, decontamination should be provided quickly in these cases. Also, HCW should wear masks, gloves, and personal protective equipment against contamination. Contaminated cases should immediately wash and clean their hands with detergent and water. Clothing should be placed in a disposable plastic bag for examination and forensic processing.

Combining a bactericidal agent with a protein synthesis inhibitor is suggested to treat inhalational anthrax. In patients with meningitis, a triple combination therapy containing two bactericidal agents from different drug groups and a protein synthesis inhibitor is recommended. While multi-drug combinations are guided for cutaneous anthrax in diffuse edema or head and neck involvement, oral ciprofloxacin or doxycycline is assumed to be adequate in other isolated cases.

Table 7. Symptoms and medical management of bacterial agents

Bacterial agents	Signs/Symptoms	Medical Management
Anthrax	Fever, shortness of breath, malaise, cough, cyanosis	Ciprofloxacin
Plague	High fever, shortness of breath, chills, headache, cough, cyanosis	Streptomycin
Brucellosis	Fever, myalgias, headache, chills, sweats	Doxycycline
Cholera	Watery diarrhea	Fluid therapy and antibiotics (Tetracyline, doxycycline/ciprofloxacin)
Tularemia	Local ulcer, fever, chills, lymphadenopathy, headache, and malaise	Streptomycin
Q fever	Fever, sputum, cough, and pleuritic chest pain	Tetracyline

Botulism

The causative agent of botulism is Clostridium botulinum, which is a gram-positive, bacillus and spore-forming anaerobic bacterium. One of the most potent poisons, botulinum neurotoxin, is more manageable to create, store and spread than other toxins; therefore, it is frequently used in bioterrorism. Clostridium botulinum can be efficiently isolated from soil, seafood, fruits, and vegetables. The obtained substrates produce heat-resistant spores, then pivot to toxin-producing bacilli. As a result of neurotoxin released by Clostridium botulinum, a life-threatening condition with neurological involvement occurs.

Clostridium botulinum causes infection with three primary forms: Infant botulism, food botulism, and wound botulism. The onset of signs after exposure to botulinum neurotoxin depends on the toxin dose and absorption kinetics. In foodborne botulism, symptoms generally emerge 12 to 72 hours after ingestion of the toxin-containing food, but it has also been demonstrated that this period can extend from two hours to eight days. The beginning of infant and wound botulism symptoms deviates according to the duration of exposure to spores, germination time, toxin serotype, bacterial species, patient age, and immunological status. The treatment contains antitoxin and supportive therapies for severe symptoms.

Plague

Yersinia pestis is a gram-negative bacillus bacterium and a member of the Enterobacteriaceae family. Furthermore, Alexandre Yersin isolated it during the Hong Kong pandemic. It is generally described as three primary forms of plague: Bubonic, pneumonic and septicemic plague. Yersinia pestis can be transmitted through flea bites (causing bubonic plague), respiratory droplets (causing alveolar plague), contaminated meat, and contact with infected animals. Although highly infectious, human-to-human transmission is infrequent. For protection, droplet precautions until antibiotics are administered for 48 to 72 hours, and then standard precautions are sufficient. However, deaths are usually very high before treatment can be started. It is potentially used in bioterrorism due to its high mortality rate and aerosol transmission (pneumonic plague). The gold standard approach for diagnosing plague is isolating and identifying the plague pathogen from clinical specimens. Initiating therapy within 24 hours is directly related to survival. Yersinia pestis is typically sensitive to streptomycin. Other than streptomycin, ciprofloxacin, doxycycline, and gentamicin are the agents administered in the cure, and supportive therapies should also be applied.

Smallpox (Variola Major)

Smallpox is caused by the Variola virus and Orthopoxvirus of the Poxviridae family. Moreover, it is highly contagious and 40% mortal in humans. The World Health Organization (WHO) declared the eradication of smallpox on 8 May 1980; then, vaccination was stopped due to serious side effects. As a result, humanity has failed immunity against this virus and other zoonotic and orthodox viruses. Advances in synthetic biology have led to a new variant of this disease possibly emerging. This situation causes humanity to worry because of the possibility of using the Variola virus in bioterrorist attacks.

Signs and symptoms are fever, myalgia, and a vesicular rash on the extremities, which usually surface within 2-4 days. Infected patients should be quarantined immediately and droplet isolation applied for 3-4 weeks until the crusts on the vesicles are separated. Although the treatment is supportive, broad-spectrum antibiotics are recommended for secondary infection.

Tularemia

Although rare in animals, Francisella tularensis is a gram-negative and facultative intracellular bacterium that causes tularemia in humans. It can survive for a long time in water and soil. Transmission to humans can occur through direct contact with an infected animal, ingesting contaminated food and drink, inhalation of aerosols, or after bites by arthropods. There is currently no vaccine available. Antibiotics such as streptomycin, gentamicin, and tetracycline can be used against Francisella tularensis. However, the presence of strains resistant to these antibiotics does not eliminate the potential of Francisella tularensis to be utilized for bioterrorism.

Viral Hemorrhagic Fever (Marburg, Ebola, Lassa, and Machupo Viruses)

Viral hemorrhagic fever is caused by viruses in the RNA virus family, such as Arenaviridae, Bunyaviridae, Filoviridae, Flaviviridae, and Rhabdoviridae. These viruses are transmitted to humans through the respiratory tract. Clinically, they progress with fever and bleeding; moreover, they can cause shock and death. The mortality rate of the Ebola virus was reported to be between 25% and 90%. Even though culturing these viruses to bacteria requires a high degree of expertise, they have the potential for bioterrorism. There is no approved treatment, and only supportive treatment is provided.

Radionuclear Warfare Agents

Nuclear weapons are described as weapons of mass destruction that can cause the death of many living things in a short period. In a nuclear war, large numbers of people are expected to die, followed by starvation and infectious diseases due to the depletion of resources. Only the United States of America has yet used two nuclear weapons in wars. As a result, approximately 120,000 people lost their lives.

Local exposure to high doses of radiation causes severe dermatological burns, including blisters, crusts, ulcerations, erythema, and necrosis, which may appear on the skin, usually 2-3 weeks after radiation exposure.

Acute radiation syndrome occurs after exposure to high amounts of ionizing radiation. A minimum dose of 1 Gy is required for acute radiation syndrome; doses greater than 10 Gy are considered to be fatal. At the 3.5 Gy dose, approximately 50% of patients are expected to die within 60 days if they are not treated. Prodromal symptoms after irradiation exposure vary according to the dose. Symptoms include dehydration with gastrointestinal manifestations. Early onset of prodromal symptoms has also been associated with increased mortality and morbidity. There are three subtypes of acute radiation syndrome: cerebrovascular, gastrointestinal, and hematopoietic. In treatment, it is recommended to treat skin involvements like thermal burns. In cases with suspected systemic involvement, chelate treatments such as hydration, gastric lavage, activated charcoal, antibiotics, and penicillamine are considered according to the symptoms.

As a result, it is worrying that it can cause numerous casualties when bioterrorism occurs. Such a disaster could affect the whole world. Health professionals should be prepared for such a possibility. Precautions should be taken to reduce mortality and morbidity when an attack occurs. The health professionals' knowledge and skill levels about potential agents should be increased.

Conclusion

CBRN events can be seen around the world with an increasing pattern due to wars and exposure in industry, both accidentally and intentionally. Workers and health authorities have to know the initial signs and symptoms and there have to be prevention measures, decontamination procedures, use of antidotes especially for time-sensitive agents, a medical transfer route for affected casualties, agent-specific medical therapy and the blocking patterns of secondary contaminations to reduce the effected number of casualties. There are many effects of CBRN agents like acute and chronic phases. Globally, newly trained, allocated and specified personnel are needed for each agent to manage and treat CBRN agent casualties. CBRN events in an environment can result in injury, illness, morbidity, and mortality through the whole society. After the exposure of CBRN threats, many victims can apply to EDs which are the main area for the decontamination and management of CBRN material effects through the human body. EDs have obligatory duties and responsibilities to prepare, decontaminate, plan and respond to CBRN threats immediately. Because of these situations, governmental and academic authorities have to focus on the preparation of emergency services (ambulances, hospital EDs, intensive care units, decontamination rooms, etc.) for CBRN incidents. ED workers should receive special training for the management of CBRN victims and maintain regular drills. New researches are needed to guide CBRN exposure with the improvement of technology.

References

Anisimov, A. P., & Amoako, K. K. (2006). Treatment of plague: Promising alternatives to antibiotics. *Journal of Medical Microbiology*, 55(Pt 11), 1461–1475.

Barelli A. B. I., Soave M., Tafani C., Bononi F. (2008). The comprehensive medical preparedness in chemical emergencies: 'the chain of chemical survival.' *Eur J Emerg Med;* 15(2): 110–118.

Barras, V., & Greub, G. (2014). History of biological warfare and bioterrorism. *Clinical Microbiology and Infection:* The Official Publication of the European Society of Clinical Microbiology and Infectious Diseases, 20(6), 497–502.

British Association 2004 Festival of Science, University of Exeter, UK, (2005); 1–9.

Cenciarelli, O., Gabbarini, V., Pietropaoli, S., Malizia, A., Tamburrini, A., Ludovici, G. M., et al. (2015). Viral bioterrorism: Learning the lesson of Ebola virus in West Africa 2013-2015. *Virus Research*, 210, 318–326.

Clarke S. F., Chilcott R. P., Wilson J. C., Kamanvire R., Baker D. J., Hallett A. (2008). Decontamination of multiple casualties who are chemically contaminated: a challenge for acute hospitals. *Prehosp Disaster Med;* 23(2): 175–181.

Domres B. D., Rashid A., Grundgeiger J., Gromer S., Kees T., Hecker N., Peter H. (2009). European survey on decontamination in mass casualty incidents. *Am J Disaster Med;* 4(3): 147–152.

Dong, M., Masuyer, G., & Stenmark, P. (2019). Botulinum and Tetanus Neurotoxins. *Annual Review of Biochemistry,* 88, 811–837. https://doi.org/10.1146/annurev-biochem-013118-111654.

Galimand, M., Guiyoule, A., Gerbaud, G., Rasoamanana, B., Chanteau, S., Carniel, E., & Courvalin, P. (1997). Multidrug resistance in Yersinia pestis mediated by a transferable plasmid. *The New England Journal of Medicine,* 337(10), 677–680. https://doi.org/10.1056/NEJM199709043371004.

Goel, A. K. (2015). Anthrax: A disease of biowarfare and public health importance. World Journal of Clinical Cases, 3(1), 20–33.

Graduated Levels of Chemical, Biological, Radiological and Nuclear Threats and Associated Protection. 8 August 2007.

Hazardous Materials Cooperative Research Program. Current Hazardous Materials Transportation Research and Future Needs. April 2012. onlinepubs.trb.org/ onlinepubs/ hmcrp /hmcrp w001.pdf.

Health Protection Agency. (2006). Heptonstall J, Gent N. CRBN incidents: clinical management & health protection. Health Protection Agency, London, November. ISBN: 0901144703. Version control: revisions

Hellmich, D., Wartenberg, K. E., Zierz, S., & Mueller, T. J. (2018). Foodborne botulism due to ingestion of home-canned green beans: Two case reports. *Journal of Medical Case Reports,* 12(1), 1.

Hilmas C. J., Smart J. K., Hill B. A. (2008). History of chemical warfare. In: Tuorinsky SD, ed. *Textbook of Military Medicine: Medical Aspects of Chemical Warfare.* Washington, DC, Office of the Surgeon General and Borden Institute, Walter Reed Army Medical Center.

http:// www.panda.org/about_wwf/ where_we_work/ europe/what_we_do/ toxics.cfm.

http:// www.panda.org/about_wwf/ where_we_work/ europe/what_we_do/ toxics.cfm.

Jansen, H. J., Breeveld, F. J., Stijnis, C., & Grobusch, M. P. (2014). Biological warfare, bioterrorism, and biocrime. *Clinical Microbiology and Infection:* The Official Publication of the European Society of Clinical Microbiology and Infectious Diseases, 20(6), 488–496.

Jeffery, I. A., & Karim, S. (2021). Botulism. In StatPearls. StatPearls Publishing. http://www.ncbi.nlm.nih.gov/books/NBK459273/.

Joseph, B., Brown, C. V., Diven, C., Bui, E., Aziz, H., & Rhee, P. (2013). Current concepts in the management of biologic and chemical warfare causalities. *The Journal of Trauma and Acute Care Surgery,* 75(4), 582–589.

Keim M. E. Industrial chemical disasters. In: Ciottone GR, Anderson PD, Auf der Heide E, et al., (2006) eds. *Disaster Medicine.* 3rd ed. Philadelphia, PA, Mosby Elsevier; 556–562.

Kreutzer K. A. Three-point Hazmat size-up. *Fire Engineering* November 2007: 119–124.

Kristi L. Koenig, Carl H. Schultz (2016), *Koenig and Schultz's disaster medicine.* New York : Cambridge University Press.

Maurin, M. (2015). Francisella tularensis as a potential agent of bioterrorism? *Expert Review of Anti-Infective Therapy,* 13(2), 141–144.

Mehta P. S., Mehta A. S., Mehta S. J., Makhijani A. B. (1990). Bhopal tragedy's health effects. *JAMA.* 264: 2781–2787.

Meyer, H., Ehmann, R., & Smith, G. L. (2020). Smallpox in the Post-Eradication Era. *Viruses,* 12(2), 138.

Mihailidou E. The 319 Major Industrial Accidents Since 1917. *Int. Rev.* 2012,4:529–540.

Miyaki K., Nishiwaki Y., Maekawa K., et al. (2005). Effects of sarin on the nervous system of subway workers seven years after the Tokyo subway sarin attack. *J Occup Health;* 47(4): 299–304.

NATO Standards of Proficiency for NBC Defence. 25 October 2002.

O'Leary, S. T., Kimberlin, D. W., & Maldonado, Y. A. (2018). Update From the Advisory Committee on Immunization Practices. *Journal of the Pediatric Infectious Diseases Society,* 7(2), 93–99.

Okumura T, Takasu N, Ishimatsu S, Miyanıki S, Mitsuhashi A, Kumada K, et al. (1996). Report on 640 victims of the Tokyo subway sarin attack. *Ann Emerg Med;* 28:129.

Olson, V. A., & Shchelkunov, S. N. (2017). Are We Prepared in Case of a Possible Smallpox-Like Disease Emergence? *Viruses,* 9(9), 242.

Patel S. S. Earliest Chemical Warfare – Dura-Europos, Syria. *Archaeology Magazine* 2010; 63(1).

Rathjen, N. A., & Shahbodaghi, S. D. (2021). Bioterrorism. *American Family Physician,* 104(4), 376–385.

Robinson J. P. P. Chemical Weapons and International Cooperation (Revision 1) in Public Discussion Meeting. Elimination of Weapons of Mass Destruction. British PugwashGroup. September 8, 2004.

Simonsen, K. A., & Chatterjee, K. (2021). Anthrax. In StatPearls. StatPearls Publishing. http://www.ncbi.nlm.nih.gov/books/NBK507773/.

Su, Z., McDonnell, D., Bentley, B. L., He, J., Shi, F., Cheshmehzangi, A., Ahmad, J., & Jia, P. (2021). Addressing Biodisaster X Threats With Artificial Intelligence and 6G Technologies: Literature Review and Critical Insights. *Journal of Medical Internet Research,* 23(5), e26109.

Suffredini, D. A., Sampath-Kumar, H., Li, Y., Ohanjanian, L., Remy, K. E., Cui, X., & Eichacker, P. Q. (2015). Does Bacillus anthracis Lethal Toxin Directly Depress Myocardial Function? A Review of Clinical Cases and Preclinical Studies. *Toxins,* 7(12), 5417–5434.

The Center For Food Security and Public Health, Iowa State University, USA, 2013.

Training of Medical Personnel for NBC Defence Operations. 12 May 2006.

Tuorinsky S. R., ed (2008). Medical Aspects of Chemical Warfare. In: *Textbook of Military Medicine series.* Washington, DC, Office of the Surgeon General and Borden Institute, Walter Reed Army Medical Center.

Tur-Kaspa I. L. E. I., Hendler I., Siebner R., et al. (1999). Preparing hospitals for toxicological mass casualties events. *Crit Care Med;* 27(5): 1004–1008.

Vietri, N. J. (2018). Does anthrax antitoxin therapy have a role in the treatment of inhalational anthrax? *Current Opinion in Infectious Diseases,* 31(3), 257–262.

Voigt, E. A., Kennedy, R. B., & Poland, G. A. (2016). Defending against smallpox: A focus on vaccines. *Expert Review of Vaccines,* 15(9), 1197–1211.

Williams, M., Armstrong, L., & Sizemore, D. C. (2021). *Biologic, Chemical, and Radiation Terrorism Review.* In StatPearls. StatPearls Publishing.

World Health Organization. *WHO Manual: The Public Health Management of Chemical Incidents.* 2009.

Yamasue H., Abe O., Kasai K., et al. (2007). Human brain structural change related to acute single exposure to sarin. *Ann Neurol;* 61(1): 37–46.

Yang, R. (2017). Plague: Recognition, Treatment, and Prevention. *Journal of Clinical Microbiology,* 56(1), e01519-17. https://doi.org/10.1128/JCM.01519-17.

Chapter 30

Crush Syndrome

Taner Şahin*, MD and Oğuzhan Bol, MD

Department of Emergency Medicine, University of Health Science Turkey,
Kayseri City Hospital, Kayseri, Turkey

Abstract

Crush syndrome is a disease that may lead to the death of many people if there is no early and proper intervention in wars and natural disasters such as earthquakes. The trauma resulting from compression imposes a functional load on the metabolism causing the destruction of cells, and this load may reach levels that cannot be tolerated by the body. In these patients, the intervention must be started while the patient is still at the scene and the treatment should be initiated by considering all foreseeable risks. It should not be forgotten that rhabdomyolysis, compartment syndrome, acute renal failure, cardiac and pulmonary side effects, sepsis and shock may occur.

Keywords: Crush syndrome, compartment, acute renal failure, rhabdomyolysis

Introduction

Crush is defined as anatomical damage caused by external crushing of the body, extremities or other parts of the body by direct physical force. As a result of physical compression, tissue trauma and ischemia-reperfusion injury occur.

When compressive forces due to the compression of the tissue disappear, muscle injury and edema occur in the affected areas due to possible muscle necrosis and neurological dysfunction. As a result of compression and nerve compression, crush syndrome (CS), traumatic rhabdomyolysis, and compartment syndrome may occur. CS, which is defined as the tissues remaining ischemic as a result of severe compression due to direct trauma and the continuation of damage due to the reperfusion of tissues, was first described in 1941 by Bywaters and Beall, who examined the casualties of World War II (Bywaters, 1942).

CS is a clinical picture that results in systemic findings, organ dysfunction or death due to crush injury. CS, by its other name "traumatic rhabdomyolysis," is the second leading cause of death after deaths resulting from direct trauma in earthquakes (Erek et al., 2002). Early

---

* Corresponding Author's Email: taner.sahin@sbu.edu.tr.

In: Environmental Emergencies and Injuries in Nature
Editors: Murat Yücel, Murat Güzel and İbrahim İkizceli
ISBN: 978-1-68507-833-1

diagnosis of renal failure resulting from CS and an early start of fluid resuscitation should be the priority of healthcare workers.

Epidemiology

Crush injuries mostly take place after natural or human-related disasters such as earthquakes, tsunamis, mining and industrial accidents and in war zones. It is difficult to statistically determine the frequency of CS since it mostly occurs after disasters such as earthquakes or tsunamis. The incidence of CS and subsequent acute renal failure (ARF) varies between 1 and 25% in various publications (Sever & Vanholder, 2013). It is reported in the literature that CS developed in 7.6% of all traumatic cases in the Spitak earthquake, 13.7% of all traumatic hospitalizations in the Kobe earthquake, and 1.4% of all hospitalized patients in the Marmara earthquake (Yokota, 2005). It was reported that approximately 80% of patients with crush injuries died of serious head injuries or suffocation. Among 20% of patients who reach the hospital, 10% recover with no problems, and the other 10% have CS (Dimitriou, 2021).

Upon examining CS after an earthquake, while rhabdomyolysis is not observed in all earthquake traumas, CS develops only in some rhabdomyolysis cases, and ARF does not occur in all CS cases. It is assumed that CS will develop in approximately 2% to 5% of all injuries after earthquakes and that ARF will develop in approximately 1.5% of all injuries. Although these ratios may initially appear to be low, when it is considered that there may be tens of thousands of casualties after disasters, it indicates that a large number of ARF cases in total may occur (Yokota, 2005).

Crush injuries are mostly observed in the extremities because head, neck, and body injuries rapidly cause death. Moreover, the incidence of crush injuries and thus the development of ARF may be affected in cases such as the prolonged time to reach the casualty, inability to initiate early fluid resuscitation by establishing proper vascular access, delayed transfer to the hospital, lack of professionals trained in this field, and lack of necessary medical equipment (such as hemodialysis). Therefore, it is necessary that healthcare professionals take the necessary measures by predicting these situations.

Etiopathogenesis

Mechanism of Injury

Crush injury may result from being run over by a vehicle, industrial accidents, being trapped in the wreckage, construction and agricultural accidents, crushing as a result of mass stampede, collapse of building walls as a result of bombing, and collapse of buildings or compression in large mass earthquakes (Sever et al., 2015).

Direct tissue damage occurs when the venous outflow is blocked by compressive force. Cellular death, tissue necrosis (myonecrosis), and crush syndrome may occur due to extended compression time (Agu & Ackroyd, 2002).

Crush Injury

Crush injury is caused by the prolonged compression of the body, extremities, or other parts of the body as a result of physical trauma. Injury to the soft tissues, muscles, and nerves may occur primarily due to the direct effect of trauma or compression-induced ischemia. In addition to a direct muscle or organ injury, after the compressive force is released, severe crush injury results in edema in the affected areas with possible muscle necrosis and neurologic dysfunction. This soft tissue injury may also be caused by a secondary injury resulting from subsequent compartment syndrome (Bywaters, 1942; Erek et al., 2002).

As a result of alcohol intoxication or prolonged immobility under anesthesia, nontraumatic crush injury may be observed. In such cases, body weight alone may lead to compartment syndrome or rhabdomyolysis. On the other hand, crush injury may also be observed in the gluteal region of the body and the regions pressing the bed due to stroke, coma, intoxication, and prolonged immobilization in the postoperative period. In such cases, there may be delays in the diagnosis and treatment of crush injury (Garner et al., 2014).

Crush Syndrome

It is possible to describe CS as a systemic condition that may result in dysfunction in the kidneys and damage to other organs or death. The symptoms of CS are systemic symptoms that usually result from ARF and rhabdomyolysis (Better, 1990). CS may also develop with prolonged immobility, burns, and electrical injury (Rajagopalan, 2010).

CS is the systemic manifestation of compression-induced muscle tissue damage (rhabdomyolysis), leading to the release of potentially toxic muscle cell components into the extracellular fluid. Hypovolemic shock, hyperkalemia, hypocalcemia, metabolic acidosis, compartment syndrome, and ARF are the typical clinical features of CS. Moreover, disseminated intravascular coagulation may be observed in peripheral neuropathy (Dimitriou, 2021).

Cases of CS were reported in World War II in Germany, during the Vietnam War and mining accidents in the 1960s, in the Nicaragua and China earthquakes in the 1970s, in the Japan Kobe earthquake, in the Iran earthquake, in the Marmara and Düzce earthquakes in Turkey, and in the Taiwan Chi-Chi earthquake in the 1990s, in the Bingol earthquake in Turkey and in the Pakistan Kashmir earthquake in the 2000s, in the 2011 Van earthquake in Turkey, and after the Elazığ earthquake in Turkey and the Iran earthquake in the 2020s (Turkdogan et al., 2021; Yokota, 2005).

Ions, such as myoglobin, potassium, magnesium, and phosphate, and enzymes, such as creatine phosphokinase, and lactate dehydrogenase, are released as a result of a crush in the muscle tissue. Later, the inclusion of these products in the blood circulation as a result of the removal of debris or reduction in tissue crushing is the underlying pathological cause in CS (Turkdogan et al., 2021). Local ischemia occurs after a crush on the muscle. Thus, sodium, calcium, and fluids are released. Muscle volume and rigidity increase. Furthermore, nitric oxide is activated and contributes to the exacerbation of hypotension by causing vasodilatation (Gunal et al., 2004). When crushed muscles are examined, they are necrotic, hard, swollen, cold, and insensitive. Myoglobin that is normally filtered through the kidney glomeruli precipitates in large amounts in the distal tubules, and myoglobin breakdown products (such as methemoglobin, acid hematin) increase the tubular damage by causing vasoconstriction in the afferent arterioles, and eventually, renal failure occurs (Agu & Ackroyd, 2002).

Reperfusion syndrome is a paradoxical phenomenon that occurs with the resumption of blood flow to ischemic tissues and leads to increased cellular degradation. It involves biochemical and cellular changes that cause oxidant production and complement activation, which trigger the inflammatory response mediated by neutrophils and platelets interacting with the vascular endothelium. Thus, the local and systemic manifestations of the inflammatory response emerge (Sellei et al., 2014).

Rhabdomyolysis

Rhabdomyolysis is a clinical entity, which leads to the release of cellular content into the vascular system as a result of muscle breakdown during crush injury and systemic complications (Better, 1990). Human-related conditions and natural disasters constitute the majority of cases of rhabdomyolysis associated with CS that have occurred with the development of life-threatening complications to date (Sever et al., 2015). In the case of rhabdomyolysis, while substances such as creatinine kinase, myoglobin, lactic acid, nucleic acids, thromboplastin, potassium, and phosphate in the striated muscle cell (myocyte) enter the blood circulation, substances such as sodium, water, and calcium enter the muscle cell (Dimitriou, 2021; Sever & Vanholder, 2012).

Compartment syndrome is one of the most common clinical manifestations of rhabdomyolysis. ARF results from various factors during rhabdomyolysis. The impairment of the renal blood supply caused by hypovolemia secondary to compartment syndrome is the most important among them.

On the other hand, myoglobin released from muscles contributes to the pathogenesis of ARF both with its direct toxic effect (iron ions released from myoglobin) and by forming tubular plugs.

Furthermore, reperfusion injury, hyperphosphatemia, hyperuricemia, disseminated intravascular coagulation, and endotoxins may also play a role in the development of ARF. Some rhabdomyolysis cases occur due to nontraumatic reasons (such as alcohol and drug use) (Agu & Ackroyd, 2002; Knochel, 1993).

Compartment Syndrome

The term compartment is the closed structure formed by the muscles and the rigid fascia surrounding them.

Compartment syndrome is the name given to an increase in the pressure of the compartments, which is normally very low (0-15mm Hg). In the case of muscle edema, capillary perfusion pressure increases along with the increase in intracompartmental pressure. In the case of perfusion pressure exceeding 30 mmHg, microvascular circulation is impaired, and ischemic damage to nerve and muscle cells and rhabdomyolysis become severe. In this case, irreversible nerve and muscle damage occurs after 4 to 6 hours. In compartment syndrome, the venous outflow is compromised as a result of the increase in fascial compartment pressure with hypoxia, which results from the increase in tissue pressure to prevent perfusion, and the exposure of muscle and nerve tissue to ischemia.

Then, edema with progressive capillary leakage leading to arteriolar inflow and skeletal muscle damage that may progress to rhabdomyolysis occurs (Sellei et al., 2014; Sever & Vanholder, 2012).

Effects of Crush Injury on Kidneys

Causes such as compartment syndrome, hypovolemia due to bleeding, and inability to reach water under debris play a role in the development of ARF during rhabdomyolysis. As a result of hypovolemia, the release of cytokines increases along with the activation of the renin-angiotensin-aldosterone system, vasopressin and the sympathetic nervous system. Thus, the renal blood flow is further disrupted. Furthermore, the fact that myoglobin, which is released as a result of muscle breakdown, has a direct toxic effect on the kidney, and its accumulation in the renal tubules also contribute to the development of ARF. Moreover, due to the reduction of myoglobin in the tubules, free iron is released, and the formation of free radicals is catalyzed. In this case, ischemic damage increases even more (Michaelson, 1992; Sahjian & Frakes, 2007).

The etiopathogenesis of the development of ARF in the course of CS is generally examined under 2 headings:

1. Emergence of rhabdomyolysis,
2. Emergence of CS and ARF.

The etiology of rhabdomyolysis includes non-physical causes such as alcohol, drugs (mostly statins), electrolyte disturbances (especially hypopotassemia and hypophosphatemia), and infections, and physical causes such as earthquakes, tsunamis, wreckage, landslides, traffic accidents, and excessive exercise.

Baromyopathy (pressure of the muscle) becomes important among physical causes. The muscle sarcolemma is stretched due to pressure. Rhabdomyolysis may occur due to the compression of the muscle, even for a very short time (30 minutes). In baromyopathy, the permeability of the sarcolemma is impaired. While substances such as potassium, myoglobin, creatine kinase, lactate dehydrogenase, ALT, AST, and uric acid that are abundant in the muscle pass into the extracellular environment and therefore into the blood circulation, water, sodium, chloride, and calcium enter the cell. Thus, cell edema and compartment syndrome occur. These elevated substances in the blood are responsible for toxic and fatal complications in crush injury (Knochel, 1993).

Muscle ischemia is another mechanism that triggers rhabdomyolysis. Within 30 minutes after a skeletal muscle crush, ischemia, and then edema and lysosome degranulation occur. Muscle ischemia and reperfusion injury that occurs during the recovery of this ischemia play a role in the pathogenesis of rhabdomyolysis (Yokota, 2005).

Cardiac Effects of Crush Injury

There is an increase in the blood concentration of potassium passing into the extracellular environment as a result of the disruption of the muscle sarcolemma during crush injury. Thus, the potassium gradient occurs between the extracellular and the intracellular compartments. While the excitability of myocytes increases along with a decrease in cell membrane potential, myocardial cells are depressed with an increase in the potassium level, and the heart stops in diastole in the following period. Furthermore, along with the development of hypovolemia, the heart attempts to compensate with tachycardia in the beginning. However, along with the deepening of hypovolemia, the heart is unable to provide hemodynamics in the following period, and ultimately, bradycardia and then asystole occur. Ischemia itself is responsible for the development of cardiomyopathy. Hypocalcemia, which occurs as a result of the entry of calcium into the cell, also contributes to the development of cardiac arrhythmia (Gonzalez, 2005; Odeh, 1991). Sudden death may be observed as a result of ventricular fibrillation resulting from the flow of potassium, phosphorus, and myoglobin from injury sites within 20 minutes after recovery, which is called "smiling death" (Agu & Ackroyd, 2002).

Management of Patients with Crush Injury

Clinical Findings and Laboratory

The clinical findings of crush syndrome are associated with the mechanism of the disease. The clinical picture appears with the duration and extent of crushing. Tension and edema are expected in the relevant extremity due to the compression injury. Along with the progression of the clinical picture, 6P signs (pain, increased pressure, paraesthesia, pulselessness, paresis, and pallor) can be detected (Sever et al., 2006). The systemic reflection of this clinical picture varies according to the affected organ. Hypotension with decreased intravascular fluid, hypovolemic shock and consequent acute heart failure, acute renal failure with renal involvement, oliguria and anuria, and arrhythmias due to electrolyte imbalance may occur. The clinical picture of shock can be observed along with the addition of the signs of infection to respiratory failure (Gonzalez, 2005).

Hyperkalemia is the most expected laboratory finding (Zhang et al., 2013). Moreover, another finding is elevated myoglobin, which can be detected at a certain level (usually 85 ng/ml) in the blood. The value may exceed 150000 ng/ml in proportion to the extent of the damage. Myoglobin can be examined in serum and urine. It can be examined by a stick in the urine. However, it should not be forgotten that there is a negative detection rate of two-thirds (Sahjian & Frakes, 2007). The urine color of the patient with high myoglobin values may be dirty brown.

Creatine kinase (CK) is present in striated muscles. In crush syndrome, especially the CK-MM form can be detected at a high rate in the blood. While the normal CK value is 25-175 U/L, it starts to increase after 2-12 hours and may reach 15000 U/L in crush syndrome (Sahjian & Frakes, 2007). High CK values are associated with ARF. However, there are publications indicating that the limit to be considered is 5000 U/L, 16000 U/L, or 76000 U/L. In a study, the risk of renal failure was found to be 41% in patients over 55 years of age, with an ISS score of over 15, and a CK value of more than 5000 U/L (Brown et al., 2004). CK cannot be removed from the blood through dialysis (Sahjian & Frakes, 2007).

Treatment

In the management of patients, the first priority is volume resuscitation, which is of critical importance to reverse hypovolemic shock, prevent acute renal failure, and minimize lactic acidosis and hyperkalemia. The second priority is systemic alkalinization to reduce acidosis and hyperkalemia. Reducing intracompartmental pressures is also important to prevent compartment syndrome (Dimitriou, 2021).

If the patient is in a disaster area, it is necessary to establish wide vascular access as soon as an extremity can be reached. If possible, central access can be established. Intraosseous access can be used because fluid resuscitation in the early period is very important, especially in terms of preventing damage to the target organ and preserving renal functions (Gunal et al., 2004). The recommended initial amount of fluid is 1 liter per hour. Here, the point to take into account is that if rescuing the patient from the wreckage exceeds 2 hours, the fluid administered should be continued at 500 ml per hour. Furthermore, it may be necessary to reduce the amount of fluid if the patient is old, the affected body mass is relatively low, the ambient temperature is low, the patient is weak, and anuria-oliguria can be detected. The target urine output should be 300-400 ml per hour (Malinoski et al., 2004). The fluids containing potassium should be avoided in patients due to the potential risk of hyperpotassemia. After the patient is rescued from the wreckage, fluid therapy can be continued with 0.45% NaCl at 1 liter per hour. Fifty ml of sodium bicarbonate fluid can be added to alkalize the urine, although this is controversial. The target urine pH is 6-7. Fifty ml of mannitol can be added to increase the intravenous volume in patients with a urine output of >20 ml/hour, which may also reduce the development of compartment syndrome (Gonzalez, 2005; Sever & Vanholder, 2013).

Along with damage to muscle tissue, a high amount of potassium from the muscles mixes into the blood, which also leads to the clinical picture called "rescue death." Various complications which may result in death occur when the electrolytes, which cannot enter the circulation while under the wreckage, quickly mix into the blood (Santangelo et al., 1982). Therefore, ECG imaging and cardiac monitoring are important in patients with suspected crush syndrome. If possible, 30 grams of kayexalate can be administered orally at the scene. In patients with suspected hyperpotassemia, 10 ml of 10% calcium gluconate should be administered IV rapidly, and 10 units of crystalline insulin should be administered together with 25 grams of dextrose (Gunal et al., 2004). Hypercalcemia is common during the recovery period of patients with crush syndrome. Therefore, it is necessary to be careful while administering calcium to patients, and it should be administered if clinical findings or laboratory results supporting hypercalcemia are available (Sever & Vanholder, 2013).

It is necessary to perform hemodialysis in patients whose target urine output cannot be achieved and whose potassium values cannot be controlled. Therefore, blood gas, creatinine, BUN, and calcium values in terms of ARF are important in the follow-up of these patients. Continuous venous-venous hemofiltration can be the most suitable option in these patients (Fernandez et al., 2005).

The intracompartmental pressure should be measured if compartment syndrome is suspected with clinical findings in the affected extremities of patients. The expected value is 0-15 mmHg. It is necessary to apply fasciotomy for decompression at values of 30 and above. The ratio of the diastolic pressure to the compartment pressure of the affected area can be guiding for tissue perfusion (Gonzalez, 2005). The increase in intraabdominal pressure can be determined when the pressure measured from the urinary catheter is 25 mmHg and above. Emergency surgery is indicated (Malinoski et al., 2004).

There are drugs, biological agents, and alternative treatments that are used experimentally in the treatment of crush syndrome and are still investigated. They are mitochondria-targeted antioxidants (SkQR1), dexamethasone, allopurinol, nitrite, anisodamine, astragaloside-IV, hydrogen sulfide, bardoxolone methyl, N-(2-hydroxyphenyl) acetamide, ulinastatin, macrophage surface molecule mac-1 inhibitor: lactoferrin (Lf), anti-HMGB1 and anti-RAGE antibody, recombinant human erythropoietin (rhEPO), mesenchymal stem cell therapy, carbon monoxide enriched red blood cell (CO-RBC), and ice and cold liquid treatment (Li et al., 2020).

Conclusion

Crush is the anatomical damage caused by external crushing of the body, extremities or other parts of the body by direct physical force.

Crush injury results from the prolonged compression of the body, extremities, or other parts of the body as a result of physical trauma.

Crush syndrome can be defined as a systemic condition that may result in dysfunction, particularly in the kidneys, damage to other organs, or death.

Rhabdomyolysis is the clinical picture that leads to the release of cellular content into the vascular system and systemic complications as a result of muscle breakdown during crush injury. Compartment syndrome is one of the most common clinical manifestations of rhabdomyolysis. Causes such as compartment syndrome, hypovolemia due to bleeding, and inability to reach water under debris play a role in the development of ARF during rhabdomyolysis. Furthermore, there is an increase in the blood concentration of potassium passing into the extracellular environment as a result of the disruption of the muscle sarcolemma during crush injury.

Clinically, compartment syndrome (6P signs), hypotension, hypovolemic shock picture and related acute heart failure, acute renal failure, and arrhythmias may occur. The clinical picture of shock can be observed along with the addition of the signs of infection to respiratory failure.

In the management of patients, the first priority is volume resuscitation. It is necessary to establish vascular access early. The treatment of hyperpotassemia should be detected early and intervened quickly. With hemodialysis in mind, transfer to a suitable center should be considered. For compartment syndrome, it is necessary to measure intracompartmental pressure and perform fasciotomy quickly.

References

Agu O & Ackroyd JS. (2002). Crush syndrome after isolated abdominal crush injury in flood water. *Journal of Trauma and Acute Care Surgery*, 53(2), 378-379.

Better OS. (1990). The crush syndrome revisited (1940-1990). *Nephron*, 55(2), 97-103.

Brown CVR, Rhee P, Chan L, Evans K, Demetriades D & Velmahos GC. (2004). Preventing renal failure in patients with rhabdomyolysis: Do bicarbonate and mannitol make a difference? *Journal of Trauma and Acute Care Surgery*, 56(6), 1191-1196.

Bywaters EGL. (1942). Crushing injury. *British Medical Journal*, 2(4273), 643.

Dimitriou N. (2021). Basics of Trauma Management: Crush Injuries. In *Emergency Medicine, Trauma and Disaster Management,* (pp. 299-309). Springer.

Erek E, Sever MS, Serdengecti K, Vanholder R, Akoğlu E, Yavuz M, Ergin H, Tekce M, Duman N & Lameire N. (2002). An overview of morbidity and mortality in patients with acute renal failure due to crush syndrome: the Marmara earthquake experience. *Nephrology Dialysis Transplantation*, 17(1), 33-40.

Fernandez WG, Hung O, Bruno GR, Galea S & Chiang WK. (2005). Factors predictive of acute renal failure and need for hemodialysis among ED patients with rhabdomyolysis. *The American Journal of Emergency Medicine*, 23(1), 1-7.

Garner MR, Taylor SA, Gausden E & Lyden JP. (2014). Compartment syndrome: Diagnosis, management, and unique concerns in the twenty-first century. *HSS Journal®*, 10(2), 143-152.

Gonzalez D. (2005). Crush syndrome. *Critical Care Medicine*, 33(1), S34-S41.

Gunal AI, Celiker H, Dogukan A, Ozalp G, Kirciman E, Simsekli H, Gunay I, Demircin M, Belhan O & Yildirim MA. (2004). Early and vigorous fluid resuscitation prevents acute renal failure in the crush victims of catastrophic earthquakes. *Journal of the American Society of Nephrology*, 15(7), 1862-1867.

Knochel JP. (1993). Mechanisms of rhabdomyolysis. *Current Opinion in Rheumatology*, 5(6), 725-731.

Li N, Wang X, Wang P, Fan H, Hou S & Gong Y. (2020). Emerging medical therapies in crush syndrome–progress report from basic sciences and potential future avenues. *Renal Failure*, 42(1), 656-666.

Malinoski DJ, Slater MS & Mullins RJ. (2004). Crush injury and rhabdomyolysis. *Critical Care Clinics*, 20(1), 171-192.

Michaelson M. (1992). Crush injury and crush syndrome. *World Journal of Surgery*, 16(5), 899-903.

Odeh M. (1991). The role of reperfusion-induced injury in the pathogenesis of the crush syndrome. *New England Journal of Medicine*, 324(20), 1417-1422.

Rajagopalan S. (2010). Crush injuries and the crush syndrome. *Medical Journal Armed Forces India*, 66(4), 317-320.

Sahjian M & Frakes M. (2007). Crush injuries: Pathophysiology and current treatment. *The Nurse Practitioner*, 32(9), 13-18.

Santangelo ML, Usberti M, Di Salvo E, Belli G, Romano G, Sassaroli C & Zotti G. (1982). A study of the pathology of the crush syndrome. *Surgery, Gynecology & Obstetrics*, 154(3), 372-374.

Sellei RM, Hildebrand F & Pape HC. (2014). Acute extremity compartment syndrome: Current concepts in diagnostics and therapy. *Der Unfallchirurg*, 117(7), 633-649.

Sever MS, Lameire N, Van Biesen W & Vanholder R. (2015). Disaster nephrology: A new concept for an old problem. *Clinical Kidney Journal*, 8(3), 300-309.

Sever MS & Vanholder R. (2012). Recommendation for the management of crush victims in mass disasters. *Nephrology, Dialysis, Transplantation : Official Publication of the European Dialysis and Transplant Association - European Renal Association*, 27 Suppl 1, i1-67. https://doi.org/10.1093/ndt/gfs156.

Sever MS & Vanholder R. (2013). Management of crush victims in mass disasters: Highlights from recently published recommendations. *Clinical Journal of the American Society of Nephrology*, 8(2), 328-335.

Sever MS, Vanholder R & Lameire N. (2006). Management of crush-related injuries after disasters. *New England Journal of Medicine*, 354(10), 1052-1063.

Turkdogan KA, Korkut S, Arslan E & Ozyavuz MK. (2021). First response of emergency health care system and logistics support in an earthquake. *Disaster and Emergency Medicine Journal*, 6(2), 63-69.

Yokota J. (2005). Crush syndrome in disaster. *Japan Medical Association Journal*, 48(7), 341.

Zhang L, Fu P, Wang L, Cai G, Zhang L, Chen D, Guo D, Sun X, Chen F & Bi W. (2013). Hyponatraemia in patients with crush syndrome during the Wenchuan earthquake. *Emergency Medicine Journal*, 30(9), 745-748.

About the Editors

Murat Yücel, MD

Associate Professor, Faculty of Medicine, Department of Emergency Medicine,
Samsun University, Samsun Training and Research Hospital, Samsun, Turkey
Email: drmrtycl@gmail.com
ORCID ID: 0000-0003-0220-9230

Murat Yücel is a medical doctor and Associate Professor in Emergency Medicine. His interests are trauma, toxicology and neurological, cardiological and surgical emergencies.

Murat Güzel, MD

Associate Professor, Department of Emergency Medicine, Health Sciences University,
Samsun Training and Research Hospital, Samsun, Turkey
Email: drmuratguzel@gmail.com
ORCID ID: 0000-0003-0276-4576

Murat Güzel is a medical doctor and Associate Professor in Emergency Medicine. His interests are toxicology, trauma and surgical emergencies.

İbrahim İkizceli, MD

Professor, Faculty of Medicine, Department of Emergency Medicine,
Istanbul University, Cerrahpasa, Istanbul, Turkey
Email: ikizceli@istanbul.edu.tr
ORCID ID: 0000-0002-9825-4716

İbrahim İkizceli is a medical doctor and Professor in Emergency Medicine. His interests are trauma, cardiologic emergencies, toxicology and disaster medicine.

Index

A

acetic acid, 52, 53, 108, 118

acetylcholine, 113, 122, 142, 152, 166, 168, 205, 213, 225, 249, 251, 252, 254, 257

acetylcholinesterase, 152, 249, 251, 254, 257

acid burns, 52, 53, 59

acids, 49, 53, 314

acute lung injury, 1, 78, 254

acute mountain sickness, 79, 81, 86, 87

acute radiation syndrome, 307

acute renal failure, 127, 170, 172, 173, 199, 282, 311, 312, 316, 317, 318, 319

air bag burns, 57

alkali burns, 54, 58

alkalis, 49, 50, 54, 55

anaphylaxis, 107, 113, 117, 118, 120, 121, 122, 127, 129, 130, 131, 132, 133, 134, 135, 136, 139, 145, 160, 167, 171, 192, 193, 194, 195

animal, vi, 92, 110, 112, 113, 123, 174, 177, 178, 179, 181, 182, 183, 184, 185, 186, 187, 189, 190, 203, 205, 206, 208, 209, 211, 216, 282, 285, 290, 304, 306

anthrax, 304, 305, 308, 309

antidotes, 57, 151, 159, 160, 171, 172, 242, 259, 273, 289, 291, 292, 294, 295, 296, 307

antivenom/anti-venom, 113, 118, 124, 137, 139, 141, 142, 143, 144, 145, 146, 147, 149, 151, 156, 158, 159, 160, 161, 162, 163, 165, 166, 167, 169, 170, 171, 172, 173, 174, 175

asphyxia, 7, 207

aspiration, 1, 2, 7, 8, 35, 37, 44, 96, 100, 113, 115, 169, 207, 254, 256

atropine, 144, 157, 227, 228, 236, 243, 247, 249, 256, 257, 259, 294, 295, 302

B

barotrauma, 73, 89, 90, 91, 95, 96, 97, 98, 99, 100, 102, 103, 104, 105

bee, 113, 134, 135, 136, 145, 244

biological, vi, 69, 124, 125, 174, 190, 198, 223, 229, 230, 244, 270, 276, 289, 304, 308, 309, 318

biological weapons, 223, 304

bite, 113, 127, 129, 137, 138, 139, 140, 142, 144, 145, 146, 147, 151, 157, 159, 162, 165, 166, 167, 168, 169, 170, 171, 172, 173, 174, 177, 178, 179,
180, 181, 182, 183, 184, 185, 186, 187, 188, 189, 190, 205, 206, 208, 209

blister, 42, 272, 291, 300

blood, 3, 5, 11, 13, 14, 15, 17, 18, 24, 30, 31, 32, 35, 37, 38, 46, 51, 63, 64, 66, 80, 82, 83, 86, 89, 93, 99, 100, 101, 112, 125, 132, 133, 134, 135, 139, 141, 142, 154, 155, 159, 167, 168, 172, 184, 191, 192, 194, 200, 201, 203, 209, 213, 219, 230, 236, 238, 246, 247, 248, 251, 254, 257, 260, 261, 262, 263, 264, 265, 267, 270, 272, 273, 274, 275, 279, 280, 281, 283, 284, 285, 286, 299, 301, 304, 313, 314, 315, 316, 317, 318

blue-ringed octopus, 107, 112, 113, 123, 125

botulism, 304, 305, 308, 309

bradycardia, 2, 9, 14, 15, 18, 19, 152, 157, 236, 243, 246, 247, 252, 300, 316

breathe, 2, 4, 13, 89, 91, 93, 95, 96, 101

burn center, 41, 43, 45, 50, 68

burn(s), 26, 28, 41, 42, 43, 44, 45, 46, 47, 49, 50, 51, 52, 54, 55, 56, 57, 58, 59, 62, 63, 64, 66, 67, 68, 69, 74, 76, 77, 212, 217, 220, 240, 286, 290, 296, 299, 301, 307, 313

C

calcium gluconate, 54, 59, 144, 147, 317

carbolic acid (Phenol), 52

carbon monoxide, vi, 18, 44, 82, 83, 95, 279, 286, 287, 288, 291, 294, 318

carbon monoxide poisoning, vi, 18, 44, 82, 83, 95, 279, 286, 287, 288

carboxyhemoglobin, 279, 280, 287

Carukia barnesi (*C. barnesi*), 116, 118

catecholamine discharge, 36, 46

Centers for Disease Control and Prevention (CDC), 8, 31, 72, 78, 140, 141, 146, 185, 189, 192, 213, 216, 220, 222, 274, 276, 304

centipede, v, 137, 145, 146, 148, 149

Cephalopoda (Octopuses), 112

chelation therapy, 261, 264, 265, 267, 273, 274

chemical, v, vi, 18, 43, 49, 50, 51, 52, 53, 54, 55, 56, 57, 58, 223, 224, 231, 245, 249, 251, 254, 267, 269, 271, 273, 274, 276, 289, 290, 291, 292, 293, 294, 295, 296, 297, 298, 299, 300, 301, 302, 303, 308, 309, 310

chemical agents, 51, 52, 53, 291, 292, 294, 296, 297

chemical burns, v, 49, 50, 51, 52, 54, 55, 57, 299

chikungunya virus (CHIKV), 197, 199, 202, 203